PROLOG

Patient Management in the Office

SEVENTH EDITION

Critique Book

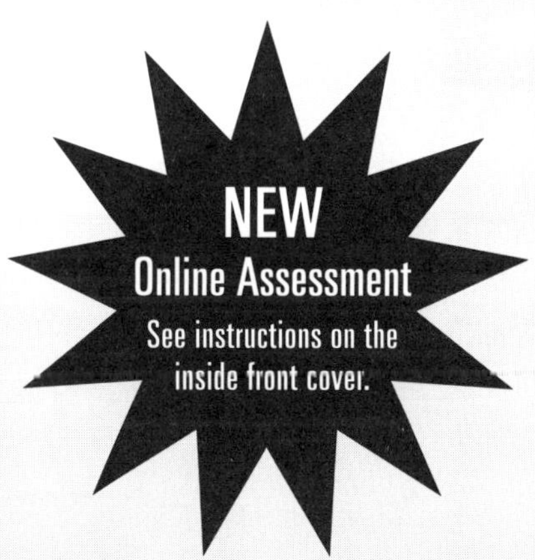

The American College of
Obstetricians and Gynecologists
WOMEN'S HEALTH CARE PHYSICIANS

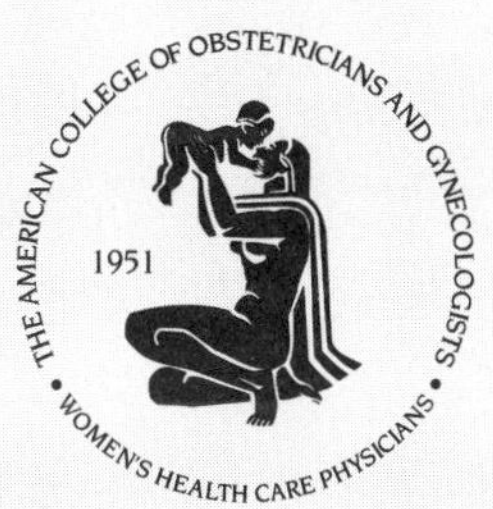

ISBN 978-1-934984-61-1

12345/10987

The American College of Obstetricians and Gynecologists
409 12th Street, SW
PO Box 96920
Washington, DC 20090-6920

Contributors

PROLOG Editorial and Advisory Committee

CHAIR

Ronald T. Burkman Jr, MD
Professor of Obstetrics and Gynecology
Department of Obstetrics and Gynecology
Division of General Obstetrics and Gynecology
Tufts University School of Medicine
Baystate Medical Center
Springfield, Massachusetts

MEMBERS

John F. Greene Jr, MD
Vice President of Medical Affairs, Hartford Region
Hartford HealthCare
Professor of Obstetrics and Gynecology
University of Connecticut School of Medicine
Farmington, Connecticut

Roger P. Smith, MD
Assistant Dean for Graduate Medical Education and Professor of Clinical Biologic Sciences
Charles E. Schmidt College of Medicine
Florida Atlantic University
Boca Raton, Florida

Linda Van Le, MD
Leonard Palumbo Distinguished Professor
Division of Gynecologic Oncology
University of North Carolina School of Medicine
Chapel Hill, North Carolina

PROLOG Task Force for *Patient Management in the Office*, Seventh Edition

COCHAIRS

Geri D. Hewitt, MD
Associate Professor of Obstetrics and Gynecology and Pediatrics
Ohio State University College of Medicine
General Division of Obstetrics and Gynecology
Department of Obstetrics and Gynecology
Chief, Obstetrics and Gynecology
Nationwide Children's Hospital
Columbus, Ohio

Heather Z. Sankey, MD, FACOG, CPE
Associate Professor
University of Massachusetts Medical School
Vice Chair and Program Director
Baystate Medical Center Department of Obstetrics and Gynecology
Springfield, Massachusetts

MEMBERS

Robert M. Abrams, MD
Associate Professor
Southern Illinois University School of Medicine
Executive Director
Southern Illinois University Division of Maternal Fetal Medicine
Director of Obstetrics
South Central Illinois Perinatal Center
Hospital Sisters Health System St. John's Hospital
Springfield, Illinois

Jeffrey S. Dungan, MD
Associate Professor
Division of Clinical Genetics
Department of Obstetrics and Gynecology
Northwestern University Feinberg School of Medicine
Chicago, Illinois

Continued on next page

PROLOG Task Force for *Patient Management in the Office*, Seventh Edition *(continued)*

Colleen M. Horan MD, MPH
Chief of Obstetrics and Gynecology
Central Vermont Medical Center
University of Vermont Health Network
Burlington, Vermont

A. Dhanya Mackeen, MD, MPH
Assistant Professor of Obstetrics and Gynecology
Temple University School of Medicine
Director of Research
Division of Maternal–Fetal Medicine
Geisinger Health System
Danville, Pennsylvania

Jessica E. Morse, MD, MPH
Assistant Professor
Division of Family Planning
Department of Obstetrics and Gynecology
University of North Carolina
Chapel Hill, North Carolina

Russell R. Snyder, MD
Associate Professor of Obstetrics and Gynecology
Vice Chair and Director, Division of Gynecology
Faculty Distinguished Chair in Obstetrics and Gynecology
University of Texas Medical Branch
Galveston, Texas

Laurie S. Swaim, MD
Associate Professor
Director, Division of Gynecologic and Obstetric Specialists
Chief of Gynecology, Pavilion for Women Texas Children's Hospital
Department of Obstetrics and Gynecology
Baylor College of Medicine
Houston, Texas

Wayne Trout, MD
Associate Professor of Obstetrics and Gynecology
Division of General Obstetrics and Gynecology
The Ohio State University Wexner Medical Center
Columbus, Ohio

Roxanne A. Vrees, MD
Assistant Professor of Obstetrics and Gynecology
Warren Alpert Medical School, Brown University
Division of Emergency Obstetrics and Gynecology
Department of Obstetrics and Gynecology
Women and Infants Hospital
Providence, Rhode Island

Katharine O'Connell White, MD, MPH
Assistant Professor
Director, Family Planning Fellowship
Department of Obstetrics and Gynecology
Boston University
Boston, Massachusetts

COLLEGE STAFF

Sandra A. Carson, MD
Vice President for Education

Erica Flynn, MBA, MS
Senior Director, Educational Development and Testing
Division of Education

Elizabeth Moran, MA
Editor, PROLOG

Disclosure Statement

The Accreditation Council for Continuing Medical Education (ACCME) requires that all faculty and planning committee members disclose any financial interests relative to topics within this edition of PROLOG. This information will be obtained in advance by staff through the American College of Obstetricians and Gynecologists' (the College) online disclosure system. There must be ample time for resolution of all potential conflicts of interest. This information (with resolution of any conflicts of interest) should be on file before honoraria are paid.

Disclosure of Faculty and Industry Relationships

In accordance with College policy, all faculty and planning committee members have signed a conflict of interest statement in which they have disclosed any financial interests or other relationships with industry relative to topics in this edition of PROLOG. Such disclosure allows for better evaluation of the objectivity of the information presented.

Conflict of Interest Disclosure

This PROLOG unit was developed under the direction of the PROLOG Advisory Committee and Task Force for *Patient Management in the Office*, Seventh Edition. PROLOG is planned and produced in accordance with the Standards for Commercial Support of the ACCME. Any discussion of unapproved use of products is clearly cited in the appropriate critique.

Current guidelines state that continuing medical education (CME) health care providers must ensure that CME activities are free from the control of any commercial interest. The task force and advisory committee members declare that neither they nor any business associate nor any member of their immediate families has material interest, financial interest, or other relationships with any company manufacturing commercial products relative to the topics included in this publication or with any provider of commercial services discussed in the unit except for **Sandra Carson, MD**, whose spouse is an employee of the March of Dimes and a consultant for Myriad Genetics; **Jeffrey S. Dungan, MD**, who is on the Speakers Bureau and Clinical Advisory Board for Sequenom Center for Molecular Medicine; **Russell R. Snyder, MD**, who is a panel member on the Medical Devices Advisory Committee for the Food and Drug Administration; and **Katharine O'Connell White, MD**, who is a consultant for Allergan for LILETTA. All potential conflicts have been resolved through the College's mechanism for resolving potential and real conflicts of interest.

Preface

Purpose

PROLOG (Personal Review of Learning in Obstetrics and Gynecology) is a voluntary, strictly confidential self-evaluation program. PROLOG was developed specifically as a personal study resource for the practicing obstetrician–gynecologist. It is presented as a self-assessment mechanism that, with its accompanying performance information, should assist the physician in designing a personal, self-directed, lifelong learning program. It may be used as a valuable study tool, a reference guide, and a means of attaining up-to-date information in the specialty. The content is carefully selected and presented in multiple-choice questions that are clinically oriented. The questions are designed to stimulate and challenge physicians in areas of medical care that they confront in their practices or when they work as consultant obstetrician–gynecologists.

PROLOG also provides the American College of Obstetricians and Gynecologists (the College) with one mechanism to identify the educational needs of the Fellows. Individual scores are reported only to the participant; however, cumulative performance data and evaluation comments obtained for each PROLOG unit help determine the direction for future educational programs offered by the College.

Process

The PROLOG series offers the most current information available in five areas of the specialty: 1) obstetrics; 2) gynecology and surgery; 3) reproductive endocrinology and infertility; 4) gynecologic oncology and critical care; and 5) patient management in the office. The series now includes a sixth volume for the subspecialty of female pelvic medicine and reconstructive surgery. A new PROLOG unit is produced annually, addressing one of those subject areas. *Patient Management in the Office*, Seventh Edition, is the fifth unit in the seventh 5-year PROLOG series.

Each unit of PROLOG represents the efforts of a task force of subject experts under the supervision of an advisory committee. PROLOG sets forth current information as viewed by recognized authorities in the field of women's health. This educational resource does not define a standard of care, nor is it intended to dictate an exclusive course of management. It presents recognized methods and techniques of clinical practice for consideration by obstetrician–gynecologists to incorporate in their practices. Variations of practice that take into account the needs of the individual patient, resources, and the limitations that are special to the institution or type of practice may be appropriate.

Each unit of PROLOG is presented as a two-part set, with performance information and cognate credit available to those who choose to submit their assessment for confidential scoring. The first part of the PROLOG set is the Assessment Book, which contains educational objectives for the unit and multiple-choice questions. The questions will be completed by taking an online assessment. Participants can work through the unit at their own pace, choosing to use PROLOG as a closed- or open-book assessment tool. Submitting the assessment is encouraged but voluntary.

The second part of PROLOG is the Critique Book, which reviews the educational objectives and questions set forth in the Assessment Book and contains a discussion or critique of each question. The critique provides the rationale for correct and incorrect options. Current, accessible references are listed for each question.

Continuing Medical Education Credit

ACCME Accreditation

The American College of Obstetricians and Gynecologists is accredited by the Accreditation Council for Continuing Medical Education (ACCME) to provide continuing medical education for physicians.

AMA PRA Category 1 Credit(s)™

The American College of Obstetricians and Gynecologists designates this enduring material for a maximum of 25 ***AMA PRA Category 1 Credits***™. Physicians should claim only the credit commensurate with the extent of their participation in the activity.

College Cognate Credit(s)

The American College of Obstetricians and Gynecologists designates this enduring material for a maximum of 25 Category 1 College Cognate Credits. The College has a reciprocity agreement with the American Medical Association that allows ***AMA PRA Category 1 Credits***™ to be equivalent to College Cognate Credits.

Participants who submit their assessment for scoring and receive a passing score will be credited with 25 continuing medical education (CME) credits for this unit. Those who complete the assessment for CME credit will receive a performance report that provides a comparison of their scores with the scores of a sample group of physicians who have taken the unit as an examination. An individual may request credit only once for each unit. Credits are available when a participant passes the online assessment with a score of 80% or higher.

Credit for PROLOG *Patient Management in the Office*, Seventh Edition, is initially available through December 2019. During that year, the unit will be reevaluated. If the content remains current, credit is extended for an additional 3 years, with credit for the unit automatically withdrawn after December 2022.

New: Electronic Assessment for CME Credit

For this edition and all future editions of PROLOG, participants will need to take the assessment electronically. Assessment results must be 80% or higher to achieve a passing score and attain CME credit. To begin the online assessment, please visit www.acog.org/PROLOGexam. Test results and the CME certificate will be available upon completion of the examination.

If you purchased a print book, use the key code located on the inside front cover of the Critique Book and follow the directions provided. If you purchased an eBook, please follow the instructions online to purchase and access the assessment. For more information about taking the assessment for *Patient Management in the Office*, Seventh Edition, please visit www.acog.org/PrologPMO or contact the Education Department via e-mail at education@acog.org.

Conclusion

PROLOG was developed specifically as a personal study resource for the practicing obstetrician–gynecologist. It is presented as a self-assessment mechanism that, with its accompanying performance information, should assist the physician in designing a personal, self-directed learning program. The many quality resources developed by the College, as detailed each year in the College's *Publications and Educational Materials Catalog*, are available to help fulfill the educational interests and needs that have been identified. PROLOG is not intended as a substitute for the certification or recertification programs of the American Board of Obstetrics and Gynecology.

PROLOG CME SCHEDULE

Patient Management in the Office, Sixth Edition	Credit through 2017
Obstetrics, Seventh Edition	Reevaluated in 2015–Credit through 2018
Gynecology and Surgery, Seventh Edition	Reevaluated in 2016–Credit through 2019
Reproductive Endocrinology and Infertility, Seventh Edition	Reevaluated in 2017–Credit through 2020
Gynecologic Oncology and Critical Care, Seventh Edition	Reevaluated in 2018–Credit through 2021
Female Pelvic Medicine and Reconstructive Surgery	Reevaluated in 2018–Credit through 2021
Patient Management in the Office, Seventh Edition	Reevaluated in 2019–Credit through 2022

PROLOG Objectives

PROLOG is a voluntary, strictly confidential, personal continuing education resource that is designed to be stimulating and enjoyable. By participating in PROLOG, obstetrician–gynecologists will be able to do the following:

- Review and update clinical knowledge.
- Recognize areas of knowledge and practice in which they excel, be stimulated to explore other areas of the specialty, and identify areas requiring further study.
- Plan continuing education activities in light of identified strengths and deficiencies.
- Compare and relate present knowledge and skills with those of other participants.
- Obtain continuing medical education credit, if desired.
- Have complete personal control of the setting and of the pace of the experience.

The obstetrician–gynecologist who completes *Patient Management in the Office*, Seventh Edition, will be able to do the following:

- Identify epidemiologic factors that contribute to women's health problems encountered in office practice.
- Determine appropriate screening approaches to identify health issues in women.
- Correlate presenting signs and symptoms with appropriate diagnostic tools in making diagnoses of a variety of women's health care needs encountered in office practice.
- Describe appropriate traditional and alternative management strategies for select conditions encountered in office practice.
- Counsel patients about the effect of health and illness throughout their lives and about risks and benefits of treatment.
- Apply professional medical ethics to the practice of obstetrics and gynecology.
- Incorporate appropriate legal, risk management, and office management guidelines and techniques in clinical practice.

Patient Management in the Office, Seventh Edition, includes the following topics (item numbers appear in parentheses):

COUNSELING

Adverse effects of tamoxifen citrate (16)
Colon cancer screening in postmenopausal women (85)
Contraceptive counseling after thrombosis (45)
Counseling for tubal sterilization (98)
Cytology screening in adolescents (127)
Date rape (10)
Depot medroxyprogesterone acetate and bone density (36)
Depression in adolescents (43)
Depression in pregnancy (13)
Diet and blood pressure (28)
Evaluation of incontinence (178–181)
Family history of intellectual and developmental disabilities (121)
In vitro fertilization and pregnancy outcome (32)
Listeria in pregnancy (130)
Oral health during pregnancy (124)
Pelvic organ prolapse (54)
Polycystic ovary syndrome (22)
Prepregnancy counseling (65)
Primary amenorrhea (95)
Risks of untreated asymptomatic bacteriuria in pregnancy (82)
Safety of breastfeeding in a patient with hepatitis C (120)

EPIDEMIOLOGY AND BIOSTATISTICS

ETHICAL AND LEGAL ISSUES

MEDICAL MANAGEMENT

OFFICE PROCEDURES

PREVENTION AND POPULATION HEALTH

SCREENING AND DIAGNOSIS

SURGICAL MANAGEMENT

A complete subject matter index appears at the end of the Critique Book.

1

Hormone therapy in patients with breast cancer

A 55-year-old woman has just completed six cycles of chemotherapy after a unilateral mastectomy for stage II breast cancer. She reports having hot flushes three times a day and severe vaginal dryness and irritation that makes intercourse painful. She has tried water-based lubricants and vaginal moisturizers with no relief. The intervention most likely to reduce her vaginal symptoms is

(A) additional lubricant
(B) oral estrogen therapy
(C) oral estrogen–progesterone therapy
(D) transdermal estrogen–progesterone patch
* (E) vaginal estrogen therapy

The described patient reports a common concern among women being treated for breast cancer. Menopausal symptoms often are secondary to either chemotherapy that has ablated ovarian function or hormonal treatments such as selective estrogen receptor modulators and aromatase inhibitors. Traditional hormone therapy (HT) to reduce vasomotor symptoms generally is avoided in women who have a recent diagnosis of breast cancer or who are actively being treated for breast cancer because of the theoretical risk of using HT in women with an endocrine-responsive tumor, such as an estrogen receptor-positive breast cancer. Therefore, oral or transdermal HT, which results in elevated serum levels of hormone, generally should be avoided. However, studies that have examined this subject have not been conclusive.

For symptoms related to vulvovaginal atrophy, first-line therapy typically is the use of moisturizers and lubricants. Studies show that approximately one half of women obtain full or partial relief of vulvovaginal atrophy symptoms when these therapies are used. However, the primary mechanism behind the symptoms is thinning of the vaginal epithelium, and reversing these changes requires the use of estrogen.

There is a lack of data to address the safety of vaginal estrogen use in women who receive a breast cancer diagnosis. Small observational studies generally do not reveal any increased risk of breast cancer recurrence, but duration and dosage of treatment varies greatly, so few generalizations can be made. A large study to examine breast cancer recurrence captured through a national database that allowed for correlation with filled prescriptions for local HT did not demonstrate an increased recurrence risk in patients who had received tamoxifen or aromatase inhibitors.

For the described patient, the primary concern is related to vulvovaginal atrophy, and focused therapy for her concerns should be the strategy. Given that nonhormonal management has not achieved relief, vaginal estrogen is a reasonable option. Using the lowest dose to provide effective relief minimizes exposure.

Systemic absorption of vaginal hormones appears to be minimal, although data are mixed. A brief treatment of regular dosage may allow the vaginal epithelium to heal; switching to less frequent application after healing is advisable. Combining low-dose vaginal estrogen with the nonhormonal measures also may result in symptom relief. Such therapy should be provided in consultation with the patient's oncologist and used for as short a duration as possible.

Drug delivery that results in the lowest systemic absorption should be the goal. Some evidence suggests that estrogen creams may be associated with increased systemic absorption. Use of a vaginal estrogen tablet or a silastic ring impregnated with estradiol would be preferable for this patient.

Antoine C, Liebens F, Carly B, Pastijn A, Neusy S, Rozenberg S. Safety of hormone therapy after breast cancer: a qualitative systematic review. Hum Reprod 2007;22:616–22.

Bakkum-Gamez JN, Laughlin SK, Jensen JR, Akogyeram CO, Pruthi S. Challenges in the gynecologic care of premenopausal women with breast cancer [published erratum appears in Mayo Clin Proc 2011;86:364]. Mayo Clin Proc 2011;86:229–40.

Le Ray I, Dell'Aniello S, Bonnetain F, Azoulay L, Suissa S. Local estrogen therapy and risk of breast cancer recurrence among hormone-treated patients: a nested case-control study. Breast Cancer Res Treat 2012;135:603–9.

Rahn DD, Carberry C, Sanses TV, Mamik MM, Ward RM, Meriwether KV, et al. Vaginal estrogen for genitourinary syndrome of menopause: a systematic review. Society of Gynecologic Surgeons Systematic Review Group. Obstet Gynecol 2014;124:1147–56.

The use of vaginal estrogen in women with a history of estrogen-dependent breast cancer. Committee Opinion No. 659. American College of Obstetricians and Gynecologists. Obstet Gynecol 2016;127:e93–6.

* Indicates correct answer.
Note: See Appendix A for a table of normal values for laboratory tests.

2
Postpartum depression

A 23-year-old woman, gravida 1, para 1, underwent a spontaneous vaginal delivery 3 weeks ago. She has no history of depression or other psychiatric disorders. She has been having difficulty sleeping, even when her baby is asleep. She has minimal energy and feels as if she is failing as a mother. Her appetite is poor, and she says her mother has to force her to eat. At times, she has crying spells with acute onset. On mental status examination, she is oriented to person, place, and time. The most likely diagnosis is

(A) postpartum psychosis
(B) postpartum blues
* (C) postpartum depression
(D) bipolar disorder

Postpartum psychiatric disorders have received much attention recently because the incidence of these conditions is increasing. According to the World Health Organization, depression accounts for $30 billion annually in direct medical costs in the United States. Depression is the leading cause of disability in women. Postpartum depression is diagnosed in up to 15% of women. The risk factors for postpartum depression include poor social support, major life events or stressors during pregnancy, history of postpartum depression, young age, history of physical or sexual abuse, and unplanned pregnancy. The etiology of postpartum depression is unclear, although it is hypothesized that the drop in estrogen and progesterone after delivery may play a role. Genetic susceptibility and major life events also may contribute to the pathogenesis.

Pregnancy and the postpartum period are ideal times to evaluate women for depression because patients have frequent contact with obstetrician–gynecologists or other health care providers at these times. The American College of Obstetricians and Gynecologists recommends that screening for depression and anxiety symptoms be done at least once during the perinatal period using a validated screening tool. The most common validated screening tool for postpartum depression is the Edinburgh Postnatal Depression Scale (Appendix B). The scale has 10 questions, and each is scored from 0 to 3. A cutoff score of 13 or more has an 86% sensitivity and a 78% specificity for diagnosing postpartum major depression. This test is easily administered and quickly scored.

Based on the criteria of the *Diagnostic and Statistical Manual of Mental Disorders*, Fifth Edition, postpartum depression falls under the diagnostic criteria for "major depressive episode with postpartum onset." Postpartum depression is diagnosed when a woman has five of the following nine symptoms that cause significant impairment in daily functioning within the first 4 weeks postpartum: 1) depressed mood, 2) decreased interest in pleasurable activities (anhedonia), 3) decreased energy, 4) changes in sleep pattern, 5) changes in weight, 6) decreased concentration or indecisiveness, 7) feelings of guilt or worthlessness, 8) psychomotor retardation or agitation, and 9) suicidal ideation. The described patient's clinical presentation meets the criteria for postpartum depression.

Treatment of postpartum depression may include nonpharmacologic treatment, pharmacologic treatment, or both. For mild-to-moderate postpartum depression, initial treatment includes interpersonal psychotherapy and cognitive behavioral therapy. This can be done either on an individual basis or in a group setting. For moderate-to-severe postpartum depression, pharmacologic therapy is recommended. In cases of suicidal or homicidal ideation, hospitalization is required. Selective serotonin reuptake inhibitors are first-line agents used for postpartum depression because of their favorable adverse effect profile; these medications also may be used while breastfeeding. Infants should be monitored for rare adverse effects, such as persistent irritability, decreased feeding, or poor weight gain. The physician should hold a thorough risk–benefit discussion with the patient before deciding on treatment for postpartum depression. In addition, appropriate follow-up is imperative.

Postpartum psychosis most commonly presents within 2 weeks postpartum; it occurs in approximately 0.1–0.2% of new mothers. Hallucinations, delusions, and profound thought disorganization usually are present. The patient may be disoriented to person, place, or time. Because this patient has a normal mental status examination, her presentation is not consistent with postpartum psychosis.

Postpartum blues begin during the first 2–3 days after delivery and resolve within 10 days. This period is characterized by mild depressive symptoms, including irritability, tearfulness, and decreased concentration. The described patient has depressive symptoms at 3 weeks postpartum, past the expected duration for postpartum blues.

Bipolar disorder is characterized by alternating episodes of major depression and mania. The overall prevalence of bipolar disorder in the postpartum period is approximately 3% among new mothers. This patient does not exhibit any manic episodes and, therefore, her symptoms are not consistent with bipolar disorder.

American Psychiatric Association. Bipolar and related disorders. Diagnostic and statistical manual of mental disorders: DSM-5. 5th ed. Washington, DC: APA; 2013.

Cox JL, Holden JM, Sagovsky R. Detection of postnatal depression. Development of the 10-item Edinburgh Postnatal Depression Scale. Br J Psychiatry 1987;150:782–6.

Hirst KP, Moutier CY. Postpartum major depression. Am Fam Physician 2010;82:926–33.

Screening for depression during and after pregnancy. Committee Opinion No. 453. American College of Obstetricians and Gynecologists. Obstet Gynecol 2010;115:394–5.

Screening for perinatal depression. Committee Opinion No. 630. American College of Obstetricians and Gynecologists. Obstet Gynecol 2015;125:1268–71.

Sit D, Rothschild AJ, Wisner KL. A review of postpartum psychosis. J Womens Health (Larchmt) 2006;15:352–68.

Use of psychiatric medications during pregnancy and lactation. ACOG Practice Bulletin No. 92. American College of Obstetricians and Gynecologists. Obstet Gynecol 2008;111:1001–20.

3

Preoperative evaluation for hypertension

A 55-year-old woman with diabetes mellitus, obesity, hypertension, and hypercholesterolemia is scheduled for a total abdominal hysterectomy, bilateral salpingo-oophorectomy, and lymph node dissection for endometrial cancer. At her preoperative visit, her body mass index (calculated as weight in kilograms divided by height in meters squared [kg/m^2]) is 45 and her blood pressure is 140/90 mm Hg. Review of systems is significant for dyspnea on minimal exertion. She states that she was not able to make it through a slow dance with her son at his recent wedding because she had some chest discomfort, which she attributed to being emotional. She has trouble walking because of pain in her knees. Her medication list consists of insulin, an angiotensin-converting enzyme inhibitor, and a statin. She has no known history of coronary artery disease. An electrocardiographic examination is unremarkable. Before proceeding with the proposed surgery, the step that you should take is to order

(A) a pulmonary function test
(B) an exercise stress test
* (C) dobutamine stress echocardiography
(D) preoperative coronary angiography

Preoperative evaluation of cardiovascular risk in a patient who is scheduled to undergo noncardiac surgery is important for several reasons. Assessment of perioperative risk may be used to inform the decision to proceed with an intended surgery, determine the need for changes in management, inform decisions about the optimal timing and location of surgery, and possibly identify cardiovascular conditions that require long-term management. Procedure-specific and patient-specific factors affect the risk of a *major adverse cardiac event*, defined as death or myocardial infarction, in the perioperative period.

The revised cardiac risk index is widely used to predict perioperative complications and discriminates moderately well between patients who are at low risk or high risk of cardiac events after noncardiac surgery. It consists of six equally weighted components: 1) coronary artery disease, 2) heart failure, 3) cerebral vascular disease, 4) diabetes requiring insulin, 5) renal insufficiency, and 6) high-risk noncardiac surgery (eg, suprainguinal vascular, intrathoracic, intraperitoneal).

The risk of a major adverse cardiac event after noncardiac surgery is elevated significantly in patients with previous coronary artery disease events, myocardial infarction, unstable angina, and heart failure. Operations for peripheral vascular disease are among those with the highest risk, whereas operations without significant fluid shifts or stress, such as plastic surgery or cataract surgery, are associated with a very low risk of major adverse cardiac events. Several validated risk precision tools can be used to estimate a patient-specific and procedure-specific risk of major adverse cardiac events. If the risk is estimated to be less than 1%, the procedure is considered low risk, and if the risk is 1% or more, the procedure is considered to be higher risk.

In 2014, the American College of Cardiology and the American Heart Association released evidence-based guidelines on perioperative evaluation and management. Table 3-1 shows a summary of how classification of recommendation and level of evidence are assigned.

Based on these guidelines, several recommendations can be made regarding the perioperative care of the described patient, who has risk factors for coronary heart

TABLE 3-1. Applying Classification of Recommendations and Level of Evidence

Estimate of Certainty (Precision) of Treatment Effect*	**Size of Treatment**			
	Class I *Benefit >>> Risk* Procedure/Treatment SHOULD be performed/ administered.	**Class IIa** *Benefit >> Risk* *Additional studies with focused objectives needed.* **IT IS REASONABLE** to perform procedure/ administer treatment.	**Class IIb** *Benefit ≥ Risk* *Additional studies with broad objectives needed; additional registry data would be helpful.* Procedure/treatment **MAY BE CONSIDERED**.	**Class III** No Benefit or **Class III** Harm (columns: — / Procedure/ Test / Treatment) COR III: No benefit / Not helpful / No proven benefit COR III: Harm / Excess cost with no benefit or harmful / Harmful to patients
Level A Multiple populations evaluated† Data derived from multiple randomized clinical trials or meta-analyses	• Recommendation that procedure or treatment is useful/effective • Sufficient evidence from multiple randomized trials or meta-analyses	• Recommendation in favor of treatment or procedure being useful/ effective • Some conflicting evidence from multiple randomized trials or meta-analyses	• Recommendation's usefulness/efficacy less well established • Greater conflicting evidence from multiple randomized trials or meta-analyses	• Recommendation that procedure or treatment is not useful/effective and may be harmful • Sufficient evidence from multiple randomized trials or meta-analyses
Level B Limited populations evaluated† Data derived from a single randomized trial or nonrandomized studies	• Recommendation that procedure or treatment is useful/effective • Evidence from single randomized trial or non-randomized studies	• Recommendation in favor of treatment or procedure being useful/ effective • Some conflicting evidence from single randomized trial or non-randomized studies	• Recommendation's usefulness/efficacy less well established • Greater conflicting evidence from single randomized trial or non-randomized studies	• Recommendation that procedure or treatment is not useful/effective and may be harmful • Evidence from single randomized trial or non-randomized studies
Level C Very limited populations evaluated† Only consensus opinion of experts, case studies, or standard of care	• Recommendation that procedure or treatment is useful/effective • Only expert opinion, case studies, or standard of care	• Recommendation in favor of treatment or procedure being useful/ effective • Only diverging expert opinion, case studies, or standard of care	• Recommendation's usefulness/efficacy less well established • Only diverging expert opinion, case studies, or standard of care	• Recommendation that procedure or treatment is not useful/effective and may be harmful • Only expert opinion, case studies, or standard of care
Suggested phrases for writing recommendations	should is recommended is indicated is useful/effective/beneficial	is reasonable can be useful/effective/ beneficial is probably recommended or indicated	may/might be considered may/might be reasonable usefulness/effectiveness is unknown/unclear/uncertain or not well established	COR III: No Benefit: is not recommended is not indicated should not be performed/ administered/ other is not useful/ beneficial/ effective COR III: Harm: potentially harmful causes harm associated with excess morbidity/mortality should not be performed/ administered/ other
Comparative effectiveness phrases‡	Treatment/strategy A is recommended/indicated in preference to treatment B. Treatment A should be chosen over treatment B.	Treatment/strategy A is probably recommended/indicated in preference to treatment B. It is reasonable to choose treatment A over treatment B.		

Abbreviation: COR, classification of recommendation.

*A recommendation with level of evidence B or C does not imply that the recommendation is weak. Many important key clinical questions addressed in the guidelines do not lend themselves to clinical trials. Although randomized trials are unavailable, there may be a very clear clinical consensus that a particular test or therapy is useful or effective.

†Data available from clinical trials or registries about the usefulness/efficacy in different subpopulations, such as sex, age, history of diabetes mellitus, history of prior myocardial infarction, history of heart failure, and prior aspirin use.

‡For comparative effectiveness recommendations (Class I and IIa; level of evidence A and B only), studies that support the use of comparator verbs should involve direct comparisons of the treatments or strategies being evaluated.

Modified from Fleisher LA, Fleischmann KE, Auerbach AD, Barnason SA, Beckman JA, Bozkurt B, et al. 2014 ACC/AHA guideline on perioperative cardiovascular evaluation and management of patients undergoing noncardiac surgery: a report of the American College of Cardiology/American Heart Association Task Force on practice guidelines. American College of Cardiology/American Heart Association. J Am Coll Cardiol 2014;64:e77–137. Copyright 2014, with permission from Elsevier.

disease and limited functional capacity. Functional status is a reliable predictor of perioperative risk and long-term cardiac events. In highly functional asymptomatic patients, it often is appropriate to proceed with planned surgery without further cardiovascular testing. Functional status is expressed in terms of metabolic equivalent tasks (METs), where 1 MET is the resting or basal oxygen consumption of a 40-year-old 70-kg (155-lb) man. In patients who have not had a recent exercise stress test, functional status can be estimated from activities of daily living. A functional capacity of greater than 10 METs is excellent, 7–10 METs is good, 4–6 METs is moderate, and fewer than 4 METs is poor. Table 3-2 lists METs for many daily activities and exercises. The described patient has limited functional status based on her intolerance for mild activity such as slow dancing. Although use of echocardiography for routine preoperative testing is not recommended in patients without signs or symptoms of cardiovascular disease, assessment of left ventricular function is reasonable in patients who have dyspnea of unknown origin, as this patient does.

It is reasonable for patients at elevated risk of noncardiac surgery with poor functional capacity to undergo either dobutamine stress echocardiography or myocardial perfusion imaging if it will change management. Given that nonsurgical palliative options are available for treatment of endometrial cancer, there is an opportunity to consider alternative management in this patient depending

Table 3-2. Energy Requirements of Selected Daily Activities*

Activities	METs
Leisure	
Mild	
Billiards	2.4
Canoeing (leisurely)	2.5
Dancing (ballroom)	2.9
Golf (with cart)	2.5
Horseback riding (walking)	2.3
Playing a musical instrument	
Accordion	1.8
Cello	2.3
Flute	2.0
Piano	2.3
Violin	2.5
Volleyball (noncompetitive)	2.9
Walking (2 mph)	2.5
Moderate	
Calisthenics (no weight)	4.0
Cycling (leisurely)	3.5
Golf (without cart)	4.4
Swimming (slow)	4.5
Walking (3 mph)	3.3
Walking (4 mph)	4.5
Vigorous	
Chopping wood	4.9
Climbing hills (no load)	6.9
Climbing hills (5 kg load)	7.4
Cycling (moderately)	5.7
Dancing	
Aerobic or ballet	6.0
Ballroom (fast) or square	5.5
Jogging (10 min mile)	10.2
Rope skipping	12.0

(continued)

Table 3-2. Energy Requirements of Selected Daily Activities* *(continued)*

Activities	METs
Leisure *(continued)*	
Vigorous *(continued)*	
Skating	
Ice	5.5
Roller	6.5
Skiing (water or downhill)	6.8
Squash	12.1
Surfing	6.0
Swimming	7.0
Tennis (doubles)	5.0
Walking (5 mph)	8.0
Activities of daily living	
Gardening (no lifting)	4.4
Household tasks, moderate effort	3.5
Lifting items continuously	4.0
Loading/unloading car	3.0
Lying quietly	1.0
Mopping	3.5
Mowing lawn (power mower)	4.5
Raking lawn	4.0
Riding in a vehicle	1.0
Sitting; light activity	1.5
Taking out trash	3.0
Vacuuming	3.5
Walking the dog	3.0
Walking from house to car or bus	2.5
Watering plants	2.5

Abbreviation: METs, metabolic equivalent tasks.

*These activities often can be done at variable intensities, assuming that the intensity is not excessive and that the courses are flat (no hills) unless so specified. Categories are based on experience or tolerance; if an activity is perceived to be more than indicated, it should be judged accordingly. MET indicates metabolic equivalent or a unit of sitting, resting oxygen uptake.

Fletcher GF, Balady GJ, Amsterdam EA, Chaitman B, et al. Exercise standards for testing and training: a statement for health professionals from the American Heart Association. Circulation 2001;104:1694–740.

on the results of her preoperative testing. Furthermore, depending on the test results, she may qualify for coronary revascularization. An exercise stress test is not the best option for her because of her limited functional capacity. Dobutamine stress echocardiography would allow assessment of left ventricular function as well as evaluation of her risk of significant underlying coronary artery disease.

In the absence of reactive airway disease, a pulmonary function test is not indicated. It is likely this patient's dyspnea is of cardiac origin.

Routine preoperative coronary angiography is not recommended. This procedure may be indicated depending on the results of pharmacologic stress testing. Lipid lowering with statin therapy is effective for primary and secondary prevention of cardiac events, and the effectiveness of statin therapy has suggested that statins may improve perioperative cardiovascular outcomes. Patients who are already taking statins should continue to do so in the perioperative period.

Fleisher LA, Fleischmann KE, Auerbach AD, Barnason SA, Beckman JA, Bozkurt B, et al. 2014 ACC/AHA guideline on perioperative cardiovascular evaluation and management of patients undergoing noncardiac surgery: a report of the American College of Cardiology/American Heart Association Task Force on practice guidelines. American College of Cardiology/American Heart Association. J Am Coll Cardiol 2014;64:e77–137.

Fletcher GF, Ades PA, Kligfield P, Arena R, Balady GJ, Bittner VA, et al. Exercise standards for testing and training: a scientific statement from the American Heart Association. American Heart Association Exercise, Cardiac Rehabilitation, and Prevention Committee of the Council on Clinical Cardiology, Council on Nutrition, Physical Activity and Metabolism, Council on Cardiovascular and Stroke Nursing, and Council on Epidemiology and Prevention. Circulation 2013;128: 873–934.

Ford MK, Beattie WS, Wijeysundera DN. Systematic review: prediction of perioperative cardiac complications and mortality by the revised cardiac risk index. Ann Intern Med 2010;152:26–35.

Wijeysundera DN, Duncan D, Nkonde-Price C, Virani SS, Washam JB, Fleischmann KE, et al. Perioperative beta blockade in noncardiac surgery: a systematic review for the 2014 ACC/AHA guideline on perioperative cardiovascular evaluation and management of patients undergoing noncardiac surgery: a report of the American College of Cardiology/American Heart Association Task Force on practice guidelines. J Am Coll Cardiol 2014;64:2406–25.

4

Emergency contraception

A 27-year-old woman, gravida 3, para 3, visits your office in a panic on Monday morning. She and her husband went away for their anniversary, and she forgot her diaphragm. The couple had unprotected intercourse twice in the past 48 hours. Her body mass index (BMI) (calculated as weight in kilograms divided by height in meters squared [kg/m^2]) is 37, but she is otherwise healthy. You tell her that the best option for preventing pregnancy is immediate use of

(A) levonorgestrel intrauterine device (IUD)
(B) levonorgestrel-only pills
(C) combination oral contraceptive pills (OCPs)
(D) ulipristal acetate
* (E) copper IUD

Unintended pregnancy is an ongoing public health problem in the United States. The rate of unintended pregnancy had remained at approximately 50% of all pregnancies over a number of years. However, data from 2011 indicates that the unintended pregnancy rate has decreased to 45%. This decrease is the most significant change in three decades. Although there are several factors that may explain this decrease, the increased use of long-acting reversible contraception, particularly IUDs, may be the most important one.

For the described patient, the most effective way to prevent an unintended pregnancy would be immediate insertion of a copper IUD. A copper IUD can be placed up to 120 hours after unprotected intercourse and has a pregnancy rate of less than 0.1%. The primary mechanism of action is thought to be inhibition of fertilization by affecting sperm and tubal motility. It has the additional benefit of providing ongoing contraception for 10 years. Many of the pregnancies seen in oral combination emergency contraception users result from repeated acts of unprotected intercourse within the same menstrual cycle. Because oral combination emergency contraception mainly works to delay or prevent ovulation, a single dose of a combined oral emergency contraception does not protect against future acts of unprotected intercourse. However, the copper IUD is effective as soon as it is in place and for the duration of its lifespan.

Many obstetrician–gynecologists and other health care providers worry that women presenting for emergency contraception will not be interested in having an IUD inserted. However, in studies assessing this topic, one in eight women presenting for emergency contraception have been interested in having an IUD placed if offered. When cost is not a barrier, almost one in five women are interested. Thus, as recommended by the American College of Obstetricians and Gynecologists, all women with no contraindications to a copper IUD should be offered immediate placement as the first-line option when requesting emergency contraception. There are currently no data to support the use of a levonorgestrel IUD for emergency contraception, although this option is being explored within a research setting.

Combined oral emergency contraception is the other option available to the described patient. Combination OCPs have been used as emergency contraception for years, in a regimen initially described in 1974 by Canadian physician Dr. A. Albert Yuzpe, based on similar regimens used in Europe at the time. The regimen involves use of routine OCPs in varied doses. Currently, 26 OCPs are approved by the U.S. Food and Drug Administration for emergency contraception in the United States. The standard regimen is two separate doses taken 12 hours apart. The number of pills taken depends on the type of progestin and dose of the OCP used. Levonorgestrel is the most studied, but there are safety and efficacy data for norethindrone as well. The initial description of using the method within 72 hours was not based on biology but instead on clinic hours (ie, to acknowledge the lack of weekend hours). The pregnancy rate is likely 2–3.5% using this regimen. However, the bigger concern with this regimen is the adverse effects. Due in large part to the estrogen, more than one half of women who use combined oral emergency contraception experience nausea and up to 15% have emesis. Many obstetrician–gynecologists and other health care providers prescribe an antiemetic along with this regimen. However, combined OCPs are considered third-line options because of lower efficacy and adverse effects.

The other commonly used oral option is a progestin-only-based regimen (typically levonorgestrel-only pills). This regimen is labeled for use for up to 72 hours after unprotected intercourse, although it has some effectiveness up to 120 hours after unprotected intercourse. The pregnancy rate after levonorgestrel regimens, which typically are a single dose, is 0.6–3.1%. Although oral levonorgestrel is superior to combination OCPs, it is less effective than ulipristal acetate.

For patients not interested in an IUD, ulipristal acetate is the next most effective option. Ulipristal acetate was approved by the U.S. Food and Drug Administration for use as emergency contraception in 2010. It is a selective progesterone receptor modulator with antagonist and partial agonist effects and is labeled for use within 120 hours of unprotected intercourse. The failure rate (or pregnancy rate) is thought to be 0.9–2.2%. The superior efficacy of ulipristal acetate over oral levonorgestrel has been well documented in randomized trials and a meta-analysis. These trials demonstrated that the risk of pregnancy is reduced by two thirds in women using ulipristal compared with those who use levonorgestrel. However, a more concerning finding is the significantly decreased effectiveness of levonorgestrel in obese women, making ulipristal acetate the preferred choice. The relative risk of pregnancy is quadrupled for obese women using levonorgestrel compared with ulipristal acetate. Some trials, although likely underpowered, suggest that levonorgestrel is no more effective than placebo in women with a BMI greater than 26. Although ulipristal acetate also has a BMI cutoff above which efficacy also is estimated to be no better than placebo, it is much higher, at 35. Even though ulipristal acetate is more effective, it has the disadvantage of requiring a prescription, unlike the levonorgestrel regimens that are available over the counter.

For the described patient, a copper IUD is the most effective way to prevent an unintended pregnancy. For all patients seeking emergency contraception, the office visit presents an ideal window of opportunity to address her immediate and long-term contraceptive needs by offering a copper IUD.

Brache V, Cochon L, Deniaud M, Croxatto HB. Ulipristal acetate prevents ovulation more effectively than levonorgestrel: analysis of pooled data from three randomized trials of emergency contraception regimens. Contraception 2013;88:611–8.

Emergency contraception. Practice Bulletin No. 152. American College of Obstetricians and Gynecologists. Obstet Gynecol 2015;126:e1–11.

Finer LB, Zolna MR. Declines in unintended pregnancy in the United States, 2008–2011. N Engl J Med 2016;374:843–52.

Glasier AF, Cameron ST, Fine PM, Logan SJ, Casale W, Van Horn J, et al. Ulipristal acetate versus levonorgestrel for emergency contraception: a randomised non-inferiority trial and meta-analysis [published erratum appears in Lancet 2014;384:1504]. Lancet 2010;375:555–62.

Trussell J, Rodriguez G, Ellertson C. New estimates of the effectiveness of the Yuzpe regimen of emergency contraception. Contraception 1998;57:363–9.

5

Graves disease

A 23-year-old woman comes to your office for a prepregnancy visit. She has unintentionally lost 9 kg (20 lb) over 2 months without any change in diet or level of activity. Your examination shows a temperature of 37°C (98.6°F), blood pressure of 142/92 mm Hg, and heart rate of 110 beats per minute. You suspect she has a thyroid disorder and order thyroid-stimulating hormone (TSH) and free thyroxine (T_4) levels. The changes in laboratory values that would support your clinical suspicion are

(A) decreased TSH; normal free T_4
* (B) decreased TSH; elevated free T_4
(C) elevated TSH; decreased free T_4
(D) elevated TSH; normal free T_4
(E) normal TSH; elevated free T_4

Thyroid disease is very common in women. Symptoms associated with hyperthyroidism and hypothyroidism are shown in Table 5-1. This patient's clinical picture of weight loss, hypertension, and tachycardia suggest thyroid disease, specifically hyperthyroidism. Although symptoms and physical findings alone may suggest thyroid disease, laboratory abnormalities are necessary to confirm the diagnosis.

The initial laboratory evaluation includes TSH and free T_4 levels. In hyperthyroidism, TSH is suppressed and the free T_4 and serum triiodothyronine (T_3) levels are elevated. Given the described patient's symptoms, these are the laboratory results most consistent with this clinical scenario. In hypothyroidism, TSH is elevated and the free T_4 is low; these results are unlikely given the patient's symptoms.

One of the most common causes of hyperthyroidism is Graves disease, an autoimmune process in which immunoglobulin G antibodies activate the thyrotropin receptor, which stimulates increased production of T_4 and T_3. Typically, serum T_3 is more elevated because of increased secretion and peripheral conversion of T_4 to T_3. The diagnosis of Graves disease may be presumed as the cause of hyperthyroidism for patients who present with goiter, ophthalmopathy, and pretibial myxedema. However, if the diagnosis is not apparent, additional testing for the following may help confirm a diagnosis of Graves disease: presence of TSH receptor antibodies or diffusely increased radioactive iodine uptake.

Graves disease usually is treated before pregnancy with antithyroid drugs (propylthiouracil or methimazole), radioiodine therapy (contraindicated in pregnancy), or subtotal thyroidectomy. Propylthiouracil and methimazole have been used safely in pregnant women with hyperthyroidism for many years, and both medications block organification of iodide, decreasing synthesis of thyroid hormone. In addition, propylthiouracil blocks the peripheral conversion of T_4 to T_3. If the described patient is managed successfully with these medications and becomes pregnant, she should continue to take them during her pregnancy. The risk to the pregnant woman and the developing fetus is likely to be greater with untreated

TABLE 5-1. Symptoms of Hyperthyroidism and Hypothyroidism

	Hyperthyroidism	Hypothyroidism
General	Fatigue	Fatigue
Weight	Loss	Gain
Heat/cold intolerance	Feel hot when others are not	Feel cold when others are not
Bowel movements	Frequent	Constipation
Other	Nervousness, tachycardia, diaphoresis, tremors	Myalgias, brittle nails, hair loss

Adapted from Thyroid disease in pregnancy. Practice Bulletin No. 148. American College of Obstetricians and Gynecologists. Obstet Gynecol 2015;125:996–1005.

hyperthyroidism than with the use of low doses of propylthiouracil or methimazole while pregnant. For patients with hyperthyroidism, the lowest effective dose that maintains maternal free T_4 within 10% above the upper limit of normal using the nonpregnant reference range should be used. In pregnant patients with tachycardia from hyperthyroidism, a β-blocker often is used. β-blockers have been associated with fetal growth restriction; therefore, serial growth assessments should be done.

Maternal risks of untreated hyperthyroidism include cardiac arrhythmias, osteoporosis, and thyroid storm. The risks to the fetus include premature delivery, preeclampsia, fetal growth restriction, and fetal demise.

Levels of TSH and free T_4 should be assessed each trimester and consideration should be given for antenatal testing starting at 32 weeks of gestation, especially in patients with uncontrolled disease. Women who have previously undergone radioiodine therapy or thyroid surgery for Graves disease should be assessed for TSH receptor antibodies in early and late pregnancy to evaluate the risk of fetal and neonatal hyperthyroidism, respectively. Those without this history who are currently euthyroid without medication do not need TSH receptor antibody assessment. Those who are currently using antithyroid drugs should have TSH receptor antibody levels assessed in late pregnancy to evaluate for neonatal hyperthyroidism risk. Patients should be counseled that propylthiouracil and methimazole can cross the placenta and result in fetal hypothyroidism, which may result in goiter formation. Thyroid-stimulating hormone receptor antibodies can cross the placenta and result in fetal hyperthyroidism, which can be evidenced by fetal arrhythmias, tachycardia, congestive heart failure, growth restriction, hydrops, and goiter. If the goiter is large enough, it may obstruct the newborn's airway. Therefore, if TSH receptor antibody levels are elevated or if the patient requires treatment with propylthiouracil or methimazole, a fetal ultrasonography at 28–32 weeks of gestation is indicated to assess fetal growth and to evaluate for the presence of a fetal goiter.

Baskin HJ, Cobin RH, Duick DS, Gharib H, Guttler RB, Kaplan MM, et al. American Association of Clinical Endocrinologists medical guidelines for clinical practice for the evaluation and treatment of hyperthyroidism and hypothyroidism. American Association of Clinical Endocrinologists [published erratum appears in Endocr Pract 2008;14:802–3]. Endocr Pract 2002;8:457–69.

Casey BM, Leveno KJ. Thyroid disease in pregnancy. Obstet Gynecol 2006;108:1283–92.

Chan GW, Mandel SJ. Therapy insight: management of Graves' disease during pregnancy. Nat Clin Pract Endocrinol Metab 2007;3:470–8.

Ladenson PW, Singer PA, Ain KB, Bagchi N, Bigos ST, Levy EG, et al. American Thyroid Association guidelines for detection of thyroid dysfunction [published erratum appears in Arch Intern Med 2001;161:284]. Arch Intern Med 2000;160:1573–5.

Laurberg P, Nygaard B, Glinoer D, Grussendorf M, Orgiazzi J. Guidelines for TSH-receptor antibody measurements in pregnancy: results of an evidence-based symposium organized by the European Thyroid Association. Eur J Endocrinol 1998;139:584–6.

Thyroid disease in pregnancy. Practice Bulletin No. 148. American College of Obstetricians and Gynecologists. Obstet Gynecol 2015;125:996–1005.

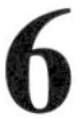

6 Nutrition deficiency in an elderly patient

An 82-year-old woman comes to your office for her annual well-woman examination. She is concerned about some recent memory decline. She reports that she has been feeling fatigued and has experienced generalized weakness for the past few months. She says she often has a "tingling sensation" in her hands and feet, which affects her ability to work in the garden. Her medications include daily omeprazole for gastroesophageal reflux disease and citalopram hydrobromide for depression. She takes no other medications or supplements and maintains a vegan diet. On examination, she has impaired position and vibratory sensation of her hands and feet bilaterally. Her complete blood count reveals a hemoglobin level of 10.4 g/dL and macrocytic indices. The most likely diagnosis is deficiency of

(A) iron
(B) folic acid
(C) calcium
(D) vitamin D
* (E) vitamin B_{12}

The described patient's use of a proton pump inhibitor (ie, omeprazole), vegan diet, manifestations of fatigue, symmetrical paresthesias, depression, and myalgias, as well as laboratory findings of macrocytic anemia, point toward a vitamin B_{12} deficiency. Iron deficiency is excluded by her complete blood count indices. Calcium deficiency is not associated with anemia, and chronic deficiency usually is mild and asymptomatic. Profound calcium deficiency can cause generalized neuromuscular irritability but does not have an insidious onset. Vitamin D deficiency typically is asymptomatic and manifests as hypocalcemia.

The nutritional status of elderly patients is an important component of their general health and well-being. Malnutrition, undernutrition, and vitamin deficiencies often are unrecognized. Vitamin B_{12} is found naturally in meat and dairy products and in some fortified foods (eg, flour, cereals). It is an essential nutrient for myelination and maintenance of the nervous system, production of red blood cells, and synthesis of DNA. The recommended dietary allowance of vitamin B_{12} for individuals older than 14 years is 2.4 micrograms daily, an amount often exceeded in daily vitamin supplements.

Vitamin B_{12} deficiency occurs in 10–24% of elderly individuals and often is first diagnosed as a macrocytic anemia. Box 6-1 lists conditions associated with macrocytosis. Figure 6-1 shows an algorithm for the workup of such patients. Vitamin B_{12} deficiency often is a result of inadequate intestinal absorption. Patients who lack intrinsic factor, as seen in pernicious anemia (autoimmune atrophic gastritis), or those with certain gastrointestinal diseases such as sprue or inflammatory bowel disease,

BOX 6-1

Conditions Associated With Macrocytosis and Macrocytic Anemia*

Nutrient deficiency
- Vitamin B_{12} deficiency
- Folate deficiency

Bone marrow disorders
- Myelodysplastic syndromes
- Congenital dyserythropoietic anemia
- Aplastic anemia
- Pure red cell aplasia
- Hematologic malignancy

Other conditions associated with macrocytosis
- Chronic liver disease
- Hypothyroidism
- Reticulocytosis
- Alcoholism

Medications
- Antineoplastic chemotherapy
  - — Cyclophosphamide
  - — Methotrexate
  - — Hydroxyurea
  - — Others
- Immunosuppressive agents
  - — Mycophenolate mofetil
  - — Azathioprine
- Antivirals
  - — Antiretroviral agents

*Mean corpuscular volume of more than $100\ mm^3$

Arcasoy MO, Telen MJ. Anemia. Clin Update Womens Health Care 2012;XI(5):1–103.

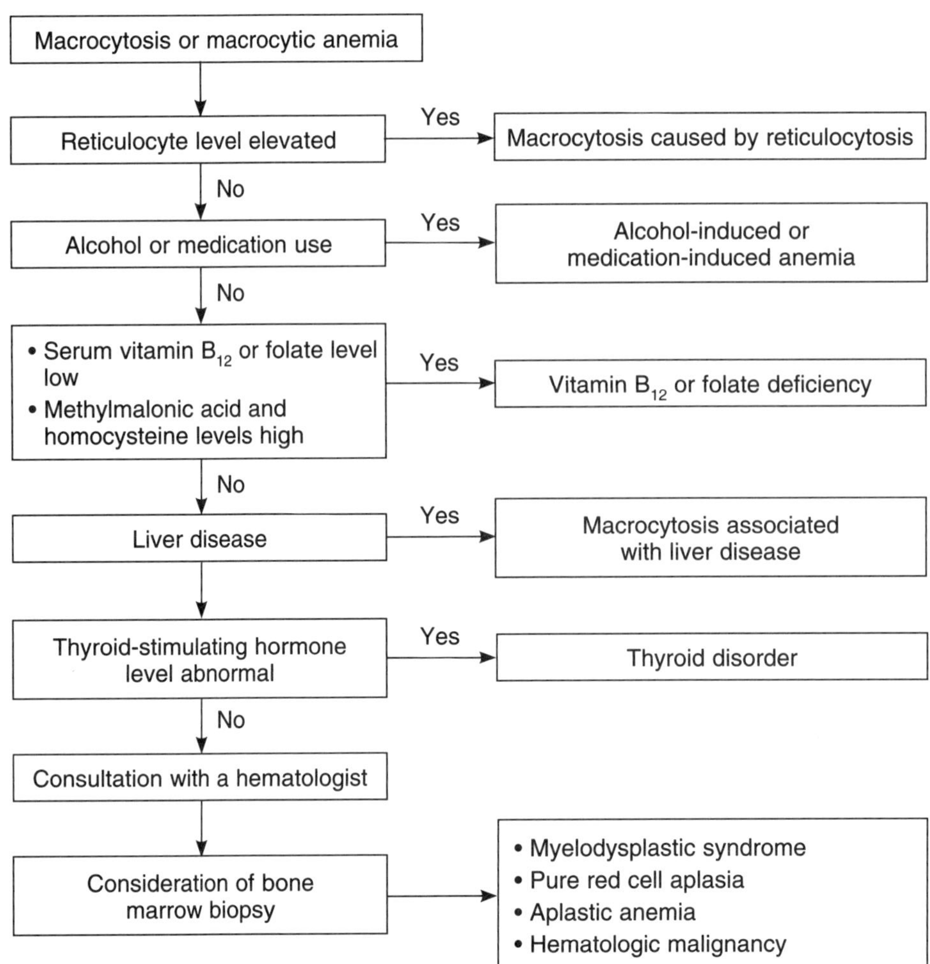

FIGURE 6-1. The evaluation of macrocytic anemia. (Arcasoy MO, Telen MJ. Anemia. Clin Update Womens Health Care 2012;XI(5):1–103.)

can have difficulties absorbing vitamin B_{12}. Other etiologies are listed in Box 6-2. Decreased absorption of vitamin B_{12} also is seen with increasing age and most likely is related to decreased separation from food in the stomach due to gastric atrophy.

The body is very efficient in storing vitamin B_{12}; therefore, symptoms may take years to develop and present subtly. Clinical manifestations of vitamin B_{12} deficiency are due to hematologic and nervous system involvement. Anemia may cause weakness, fatigue, and malaise. Nervous system symptoms, such as symmetric paresthesias of the upper and lower extremities (often more pronounced in the lower extremities), loss of balance, and ataxia, can occur. Additionally, mental status changes such as depression, confusion, impaired memory, and dementia may develop. Loss of vibratory sensation with a high-pitched tuning fork and loss of proprioception commonly are found on physical examination. In elderly patients, these symptoms and physical findings may be perceived as part of the natural aging process. Folate deficiency, another macrocytic anemia, is not a cause of neurologic symptoms.

Diagnosis of vitamin B_{12} deficiency is done through hematologic assessment. Findings include macrocytosis; hypersegmented neutrophils; and elevated levels of iron, indirect bilirubin, and lactate dehydrogenase. Serum vitamin B_{12} levels below 300 pg/mL are consistent with deficiency. Because folate and vitamin B_{12} deficiency are macrocytic anemias, assays of folic acid and red blood cell folate can distinguish between the two. If folate and vitamin B_{12} levels are equivocal and low to normal, further testing is indicated. Elevations of serum methylmalonic acid and homocysteine are specific to vitamin B_{12} deficiency. It is important to note that folic acid supplementation can actually mask vitamin B_{12} deficiency. Therefore, it is essential to exclude vitamin B_{12} deficiency before empiric treatment of a macrocytic anemia with folic acid. Lifelong oral vitamin B_{12} is necessary for those who are not found to have a reversible cause that can be eliminated.

BOX 6-2

Causes of Vitamin B_{12} Deficiency

Gastric abnormalities
Pernicious anemia
Gastrectomy/bariatric surgery
Gastritis
Autoimmune metaplastic atrophic gastritis
Small-bowel disease
- Malabsorption syndrome
- Ileal resection or bypass

Crohn disease
Blind loops
Diphyllobothrium latum (fish tapeworm) infestation
Pancreatitis
Diet
- Strict veganism
- Vegetarian diet in pregnancy

Agents that block or inhibit absorption
- Neomycin
- Biguanides (eg, metformin)

Proton pump inhibitors (eg, omeprazole)
Histamine-2 receptor antagonists (eg, cimetidine)
N_2O anesthesia inhibits methionine synthase
Inherited transcobalamin II deficiency

Abbreviation: N_2O, nitrous oxide.

Reproduced with permission from: Schrier SL. Etiology and clinical manifestations of vitamin B12 and folate deficiency. In: Post TW, editor. UpToDate. Waltham, MA: UpToDate; 2016. Accessed on April 13, 2016. Copyright 2016 UpToDate, Inc. For more information, visit www.uptodate.com.

Allen LH. How common is vitamin B-12 deficiency? Am J Clin Nutr 2009;89:693S–6S.

Arcasoy MO, Telen MJ. Anemia. Clin Update Womens Health Care 2012;XI (5):1–103.

Stabler SP. Clinical practice. Vitamin B12 deficiency. N Engl J Med 2013;368:149–60.

7

Syphilis in a pregnant patient

A 21-year-old nulligravid woman at 13 weeks of gestation comes to your office for her initial prenatal visit. She had a painless ulcer on her labia 16 months ago that resolved after 1 month, so she did not seek treatment. Prenatal laboratory results are significant for positive rapid plasma reagin (RPR) test and fluorescent treponemal antibody absorption (FTA-ABS) test. Her current titer is 1:16. She was given one dose of penicillin a week ago and experienced an anaphylactic reaction that required epinephrine in the emergency department. The most appropriate next step in management is

(A) treatment with vancomycin
(B) treatment with doxycycline
* (C) penicillin desensitization
(D) allergy skin testing
(E) repeat titers at 28 weeks of gestation

After the introduction of penicillin, the incidence of syphilis decreased drastically in the 1940s. This decrease continued until 2004, when the incidence of maternal syphilis began to increase steadily. In 2013, there were more than 56,471 cases of syphilis reported in the United States, which equates to 18 cases per 100,000 people. Syphilis is a sexually transmitted systemic infection caused by the spirochete *Treponema pallidum*. Risk factors for syphilis among pregnant women include substance abuse, limited access to health care, African American ethnicity, and poor adherence to prenatal care. The incubation period of primary syphilis is 9–90 days. Syphilis may present in various stages of the disease. Primary syphilis presents with a painless ulcer or chancre at the infection site. These chancres typically heal spontaneously within 3–6 weeks, even in the absence of treatment. Often, this lesion is not appreciated by women because it is on the vaginal or cervical mucosa. Secondary syphilis occurs in approximately 25% of untreated patients. This stage manifests with a skin rash on the palms of the hands and soles of the feet, mucocutaneous lesions, lymphadenopathy, and condyloma lata. Most women will consult their obstetrician–gynecologist or other health care provider at this stage. Tertiary syphilis is characterized by gumma formation, cardiovascular disease, or auditory deficits. Central nervous system involvement at any time during the disease is consistent with neurosyphilis.

Latent syphilis is diagnosed if an asymptomatic woman has a positive serologic test result. Latent syphilis that occurred in the past 12 months is called early latent syphilis, whereas occurrence after 12 months is called late latent syphilis. The U.S. Preventive Services Task Force and the Centers for Disease Control and Prevention strongly recommend that all pregnant women be screened for syphilis infection at their initial prenatal visit and at time of delivery. If a woman is at high risk of syphilis, she also should be tested in the third trimester.

Two types of serologic tests for syphilis are available: 1) nontreponemal and 2) treponemal. The most common nontreponemal screening tests used are the RPR test or the Venereal Disease Research Laboratory test. If the test result is positive, confirmatory testing using either the FTA-ABS test or the *T pallidum* passive particle agglutination assay is mandated. These confirmatory tests detect antibodies specifically directed at treponemal cellular components. False-positive RPR test results may be a result of autoimmune disorders such as systemic lupus erythematosus, intravenous drug use, chronic liver disease, and human immunodeficiency virus (HIV) infection. In women with confirmed syphilis infection, RPR titers should be obtained. These titers correlate with disease activity, usually decrease after treatment, and may become nonreactive over time. Therefore, titers can be monitored to evaluate the effectiveness of treatment. The FTA-ABS test result will remain positive despite treatment.

The only treatment that is indicated during pregnancy is penicillin G administered parenterally. Benzathine penicillin G 2.4 million units given intramuscularly in a single dose is recommended for primary, secondary, or early latent syphilis. Women with late latent or tertiary syphilis or syphilis of unknown duration should receive three total doses of benzathine penicillin G at 1-week intervals.

The described patient is clearly allergic to penicillin, as evidenced by an anaphylactic reaction to its administration. Because the only proven treatment for syphilis in pregnancy is penicillin, the treatment for penicillin-allergic patients is desensitization followed by penicillin therapy.

Within the first 24 hours after treatment with penicillin, the Jarisch–Herxheimer reaction may occur. In pregnancy, this may be characterized by uterine contractions, fetal heart rate decelerations, and preterm labor. Other components of the reaction include fever and myalgia. These symptoms result from the release of treponemal lipopolysaccharide from dying spirochetes and typically resolve within 24–48 hours.

Vancomycin is not an approved treatment for syphilis. Doxycycline may be an alternative treatment in nonpregnant women who are allergic to penicillin. Doxycycline is contraindicated in pregnancy because of the teratogenic risk of staining of teeth and possible effects on bone growth.

Allergy skin testing would be indicated if it was uncertain that the described woman had a true penicillin allergy. A typical indication for skin testing would be if a pregnant woman was determined to be allergic to penicillin in infancy and has never been treated with it since that time. Because the described woman had an anaphylactic reaction to penicillin, this allergy is evident; therefore, allergy skin testing would not be appropriate.

Repeating titers at 28 weeks of gestation is appropriate after treatment. However, waiting to treat this patient until 28 weeks of gestation to see if titers have decreased is not appropriate and places her and the fetus at significant risk. Besides serologic titers at 28 weeks of gestation and at delivery, detailed ultrasonography should be performed to evaluate for any fetal effects of syphilis infection. Ultrasonographic abnormalities may include nonimmune hydrops, hepatomegaly, placentomegaly, polyhydramnios, and ascites. Pediatric health care providers should be notified of the antenatal findings.

Gupta NK, Bowman CA. Managing sexually transmitted infections in pregnant women. Womens Health (Lond Engl) 2012;8:313–21.

Screening for syphilis infection in pregnancy: U.S. Preventive Services Task Force reaffirmation recommendation statement. Ann Intern Med 2009;150:705–9.

Wolff T, Shelton E, Sessions C, Miller T. Screening for syphilis infection in pregnant women: evidence for the U.S. Preventive Services Task Force reaffirmation recommendation statement. Ann Intern Med 2009;150:710–6.

Workowski KA, Bolan GA. Sexually transmitted diseases treatment guidelines, 2015. Centers for Disease Control and Prevention [published erratum appears in MMWR Recomm Rep 2015;64:924]. MMWR Recomm Rep 2015;64:1–137.

8

Female athlete triad

A 16-year-old nulligravid ballerina, who experienced menarche at age 13 years and has a 2-year history of secondary amenorrhea, presents for a physical examination. She has never been sexually active. She is not dancing this month because of a recent stress fracture in her foot. Her height is 1.65 m (65 in), and she weighs 47 kg (105 lb); her body mass index (BMI) (calculated as weight in kilograms divided by height in meters squared [kg/m^2]) is 17.4. On physical examination, she has no hirsutism. Pelvic examination reveals normal vulva, vagina, and cervix, and a small uterus is palpated. Her urine pregnancy test result is negative. Her thyroid-stimulating hormone level is 2.0 mIU/L, her follicle-stimulating hormone level is 2.0 mIU/L, and her prolactin level is 9.0 mIU/L. The best next step in management is to

(A) begin alendronate sodium
(B) start combination oral contraceptives
* (C) increase intake of dietary calories
(D) prescribe vitamin D and calcium supplements
(E) prescribe transdermal estrogen

The female athlete triad is a medical condition observed in physically active girls and is characterized by one or more of the following: menstrual dysfunction, low energy availability with or without disordered eating, and low bone density. This active patient meets all three characteristics, given her secondary amenorrhea with no other etiology, low BMI, and history of fragility fracture. Athletic activity with caloric expenditure exceeding caloric intake results in energy imbalance, leading to disordered release of luteinizing hormone and hypothalamic amenorrhea. The resulting hypoestrogenemia adversely affects bone mineralization, which can lead to low bone mineral density and an increased risk of fragility fractures. Evaluation of female athlete triad is important to protect bone health and reproductive potential, as well as to identify any psychosocial comorbidities.

All physically active female adolescents should be assessed for female athlete triad, and further evaluation is warranted if any of the three components is present. Athletes should be asked specifically about a history of amenorrhea or irregular menses, stress fractures, depression, weight concerns from parents or coaches, dietary habits, and perfectionism. This screening should occur as part of the preparticipation annual physical examination, which should review the presence and the severity of triad signs and symptoms (Box 8-1).

Infrequent cycles or secondary amenorrhea often will be the presenting symptom of female athlete triad noticed by obstetrician–gynecologists. Even when female athlete triad is suspected, all patients with menstrual abnormalities require standard evaluation because female athlete triad is a diagnosis of exclusion. A patient with secondary amenorrhea should have a pregnancy test and an assessment of thyroid-stimulating hormone, prolactin, and follicle-stimulating hormone levels.

BOX 8-1

Triad Consensus Panel Screening Questions

Have you ever had a menstrual period?

How old were you when you had your first menstrual period?

When was your most recent menstrual period?

How many periods have you had in the past 12 months?

Are you presently taking any female hormones (estrogen, progesterone, birth control pills)?

Do you worry about your weight?

Are you trying to or has anyone recommended that you gain or lose weight?

Are you on a special diet or do you avoid certain types of foods or food groups?

Have you ever had an eating disorder?

Have you ever had a stress fracture?

Have you ever been told you have low bone density (osteopenia or osteoporosis)?

De Souza MJ, Nattiv A, Joy E, Misra M, Williams NL, Mallinson RJ, et al. 2014 female athlete triad coalition consensus statement on treatment and return to play of the female athlete triad. Curr Sports Med Rep 2014;13(4):219–32.

A panel of experts at the 2014 Female Athlete Triad Coalition recommended dual-energy X-ray absorptiometry for women or adolescent athletes based on risk stratification that considers the following variables: diagnosed eating disorder, low BMI, weight as a percentage of estimated weight, percentage of recent weight loss in 1 month, age at beginning of menarche, frequency of menses, and history of stress fractures. Low bone mineral density (Z-score is less than –2.0 in nonweight-bearing athletes) and a history of long bone (one leg or two arm) or vertebral fracture are required to make a diagnosis of osteoporosis in adolescents. Athletes diagnosed with female athlete triad also should be screened for psychosocial comorbidities such as eating disorders and depression.

First-line therapy for girls with female athlete triad is correction of the energy imbalance by increasing caloric intake, decreasing activity level, or both. Collaboration amongst the patient, family, coaches, sport nutritionist, and health care providers may be required. Correction of the energy imbalance leads to resumption of menses, correction of the hypoestrogenemia, and improvement in bone mineral density. Pharmacologic therapy for the treatment of female athlete triad is not first-line therapy. Currently, bisphosphonates are not indicated for treatment of low bone mineral density seen in female athlete triad. Combination oral contraceptive pills are not primary therapy but are reasonable for patients who are sexually active and seeking birth control. There is growing evidence that oral contraceptive pills may stop further bone mineral loss but no evidence that they will improve bone mineral density. Use of hormonal contraception also makes it difficult to judge whether there has been a spontaneous resumption of menses. Appropriate intake of vitamin D and calcium is necessary for bone health and improvement in bone mineral density, but their use as a single therapy will not result in a return to normal bone density or the resumption of menses. Transdermal estrogen has been shown to maintain bone density in patients with anorexia but is not first-line therapy for female athlete triad. The best next step for the described patient is for her to increase her intake of dietary calories to exceed and then match the calories she expends.

De Souza MJ, Nattiv A, Joy E, Misra M, Williams NI, Mallinson RJ, et al. 2014 Female Athlete Triad Coalition Consensus Statement on Treatment and Return to Play of the Female Athlete Triad: 1st International Conference held in San Francisco, California, May 2012 and 2nd International Conference held in Indianapolis, Indiana, May 2013. Expert Panel. Br J Sports Med 2014;48:289,2013-093218.

De Souza MJ, West SL, Jamal SA, Hawker GA, Gundberg CM, Williams NI. The presence of both an energy deficiency and estrogen deficiency exacerbate alterations of bone metabolism in exercising women. Bone 2008;43:140–8.

9

Care of a nonpregnant patient who has syphilis

A 16-year-old nulligravid girl comes to your office with a vulvar lesion. She had menarche at age 12 years and reports regular cycles. She is sexually active and started a new relationship 2 weeks ago; for contraception, she is using a contraceptive implant. She tells you that she has not experienced dysuria, fever, myalgia, or rash. The area of the lesion has a raised indurated border and is nontender (Fig. 9-1; see color plate). The test most likely to confirm the diagnosis at this time is

(A) serum rapid plasma reagin (RPR) titer
(B) herpes simplex polymerase chain reaction test of lesion
(C) Gram stain of fluid
* (D) fluorescent antibody staining of fluid

Genital ulcerative lesions are either infectious or noninfectious. Ulcerations due to infections can be caused by primary or recurrent herpes simplex, primary syphilis, or *Haemophilus ducreyi* (chancroid). Noninfectious ulceration can be caused by trauma, carcinoma, aphthae, fixed drug reaction, or psoriasis. In the United States, most young, sexually active patients who have genital ulcerative lesions have either genital herpes or syphilis. Table 9-1 shows diseases characterized by genital ulcers.

Chancroid will present as a genital ulceration that is painful and associated with tender suppurative inguinal adenopathy. The incidence of this infection has decreased in the United States. Patients who have recently traveled to regions of Africa or the Caribbean may be at increased risk of acquiring this infection. Diagnosis of chancroid requires culture of *H ducreyi* on special culture media. Gram staining of the ulcer will demonstrate the classic "school of fish" appearance.

Genital herpes is caused by infection with herpes simplex virus type 1 (HSV-1) or type 2 (HSV-2). It is estimated that at least 45 million people in the United States have genital herpes. Historically, genital herpes has been caused by infections with HSV-2, which has a predilection for the sacral ganglion, where it remains dormant after a primary infection. The National Health and Nutrition Examination Survey reported an overall prevalence in women of 20.9% for HSV-2; however, there was great racial disparity, with non-Hispanic black women having a prevalence of 39.2% compared with a prevalence of 12.3% in non-Hispanic white women. Increasingly, HSV-1 has become a common cause of genital herpes. Traditionally, HSV-1, which has a predilection for the trigeminal ganglion, has been viewed as mostly responsible for oral labial infections (cold sores); however, it is now recognized that HSV-1 also has a role in genital herpes. The overall prevalence of HSV-1 in the population approaches 80%. Genital herpes, whether primary or recurrent, typically results in a painful ulcerative lesion. Primary infection often is associated with fever, headaches, malaise, and myalgia after a 4-day incubation period. Genital lesions start with a blister that quickly ulcerates. Primary lesions frequently have multiple sites of ulceration. Testing of primary or recurrent lesions will demonstrate herpes simplex.

Syphilis is caused by infection with the spirochete *Treponema pallidum*. The rates of primary and secondary syphilis have almost doubled in the past decade, with more than 16,000 cases identified in the United States each year. Syphilis is more common in men who have sex with men, but the rates are increasing in women as well. Syphilis is classified as early (primary and secondary) and latent (early and late) syphilis. Primary syphilis will present 2–3 weeks after exposure as a painless ulcerative lesion with a raised indurated margin that heals spontaneously in 3–6 weeks even in the absence of treatment. Secondary syphilis represents a systemic illness that may be associated with a diffuse macular papular rash involving the entire trunk or extremities, including the palms of the hands and soles of the feet. Latent syphilis is asymptomatic and usually diagnosed by serologic testing. Rapid plasma reagin is a test for anticardiolipin antibodies and is a nonspecific nontreponemal test. Because these antibodies are not specific to syphilis, a reactive RPR result must be confirmed with an assay that detects antibodies produced against *T pallidum*. False-positive RPR test results occur approximately 1–2% of the time. A traditional treponemal assay used for confirmatory testing is the fluorescent treponemal antibody absorption test. Some laboratories employ a reversed screening algorithm, using the *T pallidum* antibody screen as the initial test because this can be an automated test, and perform the nonspecific test—the RPR—as the second test for positive test results.

Treponemal antibody tests will remain positive after treatment and are ineffective for primary screening in women with previous infection.

For the described patient, the RPR test could be appropriate; however, in primary syphilis, seroconversion may not have occurred, and the test would likely be negative. The RPR test is useful for tracking the disease after initial treatment and identifying cases that may have failed treatment. The spirochete may be visualized by dark field microscopic examination, which is a specialized test that requires dedicated equipment. Detection may be aided by the use of direct fluorescent antibodies that will adhere to

TABLE 9-1. Diseases Characterized By Genital Ulcers*

- Differential diagnosis: genital herpes, syphilis, chancroid, and nonsexually transmitted infections
- Diagnosis: history and physical examination frequently inaccurate; all patients should be tested for syphilis and herpes; consideration given to chancroid

Herpes	Syphilis	Chancroid
Prevalence: • At least 45 million individuals in the United States have HSV infection	Prevalence: • Decreasing; more prevalent in metropolitan areas	Prevalence: • Decreasing in the United States • Usually in discrete outbreaks—high rates of HIV coinfection
Presentation: • Classic presentation of vesicles/ulcers absent in many cases • Many women with either HSV-1 or HSV-2 infection are asymptomatic. • Recurrences much less common with HSV-1; important fact for counseling	Common presentations: • Primary: ulcer or chancre • Secondary: skin rash, lymphadenopathy, mucocutaneous lesions • Tertiary: cardiac or ophthalmic manifestations, auditory abnormalities, gummatous lesions • Latent: no symptoms, diagnosed by serology	Presentation: • Combination of a painful genital ulcer and tender suppurative inguinal adenopathy
Diagnostic tests: • Clinical diagnosis should be confirmed by laboratory testing. • Isolation of HSV in cell culture or PCR are the preferred virologic tests. • Viral culture isolates should be typed to determine if HSV-1 or HSV-2 is the cause of the infection. • The serologic type-specific glycoprotein G-based assays should be specifically requested when serology is performed.	Diagnostic tests: • Dark-field examinations and direct fluorescent antibody tests of lesion exudate or tissue are the definitive methods for diagnosing early syphilis. • Presumptive diagnosis is possible with nontreponemal tests (VDRL and RPR) and treponemal tests (eg, FTA-ABS and TP-PA). • The use of only one type of serologic test is insufficient; false-positive nontreponemal test results are sometimes associated with medical conditions unrelated to syphilis.	Diagnosis: • Culture media • No FDA-approved test is available • Probable diagnosis: patient with painful ulcers, no evidence of syphilis, typical chancroid presentation, and diagnostic tests negative for herpes

Abbreviations: FDA, U.S. Food and Drug Administration; FTA-ABS, fluorescent treponemal antibody absorbed; HIV, human immunodeficiency virus; HSV, herpes simplex virus; PCR, polymerase chain reaction; RPR, rapid plasma reagin; TP-PA, *T pallidum* particle agglutination; VDRL, Venereal Disease Research Laboratory.

*The information in this table is from the 2010 *Sexually Transmitted Diseases Treatment Guidelines* from the Centers for Disease Control and Prevention. A revision of these guidelines was underway during the production of the fourth edition of *Guidelines for Women's Health Care*. For the most up-to-date guidance, please refer to the current Centers for Disease Control and Prevention guidelines, available at www.cdc.gov/std/.

Data from Workowski KA, Berman S. Sexually transmitted diseases treatment guidelines, 2010. Centers for Disease Control and Prevention [published erratum appears in MMWR Morb Mortal Wkly Rep 2011;60:18]. MMWR Recomm Rep 2010;59:1–110.

the spirochetes, facilitating their detection. In this patient, the ulcerative lesion is painless, which is characteristic of primary syphilis, and the test most likely to detect the spirochete is a fluorescent antibody test for *T pallidum*. A negative RPR test at this time would not exclude syphilis because there may not have been enough time for seroconversion.

American College of Obstetricians and Gynecologists. Guidelines for women's health care: a resource manual. 4th edition. Washington, DC: American College of Obstetricians and Gynecologists; 2014.

Binnicker MJ. Which algorithm should be used to screen for syphilis? Curr Opin Infect Dis 2012;25:79–85.

Workowski KA, Bolan GA. Sexually transmitted diseases treatment guidelines, 2015. Centers for Disease Control and Prevention [published erratum appears in MMWR Recomm Rep 2015;64:924]. MMWR Recomm Rep 2015;64:1–137.

10
Date rape

A 20-year-old female student comes to campus health services escorted by her roommate, who reports that they were at a fraternity party together earlier in the evening but got separated halfway through the party. Later that evening, she found her friend unconscious, face down in the bathroom without any clothes on. She remembers that her friend was "very unsteady and somewhat disoriented" when she last saw her. She is concerned that someone may have drugged and raped her. The drug most likely to be implicated is

(A) rohypnol
* (B) alcohol
(C) gamma-hydroxybutyrate
(D) ketamine

Sexual assault is a common problem that affects women worldwide. According to the National Violence Against Women Survey, 13–39% of women report sexual assault during their lifetime. Risk factors for sexual assault include age younger than 24 years; female gender; female college student; prior assault; gay, lesbian, or transgender identity; military status; homelessness; physical or mental disability; and use of drugs and alcohol. Among those at risk, adolescents and young women are disproportionately affected and are four times more likely to be sexually assaulted than women in other age groups. Sexual assault is a significant public health concern. Based on epidemiologic data from the National Intimate Partner and Sexual Violence Survey, the lifetime prevalence of sexual assault among women is approximately 19.3%; that is, more than 23 million U.S. women will experience sexual assault.

Sexual assault is defined as any type of sexual contact that occurs without the explicit consent of the recipient and can be further characterized based on the nature of the assault (eg, oral, vaginal, or anal contact or penetration), characteristics of the victim (eg, age), as well as the victim's relationship to the perpetrator (eg, acquaintance). Date rape is the most commonly encountered form of sexual assault, with alcohol and drug use being important risk factors.

Drug-facilitated sexual assault is rape or sexual assault facilitated by the use of drugs to incapacitate the victim. This form of sexual assault ultimately depends on the vulnerability of a victim who either willingly consumes alcohol or drugs or is surreptitiously given a substance by the perpetrator. As a result, the victim is rendered mentally incapacitated or physically helpless and is unable to consciously give consent. Up to 50% of cases of acquaintance rape involve alcohol consumption by the perpetrator, victim, or both. Alcohol use remains the leading risk factor for date rape on college campuses, partly because of its common use but also because of the profound effects it has on victims. The use of alcohol can lead to loss of inhibition, diminished coping, and a blunted response that renders the victim unable to ward off a potential attack. Characteristics that have been shown to increase a victim's vulnerability to date rape include younger age at first date, early age at menarche, early age at first sexual encounter, and a history of sexual abuse. Additionally, it has been suggested that there is a curvilinear relationship between the perpetrator's level of aggression and the perpetrator's alcohol consumption. Perpetrators in general have a tendency toward aggressiveness in intimate relationships, are often demanding of partners, and problem solve by way of aggression.

Broad categories of intoxicants include benzodiazepines, nonbenzodiazepine hypnotics, barbiturates, antidepressants, dissociative hypnotics, opioids, and antihistamines. In addition to alcohol, other substances that have been implicated commonly in the facilitation of rape include rohypnol, gamma-hydroxybutyrate, and ketamine. When combined with alcohol, these substances can lead to blackouts and subsequently predispose a woman to rape. Furthermore, upon regaining consciousness, victims may experience amnesia. Additionally, victims typically describe a degree of intoxication inconsistent with the quantity of the substance ingested. Although the described patient in this case could have been drugged, it is far more likely that she was incapacitated by binge drinking alcohol at the fraternity party. Her symptoms of drowsiness and disorientation correlate with her extent of intoxication, and as a result of her diminished level of consciousness and response, she probably was incapacitated and, by definition, unable to consent to sexual activity.

Black MC, Basile KC, Breiding MJ, Smith SG, Walters ML, Merrick MT, et al. The National Intimate Partner and Sexual Violence Survey (NISVS) 2010 summary report. National Center for Injury Prevention and Control. Atlanta (GA): Centers for Disease Control and Prevention; 2011. Available at: https://www.cdc.gov/violenceprevention/pdf/nisvs_executive_summary-a.pdf. Retrieved June 15, 2016.

Breiding MJ, Smith SG, Basile KC, Walters ML, Chen J, Merrick MT. Prevalence and characteristics of sexual violence, stalking, and intimate partner violence victimization —National Intimate Partner and Sexual Violence Survey, United States, 2011. MMWR Surveill Summ 2014;63:1–18.

Hall JA, Moore CB. Drug facilitated sexual assault—a review. J Forensic Leg Med 2008;15:291–7.

Rickert VI, Wiemann CM, Vaughan RD, White JW. Rates and risk factors for sexual violence among an ethnically diverse sample of adolescents. Arch Pediatr Adolesc Med 2004;158:1132–9.

Sexual assault. Committee Opinion No. 592. American College of Obstetricians and Gynecologists. Obstet Gynecol 2014;123:905–9.

11

Cervical cancer in pregnancy

A 26-year-old woman comes to your office for her second prenatal visit at 14 weeks of gestation. Cytologic screening at her initial visit showed high-grade squamous intraepithelial lesion (HSIL). The best next step in management is colposcopy

(A) at 6 weeks postpartum
(B) without biopsies
* (C) with biopsies
(D) with endocervical curettage

Cervical cancer is one of the most common malignancies in pregnancy, with an estimated incidence of 0.8–1.5 cases per 10,000 births. Most patients are diagnosed at an early stage; the disease course and prognosis in pregnant women are similar to those in nonpregnant women. Treatment of preinvasive disease can be deferred to the postpartum period, but further evaluation of the cervix to rule out invasive disease is recommended.

A number of factors can complicate the sampling and analysis of cytologic testing in pregnancy, such as a large ectropion, inflammatory changes, and decidua cells that may mimic low-grade squamous intraepithelial lesion (LSIL), HSIL, and carcinoma. Care must be taken to provide the cytopathologist with an accurate patient history to minimize these errors. Overall, cytologic testing in pregnant women approximates the sensitivity of testing in nonpregnant women. Because the described patient has a test result of HSIL, she needs further evaluation.

Colposcopy in pregnancy can be complicated by increased pelvic congestion and vaginal wall redundancy, an enlarged cervix, and greater cervical vascularity. Recommendations for evaluation of abnormal cervical cytology in pregnancy are dependent on the result. For a finding of atypical squamous cells of undetermined significance or LSIL, colposcopy can be deferred until postpartum (American Society for Colposcopy and Cervical Pathology consensus conference level C3 evidence; Table 11-1), although colposcopy is preferred for pregnant women with LSIL (level B evidence). There is no change in the recommendation for colposcopy for a finding of atypical squamous cells cannot exclude high-grade squamous intraepithelial lesion or HSIL, even if the woman is pregnant. Endocervical curettage (ECC) is not recommended in pregnancy, although no evidence is available that performing ECC increases the risk of pregnancy disruption.

Microinvasive cervical cancer is found at colposcopy in 2% of women with HSIL, although risk increases with age. Small and focal microinvasive lesions may even be hidden within large cervical intraepithelial neoplasia (CIN) 3 lesions. Additionally, the most severe lesions do not always demonstrate the most abnormal colposcopic

TABLE 11-1. Infectious Diseases Society of America—United States Public Health Service Grading System for Ranking Recommendations in Clinical Guidelines

Category, grade	Definition
Strength of Recommendation	
A	Good evidence to support a recommendation for use
B	Moderate evidence to support a recommendation for use
C	Poor evidence to support a recommendation for use
D	Moderate evidence to support a recommendation against use
E	Good evidence to support a recommendation against use
Quality of Evidence	
I	Evidence from ≥1 properly randomized, controlled trial
II	Evidence from ≥1 well-designed clinical trial, without randomization; from cohort or case-controlled analytic studies (preferably from >1 center); from multiple time-series; or from dramatic results from uncontrolled experiments
III	Evidence from opinions of respected authorities, based on clinical experience, descriptive studies, or reports of expert committees

Kish MA. Guide to development of practice guidelines. Clin Infect Dis. 2001;32(6):851–4. Reprinted by permission from Clinical Infectious Diseases.

findings, and lack of abnormal colposcopic findings does not always indicate an absence of cervical pathology. For these reasons, performing colposcopy only if the patient's examination is abnormal is insufficient. Biopsies should be performed even in the absence of colposcopic findings.

The described patient's pregnancy status does not alter the recommendation for immediate colposcopy with biopsy; however, ECC should be avoided. Because she had a cytologic result of HSIL, colposcopic evaluation is required, so she should not have colposcopy deferred until the postpartum period. Concerns of bleeding from a pregnant, hyperemic cervix prevent many clinicians from performing cervical biopsies; however, pregnancy is not a contraindication to biopsy of a suspected high-grade lesion. No significant bleeding complications or adverse pregnancy outcomes have been reported from cervical biopsies in pregnancy. Obstetrician–gynecologists and other health care providers should be prepared for bleeding, as with any patient who undergoes colposcopy with biopsies, by having scopettes, with available silver nitrate, ferric subsulfate, and equipment for suturing.

The sensitivity of colposcopy increases when more biopsies are taken; each additional biopsy significantly increases the detection of CIN 2 and CIN 3. Even experts in performing colposcopies cannot always visually distinguish CIN 2 from CIN 3. Colposcopically directed biopsies are more accurate than random biopsies, but random biopsies are better than no biopsies for detecting dysplasia. Because no other approach equals the level of detection of CIN 2 or 3, the described patient should undergo colposcopy with biopsies.

Creasman WT. Cancer and pregnancy. Ann N Y Acad Sci 2001;943: 281–6.

Hunter MI, Monk BJ, Tewari KS. Cervical neoplasia in pregnancy. Part 1: screening and management of preinvasive disease. Am J Obstet Gynecol 2008;199:3–9.

Massad LS, Einstein MH, Huh WK, Katki HA, Kinney WK, Schiffman M, et al. 2012 updated consensus guidelines for the management of abnormal cervical cancer screening tests and cancer precursors. 2012 ASCCP Consensus Guidelines Conference. Obstet Gynecol 2013;121:829–46.

Van Calsteren K, Vergote I, Amant F. Cervical neoplasia during pregnancy: diagnosis, management and prognosis. Best Pract Res Clin Obstet Gynaecol 2005;19:611–30.

12

Mortality data in adolescents

A 16-year-old girl visits your office for her first annual well-woman examination. She is healthy, has regular menstrual cycles, and is newly sexually active with one male partner. She uses condoms sporadically and has yet to initiate human papillomavirus vaccination. She feels safe at home but discloses that her boyfriend carries a gun. She does well in school and is planning to attend college. She recently obtained her driver's license and has a part-time job. She occasionally smokes cigarettes but states that she does not indulge in illicit drug or alcohol use, although she sometimes uses oxycodone to alleviate her menstrual cramps. The oxycodone was prescribed to her mother for her chronic back pain. In order to address her most likely cause of mortality in adolescence, it is important to counsel her in regard to

(A) gun violence
(B) smoking cessation
(C) prescription drugs
(D) recreational drugs and alcohol
* (E) motor vehicle safety

Unintentional injury is the leading cause of mortality in adolescents in the United States and worldwide, followed by homicide, suicide, cancer, and heart disease. The U.S. adolescent mortality rate was 44.8 per 100,000 in 2013. Unintentional injury deaths are classified by the Centers for Disease Control and Prevention into drowning, falling, fire or burn, motor vehicle traffic-related causes, other transportation-related causes, poisoning, suffocation, and all other causes. Within the category of unintentional injury death, the primary cause of death for adolescents is motor vehicle accidents. Therefore, it is most important to provide the described patient with counseling on motor vehicle safety. Bright Futures, the national health promotion initiative of the American Academy of Pediatrics and the Health Resources and Services Administration's Maternal and Child Health Bureau, recommends discussion of violence and injury prevention as one of the priority issues to be addressed during middle adolescence (age 15–17 years).

Unintentional injury accounts for 37% of all deaths in individuals aged 1–19 years and accounts for more potential life lost before age 65 years than any other cause of death. Furthermore, for every childhood death due to unintentional injury, more than 1,000 children are treated or receive medical consultation for a nonfatal injury. In 2009, unintentional injuries among children and adolescents resulted in 9,000 deaths, 225,000 hospitalizations, and 8.4 million patients treated and released from emergency departments. This results in costs as high as $11.5 billion in a single year.

Rates of unintentional injury deaths show significant disparities by gender, race, and state of residence. Table 12-1 shows 2014 adolescent mortality rates for all races and both genders for those aged 15–19 years. Death rates from unintentional injury by state range from 4 per 100,000 in Massachusetts to 25.1 per 100,000 in Mississippi. These disparities suggest that environment, exposure to hazards, and public policy may play a role in risk of death due to injury, and they highlight the opportunity for public health action.

Public health efforts that have targeted unintentional injury avoidance have been successful in decreasing adolescent mortality. From 2000 to 2010 the rate of adolescent mortality decreased by 26.4%, largely because of decreases in unintentional injury. It has been estimated that seat belts prevented 275,000 deaths between 1975 and 2008. Still, a significant number of adolescents do not wear seatbelts. As of 2012, one half of teenagers who died in motor vehicle accidents were unrestrained. Graduated driver licensing programs are estimated to decrease crashes in 16-year-olds and 17-year-olds by 20–50%. Additional public health campaigns have targeted the dangers of distracted driving, such as texting while driving. The Centers for Disease Control and Prevention has identified eight "danger zones" for teenagers who drive (Box 12-1).

Motor vehicle accidents are followed by homicide because of the use of firearms and unintentional poisoning as the most common cause of death in individuals aged 15–24 years. Homicide and suicide combined account for almost as many deaths as unintentional injuries among male adolescents.

Poisoning, including recreational and prescription drug overdose, is the only unintentional injury mechanism to increase over the past decade. From 2002 to 2004, an estimated 13.5% of those aged 12–17 years reported having

TABLE 12-1. Death, Percentage of Total Deaths, and Death Rates for the 15 Leading Causes of Death in 5-Year Age Groups, By Race and Sex: United States, 2014*

Rank†	Cause of Death (Based on the *International Classification of Diseases, Tenth Revision*), Race, Sex, and Age	Number	Percentage of Total Deaths	Rate
	All races, both sexes, ages 15–19 years			
...	All causes	9,586	100.0	45.5
1	Accidents (unintentional injuries)	3,736	39.0	17.7
2	Intentional self-harm (suicide)	1,834	19.1	8.7
3	Assault (homicide)	1,397	14.6	6.6
4	Malignant neoplasms	612	6.4	2.9
5	Diseases of heart	299	3.1	1.4
6	Congenital malformations, deformations, and chromosomal abnormalities	179	1.9	0.8
7	Influenza and pneumonia	64	0.7	0.3
8	Cerebrovascular diseases	58	0.6	0.3
9	Chronic lower respiratory diseases	55	0.6	0.3
10	Septicemia	39	0.4	0.2
11	In situ neoplasms, benign neoplasms, and neoplasms of uncertain or unknown behavior	38	0.4	0.2
12	Diabetes mellitus	34	0.4	0.2
13	Pregnancy, childbirth, and the puerperium	31	0.3	0.1
14	Anemias	27	0.3	0.1
15	Legal intervention	24	0.3	0.1
...	All other causes (residual)	1,159	12.1	5.5

*Rates per 100,000 population in a specified group. Rates are not shown for age groups older than 85 years. Rates for "all ages" include deaths for age "under 1 year." Figures for "age not stated" are included in "all ages" but are not distributed among age groups. Data for races other than white and black should be interpreted with caution because of inconsistencies between the reporting of race on death certificates and on censuses and surveys.

†Based on number of deaths.

National Center for Health Statistics. LCWK1. Deaths, percent of total deaths, and death rates for the 15 leading causes of death in 5-year age groups, by race and sex: United States, 2014. Hyattsville (MD): NCHS; 2015. Available at: http://www.cdc.gov/nchs/data/dvs/lcwk1_2014.pdf. Retrieved June 13, 2016.

BOX 12-1

Danger Zones for Teenagers Behind the Wheel

- Driver inexperience
- Driving with teen passengers
- Nighttime driving
- Not using seat belts
- Distracted driving
- Drowsy driving
- Reckless driving
- Impaired driving

Centers for Disease Control and Prevention. Parents are the key to safe teen drivers. Atlanta (GA): CDC; 2015. Available at: https://www.cdc.gov/parentsarethekey/. Retrieved June 13, 2016.

misused prescription drugs. The percentage of poisoning deaths among adolescents in which prescription drugs were contributory increased from 30% in 2000 to 57% in 2009. Strategies to reduce the misuse of prescription drugs include appropriate prescribing, proper storage and disposal, discouraging medication sharing, and state-based prescription drug monitoring programs.

Tobacco use is the leading preventable cause of death in the United States. Causes of premature death attributable to smoking include smoking-related cancer, cardiovascular and metabolic disease, pulmonary diseases, complications of pregnancy, and residential fires. Although rates of smoking in general and among adolescents and young adults have decreased significantly in the past 50 years, the rate of decrease has slowed. Most smokers will have their first cigarette before age 18 years.

Centers for Disease Control and Prevention. Parents are the key to safe teen drivers. Atlanta (GA): CDC; 2015. Available at: https://www.cdc.gov/parentsarethekey/. Retrieved June 13, 2016.

Centers for Disease Control and Prevention. Vital signs: unintentional injury deaths among persons aged 0–19 years—United States, 2000–2009. MMWR Morb Mortal Wkly Rep 2012;61:270–6.

Hagan JF, Shaw JS, Duncan PM, editors. Bright futures: guidelines for health supervision of infants, children, and adolescents. 3rd ed. Elk Grove Village (IL): American Academy of Pediatrics; 2008.

Health Resources and Services Administration, Maternal and Child Health Bureau. Child health USA 2014. Rockville (MD): U.S. Department of Health and Human Services; 2015. Available at: http://mchb.hrsa.gov/chusa14/dl/chusa14.pdf. Retrieved June 13, 2016.

National Center for Health Statistics. Adolescent health. Hyattsville (MD): NCHS; 2016. Available at: http://www.cdc.gov/nchs/fastats/adolescent-health.htm. Retrieved June 13, 2016.

National Center for Health Statistics. LCWK1. Deaths, percent of total deaths, and death rates for the 15 leading causes of death in 5-year age groups, by race and sex: United States, 2014. Hyattsville (MD): NCHS; 2015. Available at: http://www.cdc.gov/nchs/data/dvs/lcwk1_2014.pdf. Retrieved June 13, 2016.

National Center for Statistics and Analysis. Young drivers: 2013 data. traffic safety facts report no. DOT HS 812 200. Washington, DC: National Highway Traffic Safety Administration; 2015. Available at: http://www-nrd.nhtsa.dot.gov/Pubs/812200.pdf. Retrieved June 13, 2016.

U.S. Department of Health and Human Services. The health consequences of smoking: 50 years of progress. A report of the surgeon general. Atlanta (GA): U.S. Department of Health and Human Services, Centers for Disease Control and Prevention, National Center for Chronic Disease Prevention and Health Promotion, Office on Smoking and Health; 2014. Available at: http://www.surgeongeneral.gov/library/reports/50-years-of-progress/full-report.pdf. Retrieved June 13, 2016.

13

Depression in pregnancy

A 33-year-old nulligravid woman presents for prepregnancy counseling. She has depression that is well controlled on paroxetine. You counsel her that the birth defect with which paroxetine has been associated is

(A) renal disorders
(B) hypospadias
(C) orofacial clefts
* (D) cardiac defects
(E) extremity malformations

The estimated prevalence of depression is 17% in U.S. adults, and women are twice as likely as men to experience depression. The highest depression rates occur during the reproductive years, between ages 25 years and 44 years. Up to 70% of pregnant women report depressive symptoms, including depressed mood; anhedonia; changes in sleep, appetite and weight; decreased energy; feelings of guilt or worthlessness; psychomotor retardation or agitation; and suicidal ideation.

Depression can and should be treated during pregnancy when the benefits of treatment outweigh potential risks. Untreated or undertreated maternal depression is associated with serious risks, including suicide and homicide. Treatment for depression during pregnancy should be determined on an individualized basis and should be handled in a multidisciplinary fashion, including involving a mental health specialist. Approximately 60% of women who are taking antidepressants when they become pregnant experience depressive symptoms during pregnancy; women who discontinue their antidepressants are five times more likely to relapse than those who continue their antidepressant regimen during pregnancy.

Selective serotonin reuptake inhibitors (SSRIs) are the most commonly used antidepressants in pregnancy. Two large case-control studies assessed SSRI use in pregnancy and found conflicting results regarding fetal abnormalities. Positive findings were found only after more than 40 statistical tests were performed; therefore, the results may have been due to chance. Previous reports have suggested that antidepressant therapy use in pregnancy may be associated with fetal abnormalities. However, according to the U.S. Food and Drug Administration, only paroxetine increases the incidence of fetal anomalies. Multiple studies have shown an up to twofold increased risk of cardiac malformations in fetuses of women who used paroxetine. Although paroxetine has been shown to increase the risk of fetal cardiac defects, it has not been shown to increase the risk of the other potential anomalies listed: renal disorders, hypospadias, orofacial clefts, and extremity malformations. Because of the increased incidence of fetal cardiac anomalies, paroxetine use is best avoided in pregnancy. A patient whose fetus has been exposed to paroxetine should be counseled about the risk and offered fetal echocardiography. Because abrupt discontinuation of paroxetine has been associated with maternal withdrawal symptoms, discontinuation should be done according to the product's prescribing information.

Antidepressant use has been associated with transient neonatal complications, including jitteriness, transient tachypnea of the newborn, mild respiratory distress, and neonatal intensive care unit admission. Additionally, more recent studies have suggested that SSRIs may be associated with persistent pulmonary hypertension of the newborn. Infants with this condition are not able to oxygenate well and require intensive medical care. This condition was noted to be six times more common in infants of women who took an SSRI after midpregnancy than those who did not take any antidepressants. However, the absolute risk of this complication remains low. Therefore, at this time, the U.S. Food and Drug Administration advises obstetrician–gynecologists and health care providers to continue current clinical practice and to report any adverse events. Regardless, the described patient should be well informed about the importance of balancing the potential risks to the fetus by taking medications versus the risk of relapse of depression if therapy is discontinued.

Alwan S, Reefhuis J, Rasmussen SA, Olney RS, Friedman JM. Use of selective serotonin-reuptake inhibitors in pregnancy and the risk of birth defects. National Birth Defects Prevention Study. N Engl J Med 2007;356:2684–92.

Chambers CD, Hernandez-Diaz S, Van Marter LJ, Werler MM, Louik C, Jones KL, et al. Selective serotonin-reuptake inhibitors and risk of persistent pulmonary hypertension of the newborn. N Engl J Med 2006;354:579–87.

Cohen LS, Altshuler LL, Harlow BL, Nonacs R, Newport DJ, Viguera AC, et al. Relapse of major depression during pregnancy in women who maintain or discontinue antidepressant treatment [published erratum appears in JAMA 2006;296:170]. JAMA 2006;295:499–507.

Diav-Citrin O, Shechtman S, Weinbaum D, Wajnberg R, Avgil M, Di Gianantonio E, et al. Paroxetine and fluoxetine in pregnancy: a prospective, multicentre, controlled, observational study. Br J Clin Pharmacol 2008;66:695–705.

Louik C, Lin AE, Werler MM, Hernandez-Diaz S, Mitchell AA. First-trimester use of selective serotonin-reuptake inhibitors and the risk of birth defects [published erratum appears in N Engl J Med 2015;373:686]. N Engl J Med 2007;356:2675–83.

Moses-Kolko EL, Bogen D, Perel J, Bregar A, Uhl K, Levin B, et al. Neonatal signs after late in utero exposure to serotonin reuptake inhibitors: literature review and implications for clinical applications. JAMA 2005;293:2372–83.

Use of psychiatric medications during pregnancy and lactation. ACOG Practice Bulletin No. 92. American College of Obstetricians and Gynecologists. Obstet Gynecol 2008;111:1001–20.

14

Screening for thyroid disease

A 33-year-old woman, gravida 2, para 2, presents for her annual well-woman examination. Her only concern is related to thyroid disease. She is worried that she could have thyroid problems because her paternal grandmother did. Her body mass index (calculated as weight in kilograms divided by height in meters squared [kg/m^2]) is 21. She denies any hair or skin changes and reports feeling tired but proud of her new exercise routine. Physical examination findings are all within normal limits. The best next course of action is

(A) thyroid-stimulating hormone (TSH) testing
(B) thyroid ultrasonography
* (C) routine follow-up in 1 year
(D) serum iodine level testing
(E) antithyroid peroxidase antibodies testing

The thyroid gland controls metabolic homeostasis through the secretion of triiodothyronine (T_3) and thyroxine (T_4). Triiodothyronine and T_4 are regulated by TSH, which is secreted by the anterior pituitary. Hypothyroidism, or undersecretion of T_3 and T_4, is marked by fatigue, feeling cold, weight gain, hair loss, poor concentration, dry skin, and constipation. Because some of these symptoms are quite common, the diagnosis is easily missed. In extreme disease states, mainly seen only in the elderly, hypothyroidism can lead to myxedema coma, a rare but life-threatening condition. In the United States, the most common cause of hypothyroidism is autoimmune thyroiditis (Hashimoto disease).

Hyperthyroidism is distinguished by signs and symptoms such as heart palpitations, heat intolerance, sweating, weight loss, hyperactivity, and fatigue. Thyroid storm, also a life-threatening condition, can result from an added stressor, such as illness or trauma, in cases of undiagnosed or undertreated hyperthyroidism. Hyperthyroidism can be caused by Graves disease, autoimmune thyroiditis, or functional thyroid nodules.

Subclinical thyroid dysfunction affects an estimated 5% of women in the United States. Approximately 0.5% of the population is thought to have undiagnosed overt thyroid disease. Subclinical hypothyroidism has been associated with increased risk of coronary artery disease and congestive heart failure, whereas subclinical hyperthyroidism has been associated with increased risk of all-cause and coronary heart disease mortality, atrial fibrillation, and decreased bone density. Overt thyroid disease can cause problems with the cardiovascular, musculoskeletal, dermatologic, and gastrointestinal systems, with the signs and symptoms being highly variable depending on the severity of disease. Approximately 1–5% of patients with subclinical thyroid dysfunction will develop overt thyroid disease and as many as 40% will revert to normal function with no intervention.

The U.S. Preventive Services Task Force (USPSTF) found insufficient evidence to recommend for or against routine screening in asymptomatic patients. Although screening can accurately identify patients with subclinical thyroid dysfunction or those who are asymptomatic but have overt thyroid disease, there is not enough evidence to clearly understand and weigh the benefits and harms of routine screening. Thus, in this patient who is asymptomatic, there is no indication for screening at this time. The described patient has no concerning symptoms and a weak family history of thyroid disease, so she should return in 1 year for her annual examination.

Despite these recommendations, thyroid medication prescription rates have increased significantly over the past several years. In community-living adults older than 65 years who have subclinical hypothyroidism, the percentage taking thyroid hormone replacement more than doubled to 20% from 1989 to 2005. This reflects, in part, increased patient, obstetrician–gynecologist, and other health care provider concern and likely increased screening in certain high-risk groups. Although there are certain high-risk groups (eg, postpartum women, elderly patients) in whom the yield of screening is higher because of a higher pretest probability of dysfunction, the USPSTF found poor evidence regarding clinically significant benefits of screening, even in these groups.

The American College of Obstetricians and Gynecologists is in agreement with the USPSTF's recommendation, although it does recommend screening in high-risk groups (those with a strong family history of thyroid disease and autoimmune disease). The American College of Obstetricians and Gynecologists does not recommend routine screening in women who are trying to become pregnant or who are already pregnant unless they have a personal history of thyroid disease or symptoms. Even routine palpation of an enlarged thyroid in pregnancy does not necessitate screening in an asymptomatic patient because the thyroid is known to increase in size by 30% during pregnancy. However, for women with clear symptoms of thyroid dysfunction, especially in those trying to become pregnant, screening is recommended. Overt thyroid disease diagnosed before or during pregnancy requires more frequent testing to appropriately monitor treatment to decrease fetal risk.

If the described patient did need thyroid screening, TSH is the recommended initial screening tool (Fig. 14-1 and Fig. 14-2). The assays currently used for TSH are quite

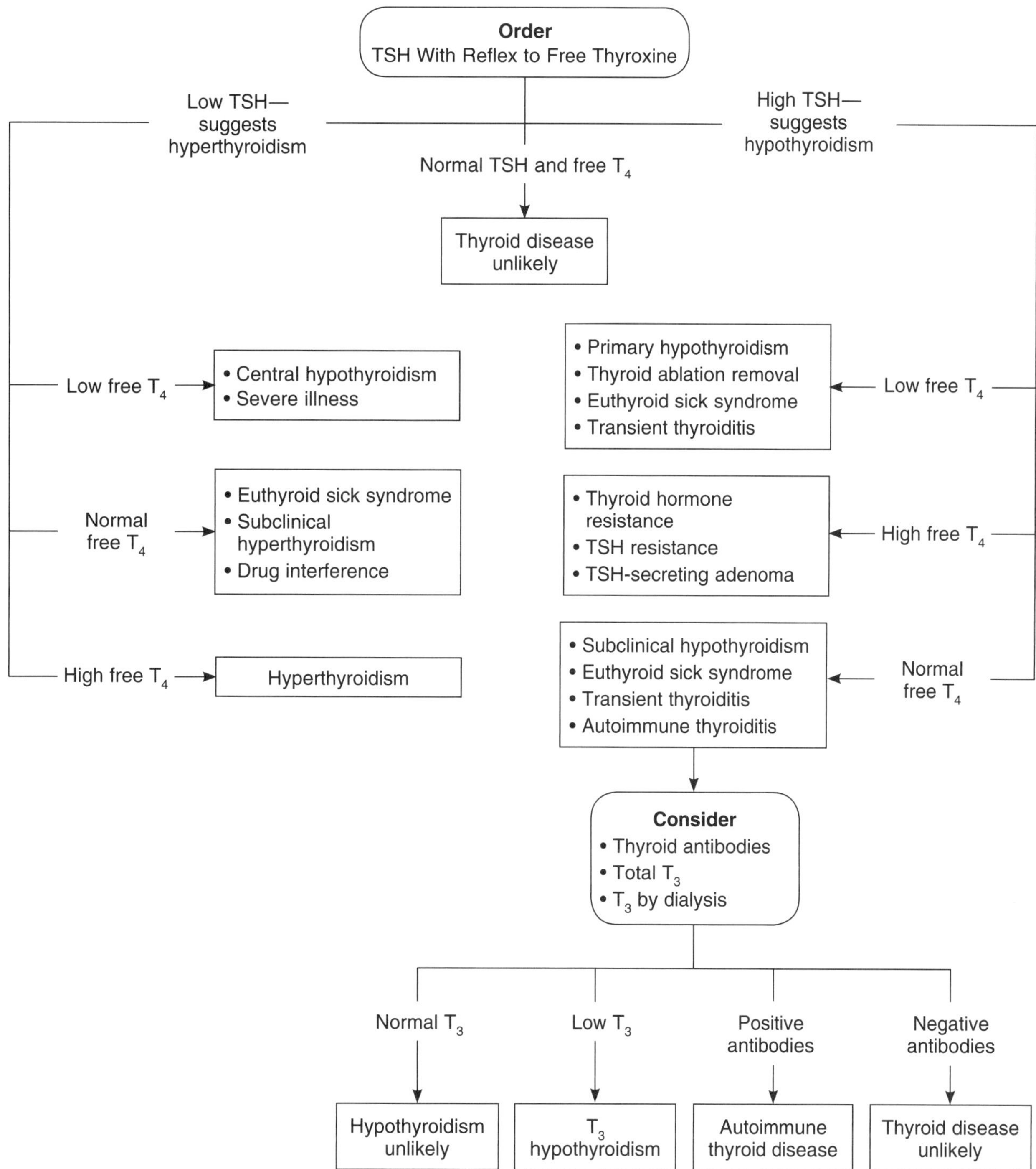

FIGURE 14-1. Thyroid disorders testing algorithm. Abbreviations: T_3, triiodothyronine; T_4, thyroxine; TSH, thyroid-stimulating hormone. (Modified with permission of ARUP Consult [http://www.arupconsult.com], an ARUP Laboratories test selection tool for healthcare professionals. Thyroid Disorders Testing Algorithm. Copyright 2006 ARUP Laboratories. All Rights Reserved. Revised 05/07/2014.)

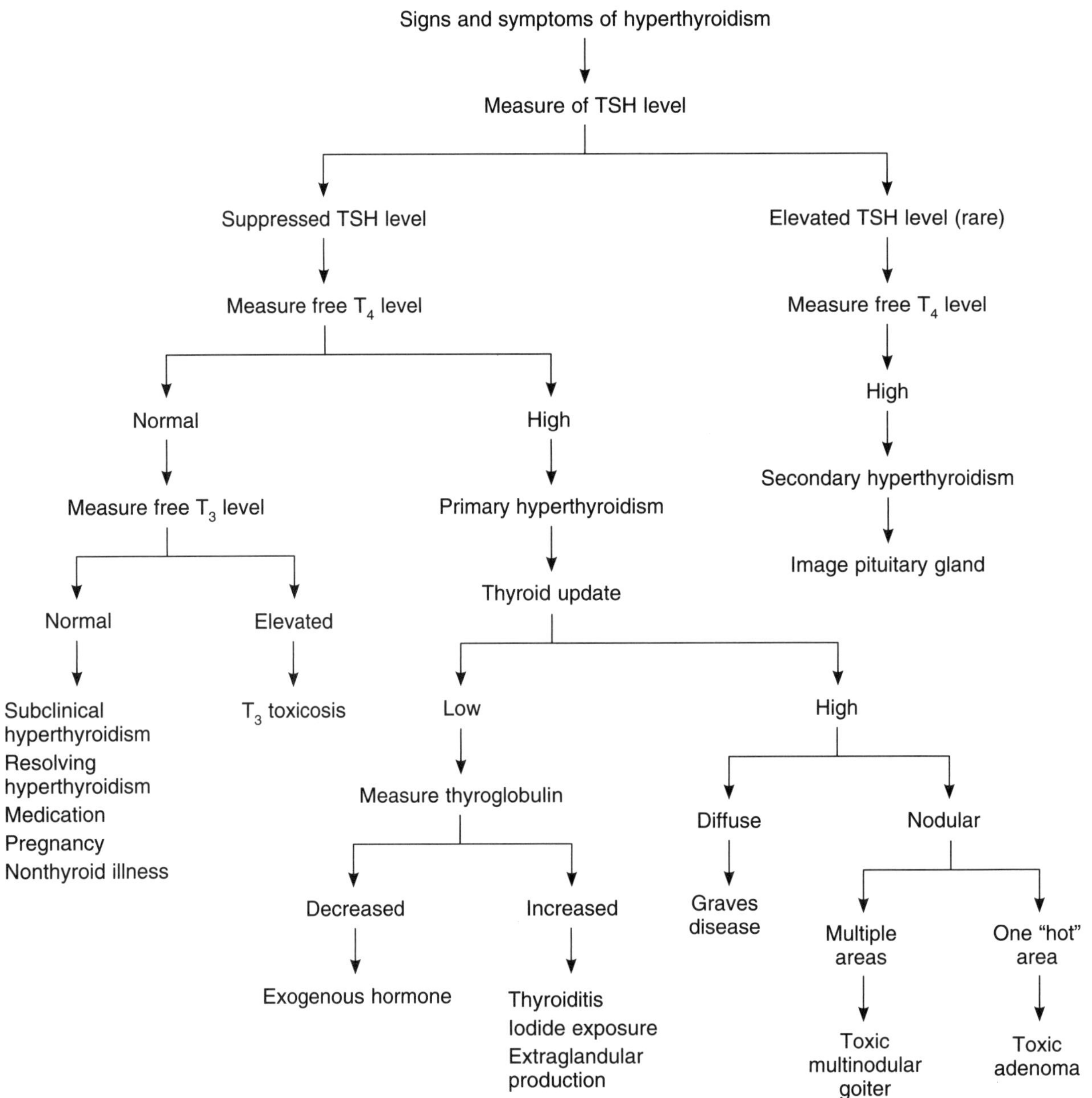

FIGURE 14-2. Algorithm for diagnosing hyperthyroidism. Abbreviations: T_3, triiodothyronine; T_4, thyroxine; TSH, thyroid-stimulating hormone. (Adapted or reprinted with permission from Reid JR, Wheeler SF. Hyperthyroidism: diagnosis and treatment. Am Fam Physician 2005;72:623–30. Copyright 2005 American Academy of Family Physicians. All Rights Reserved.)

sensitive and can detect changes before abnormalities in T_3 and T_4 can be detected. *Subclinical hypothyroidism* is defined as an elevated TSH level in a patient with a normal T_4 level. In patients with normal TSH, no additional testing is needed. If TSH is high, T_4 levels are needed to determine the degree of hypothyroidism. If TSH levels are low, T_3 and T_4 levels are needed to evaluate the degree of hyperthyroidism. Thyroid ultrasonography is reserved for patients with palpable nodules to further evaluate the mass.

Assessing serum iodine levels is rarely necessary for hypothyroid patients in the United States. The thyroid gland converts dietary iodine to T_3 and T_4. Iodine deficiency is rare in the United States, in part because salt is iodized, which helps to ensure that the population gets adequate dietary iodine. However, in much of the developing world, iodine deficiency is common and leads to impaired thyroid function, thyroid enlargement (goiter), or both. Although iodine levels are unlikely to be of any value in this asymptomatic patient, they can help elucidate the etiology of severe hypothyroidism in some immigrant populations.

Antithyroid antibodies are a group of autoantibodies targeted at the thyroid. Antithyroid peroxidase antibodies are associated with Hashimoto thyroiditis, whereas the activating autoantibodies (thyrotropin receptor antibodies and thyroglobulin antibodies) are associated with Graves disease. These antibodies do not need to be checked in a patient without thyroid dysfunction.

American College of Obstetricians and Gynecologists. Annual women's health care. Washington, DC: American College of Obstetricians and Gynecologists; 2016. Available at: http://www.acog.org/About_ACOG/ACOG_Departments/Annual_Womens_Health_Care. Retrieved June 16, 2016.

Rugge JB, Bougatsos C, Chou R. Screening for and treatment of thyroid dysfunction: An evidence review for the U.S. Preventive Service Task Force. Evidence Synthesis No. 118. Rockville (MD): Agency for Healthcare Research and Quality; 2014.

Thyroid disease in pregnancy. Practice Bulletin No. 148. American College of Obstetricians and Gynecologists. Obstet Gynecol 2015;125: 996–1005.

15

Bacterial vaginosis

A 38-year-old woman comes to your office for her annual well-woman examination. She has no significant medical history, and her review of symptoms is negative. Pelvic examination shows no vaginal discharge. Liquid-based cervical cytology is negative for intraepithelial lesion and malignancy, but a shift in vaginal flora suggests bacterial vaginosis. The best next step is

(A) treatment with antibiotics
(B) evaluation with a wet mount
* (C) assessment for symptoms
(D) testing with a DNA probe
(E) vaginal culture

Asymptomatic bacterial vaginosis is not routinely treated because most patients will have spontaneous resolution or never develop symptoms. One study that randomized women to treatment or placebo for asymptomatic bacterial vaginosis failed to find any subjective improvement in discharge or odor in those treated. Up to 20% of women treated for bacterial vaginosis will subsequently develop vaginal candidiasis, so unnecessary treatment can have untoward consequences in addition to causing allergic reactions.

The most common cause of vaginitis, bacterial vaginosis is caused by an overgrowth of facultative or strictly anaerobic microorganisms, such as *Gardnerella vaginalis, Peptostreptococcus, Prevotella, Mobiluncus, Bacteroides, Fusobacterium, Atopobium vaginae,* and *Mycoplasma hominis*. Normal vaginal flora is maintained by adequate lactobacilli species, some of which produce hydrogen peroxide to maintain a normal vaginal pH of 4.5–5.0. When the concentration of lactobacilli becomes overwhelmed by an overgrowth of vaginal anaerobes, the vaginal pH rises further and favors more anaerobe growth. Anaerobes produce proteolytic enzymes that release amines, which results in a "fishy" odor. An off-white to gray-colored, thin, and homogenous vaginal discharge that coats the vaginal walls is typical. Symptoms can worsen after intercourse, during menses, and with douching. Rarely does bacterial vaginosis cause sufficient inflammation to result in symptoms of vulvitis, such as dysuria, pruritus, burning, or dyspareunia. It is estimated that 50–75% of women have asymptomatic bacterial vaginosis.

Although the Nugent score, which is based on Gram staining of vaginal discharge, is considered the criterion standard for the diagnosis of bacterial vaginosis, the procedure requires more time and special expertise than the readily available wet mount. Therefore, the diagnosis of bacterial vaginosis is best made with a wet mount and microscopy. At least three of four Amsel criteria are required for the diagnosis: 1) characteristic vaginal discharge, 2) pH greater than 4.5, 3) fishy odor before or after a positive 10% potassium hydroxide amine test (whiff test), and 4) presence of greater than 20% clue cells on saline wet mount. Clue cells are characteristic of bacterial vaginosis and are vaginal epithelial cells coated with coccobacilli. Although there are now commercially available tests that include DNA probes, it is important to note that the mere presence of *Gardnerella* or other species of bacteria is not necessarily diagnostic of bacterial vaginosis because greater than 50% of women who are colonized with *Gardnerella* do not have symptoms. Use of vaginal culture in women with vaginitis has not been shown to be useful diagnostically.

Cytologic criteria for reporting bacterial vaginosis include filmy background of small coccobacilli, clue cells, and absence of lactobacilli. If these findings are present, the normal reporting nomenclature is "shift in flora suggestive of bacterial vaginosis." Cytology, however, is not considered to be a reliable method for diagnosing bacterial vaginosis. If bacterial vaginosis is present on the Pap test report, the obstetrician–gynecologist or other health care provider should inquire about the presence of symptoms; the patient need not have confirmatory testing if she has no symptoms. In one study that used the Nugent score as diagnostic for bacterial vaginosis, the cytology specimen had 43% sensitivity, 94% specificity, a positive predictive value of 74%, and a negative predictive value of 80%. The true sensitivity most likely was overestimated because the investigators did not report the number of patients who actually had symptomatic infection. Standard wet mount using the Amsel criteria or DNA probe testing should be undertaken in symptomatic women. It is reasonable to treat patients with symptoms if a Pap smear suggests infection.

Heller DS, Pitsos M, Skurnick J. Does the presence of vaginitis on a Pap smear correlate with clinical symptoms in the patient? J Reprod Med 2008;53:429–34.

Prediction and prevention of preterm birth. Practice Bulletin No. 130. American College of Obstetricians and Gynecologists. Obstet Gynecol 2012;120:964–73.

Schwebke JR. Asymptomatic bacterial vaginosis: response to therapy. Am J Obstet Gynecol 2000;183:1434–9.

Schwebke JR, Desmond R. A randomized trial of metronidazole in asymptomatic bacterial vaginosis to prevent the acquisition of sexually transmitted diseases. Am J Obstet Gynecol 2007;196:517.e1–6.

Tokyol C, Aktepe OC, Cevrioglu AS, Altindis M, Dilek FH. Bacterial vaginosis: comparison of Pap smear and microbiological test results. Mod Pathol 2004;17:857–60.

Vaginitis. ACOG Practice Bulletin No. 72. American College of Obstetricians and Gynecologists. Obstet Gynecol 2006;107:1195–206.

16

Adverse effects of tamoxifen citrate

A 41-year-old woman comes to your office for a well-woman examination. She reports that her 52-year-old sister was just diagnosed with breast cancer and that her mother was diagnosed with breast cancer at age 56 years. She has read that tamoxifen citrate has been shown to help reduce the chances of developing breast cancer and wants more information about possible adverse effects. Her use of tamoxifen is most likely to increase her risk of

(A) myocardial infarction
(B) endometrial cancer
(C) colon cancer
* (D) venous thromboembolism
(E) osteoporosis

Tamoxifen is a selective estrogen receptor modulator that has stimulatory effects on some estrogen receptors (ERs) but not on others. Tamoxifen is a prodrug and only its metabolites, such as endoxifen, bind to ERs. Tamoxifen is metabolized by the cytochrome P450 system, which is important in identifying drug-to-drug interactions. Specifically, the metabolites of tamoxifen block the effect of native estrogen in breast tissue but are stimulatory to ERs in the endometrium.

Tamoxifen is labelled for use in women to reduce the risk of breast cancer if their personal or family history places them in an elevated risk category. One of the most popular models for determining the risk of breast cancer is the Gail model, which is available online (www.cancer.gov/bcrisktool/). If a woman's lifetime risk of breast cancer is calculated as greater than 1.6% for the next 5 years, then she is a candidate for tamoxifen chemoprevention. However, its use to increase the likelihood of breast cancer survival has not been demonstrated in large trials. A meta-analysis calculated a 38% reduction in breast cancer incidence in women who used tamoxifen for 5 years. Risk reduction for ER-positive and ductal carcinoma in situ has been demonstrated, but no risk reduction occurs in the incidence of ER-negative breast cancer.

Additionally, tamoxifen has other estrogenic properties, specifically procoagulant effects, which exist partly because of lowered levels of antithrombin III and protein C. Tamoxifen is associated with an elevated risk of venous thromboembolism. Women of any age who use tamoxifen are at higher risk of developing this condition. Tamoxifen is not recommended in women with a history of venous thromboembolism. The risk is increased twofold to threefold in older women who use tamoxifen. Because of the patient's use of tamoxifen, the adverse event for which she would be most at risk is venous thromboembolism.

Tamoxifen's effect on endometrial proliferation appears to be somewhat dependent on age. In the large National Surgical Adjuvant Breast and Bowel Project P-1 trial, premenopausal women who used tamoxifen had no increased risk of endometrial neoplasia, but postmenopausal women had a relative risk of 4.0 for developing endometrial neoplasia. Because the described patient is premenopausal, she is not at increased risk of developing endometrial cancer. However, the risk of endometrial neoplasia should be discussed with women who are considering using tamoxifen. No specific surveillance for development of endometrial carcinoma is recommended in either premenopausal or postmenopausal women who use tamoxifen. In the absence of abnormal vaginal bleeding, neither endometrial stripe thickness measured by ultrasonography nor tissue sampling by endometrial biopsy is recommended. If a woman taking tamoxifen therapy develops abnormal bleeding, then an appropriate diagnostic workup is warranted. The increased risk of endometrial carcinoma appears to diminish when tamoxifen is stopped.

The use of a levonorgestrel intrauterine device (IUD) has been proposed as a method to reduce endometrial proliferation in women who take tamoxifen. However, in studies of breast cancer patients who take tamoxifen, use of this IUD was associated with a reduction in incidence of polyps but not with reduced incidence of hyperplasia or malignancy. Therefore, the routine use of a levonorgestrel IUD for endometrial protection in women using tamoxifen is not recommended.

Other adverse effects of tamoxifen include vaginal discharge, sleep problems, and cataracts (albeit the absolute risk is low). There is no evidence that tamoxifen increases the risk of myocardial infarction or colon cancer. A slightly increased rate of diabetes mellitus has been observed among breast cancer patients who take tamoxifen.

Postmenopausal tamoxifen users have lower rates of osteoporosis because of tamoxifen's antiosteoclast activity. Premenopausal users have been shown in some studies to have some decrease in bone mineral density compared with nonusers, but no increased fracture risk has been demonstrated.

Breast cancer risk assessment tool. Available at: http://www.cancer.gov/bcrisktool/. Retrieved March 20, 2014; June 11, 2016.

Cuzick J, Sestak I, Bonanni B, Costantino JP, Cummings S, DeCensi A, et al. Selective oestrogen receptor modulators in prevention of breast cancer: an updated meta-analysis of individual participant data. SERM Chemoprevention of Breast Cancer Overview Group. Lancet 2013;381:1827–34.

Nelson HD, Smith ME, Griffin JC, Fu R. Use of medications to reduce risk for primary breast cancer: a systematic review for the U.S. Preventive Services Task Force. Ann Intern Med 2013;158:604–14.

Tamoxifen and uterine cancer. Committee Opinion No. 601. American College of Obstetricians and Gynecologists. Obstet Gynecol 2014;123:1394–7.

17
Primary dysmenorrhea in adolescents

A 15-year-old adolescent girl has had persistent dysmenorrhea despite 6 months of use of combination oral contraceptives and nonsteroidal antiinflammatory drugs. She has regular bleeding episodes that last 3–4 days during which she uses three tampons a day. The patient states that the pain is severe and is sometimes associated with defecation. She has been missing school because of the pain. She reports no intermenstrual pain. The patient has had intercourse with one partner. Abdominal and pelvic examinations are normal with the exception of mild tenderness of the left adnexa. No masses are palpated. Her gonorrhea, chlamydial infection, and pregnancy tests are all negative. Transvaginal ultrasonography is normal. The best next step is

(A) pelvic magnetic resonance imaging (MRI) scan
(B) colonoscopy
(C) prescribe oral narcotics
(D) leuprolide acetate
* (E) diagnostic laparoscopy

A secondary cause should be sought for women and adolescents with dysmenorrhea that does not resolve after a trial of medical management. Worsening dysmenorrhea despite adequate medical therapy is a common finding in adolescents with endometriosis, and the incidence of endometriosis can be as high as 70% in teenagers with chronic pain that is unresponsive to medical management. Other potential etiologies of pelvic pain, such as ovarian cysts; pelvic infection; pregnancy; uterine anomalies; and psychosocial, urologic, and gastrointestinal (GI) disorders, should be considered. In the described patient, however, the progressive nature of her pain despite medical interventions suggests endometriosis as the most likely etiology.

A müllerian anomaly is an important consideration in adolescents with progressive pelvic pain; however, a pelvic MRI is unlikely to reveal the etiology of pain in this patient with normal physical and ultrasonographic findings. Furthermore, endometriomas are rare in adolescents and, thus, an MRI is not recommended as an additional imaging study because of the expense and lack of sensitivity for the detection of small endometriosis implants.

Associated GI symptoms and pain are noted in up to one third of adolescents with endometriosis. Women may experience such symptoms even when endometriosis implants are not identified on the bowel. Colonoscopy is indicated for adolescents with significant GI signs and symptoms. The described patient's constellation of symptoms, which includes dyschezia and pain with predefecation, is most consistent with pelvic endometriosis.

A trial of leuprolide acetate is an acceptable alternative to diagnostic laparoscopy in adults with symptoms consistent with endometriosis; however, this empiric approach is not recommended in adolescents. Diagnostic laparoscopy is indicated in adolescents with severe dysmenorrhea who do not improve after a 3–6-month course of nonsteroidal antiinflammatory drugs and oral contraceptives (Box 17-1). Gastrointestinal, genitourinary, musculoskeletal, and psychosocial evaluations, as well as ultrasonography, should be undertaken before surgery. The risk profile of medications used for the treatment of endometriosis differs in adolescents and adults. For this reason, definitive diagnosis is essential to tailor long-term therapy for adolescents with endometriosis. Laparoscopic findings of endometriosis in adolescents include red or white implants as opposed to brown "powder burn" lesions more commonly seen in adults. Laparoscopy with liberal peritoneal biopsy is the best option to determine the etiology of pelvic pain in this patient. In the absence of a diagnosis, empiric use of oral narcotics would be contraindicated.

BOX 17-1

Indications for Laparoscopy in an Adolescent With Pelvic Pain

Chronic pelvic pain unresponsive to oral contraceptives and nonsteroidal antiinflammatory drugs
Diagnostic dilemma (eg, suspected chronic pelvic inflammatory disease or appendicitis)
Identified pelvic mass
Painful irregular vaginal bleeding
Progressive dysmenorrhea

Hewitt GD, Brown RT. Chronic pelvic pain in the adolescent differential diagnosis and evaluation. Female Pat 2000;25(1):38, 43–4, 47–8.

Laufer MR. Gynecolgic pain: Dysmenorrhea, acute and chronic pelvic pain, endometriosis, and premenstrual syndrome. In: Emans SJ, Laufer MR, editors. Emans, Laufer, Goldstein's pediatric & adolescent gynecology. 6th ed. Philadelphia (PA): Wolters Kluwer Lippincott Williams & Wilkins; 2012. p. 238–71.

Park JH. Role of colonoscopy in the diagnosis and treatment of pediatric lower gastrointestinal disorders. Korean J Pediatr 2010;53:824–9.

Song AH, Advincula AP. Adolescent chronic pelvic pain. J Pediatr Adolesc Gynecol 2005;18:371–7.

Stratton P, Winkel C, Premkumar A, Chow C, Wilson J, Hearns-Stokes R, et al. Diagnostic accuracy of laparoscopy, magnetic resonance imaging, and histopathologic examination for the detection of endometriosis. Fertil Steril 2003;79:1078–85.

Vendrig AA. The Minnesota Multiphasic Personality Inventory and chronic pain: a conceptual analysis of a long-standing but complicated relationship. Clin Psychol Rev 2000;20:533–59.

Wright KN, Laufer MR. Endometriomas in adolescents. Fertil Steril 2010;94:1529.e7–9.

18

Headache

A 32-year-old woman, gravida 1, comes to your office at 12 weeks of gestation with what she describes as a severe headache that is not like her usual headaches. The only medication she takes is a prenatal vitamin. She reports no other medical problems except for complex migraines, which have been well controlled during the pregnancy. Her headache is described as a unilateral intense pressure, abrupt in onset, and is associated with blurry vision, numbness in her arm, lightheadedness, and nausea with one episode of emesis. It did improve without intervention but has not resolved completely. Her arm numbness resolved 90 minutes after onset of her symptoms, but dizziness and blurry vision persist. She reports no fever, trauma, or loss of consciousness. Physical examination reveals a temperature of 37.2°C (99°F), a heart rate of 92 beats per minute, and blood pressure of 138/74 mm Hg. On examination, she appears well, with no apparent neurologic deficits. Laboratory studies show a white blood cell count of 14 g/dL and a hemoglobin level of 11.5 g/dL. The best next step in management is

(A) reassurance with follow-up
(B) lumbar puncture
* (C) head computed tomography (CT) scan
(D) head magnetic resonance imaging (MRI) scan
(E) head magnetic resonance angiography scan

Headaches represent the most common constellation of symptoms of neurologic disorders seen in the outpatient setting and can be associated with significant morbidity, including diminished quality of life and prolonged absences from work. According to the National Health Interview Survey put forth by the Centers for Disease Control and Prevention, 25% of women aged 18–44 years reported a severe headache within the previous 3 months. Headache also is the most common neurologic concern during pregnancy.

Migraine headaches represent a prevalent, genetically influenced, chronic neurologic brain disorder. The World Health Organization estimates that migraines affect 324 million individuals worldwide. However, despite the prevalence of migraines, the condition remains underrecognized by patients and clinicians. One large population-based survey showed that only one half of all individuals identified with migraine headaches were aware of their diagnosis. Symptoms generally begin in adolescence or early adulthood and peak during middle age, for a lifetime prevalence of 43% in women. *Migraine without aura* is defined as episodic attacks, lasting 4–72 hours, with characteristic features including unilateral location, pulsating quality, moderate-to-severe intensity, exacerbation because of physical activity, and possible association with nausea with or without photophobia and phonophobia. In contrast, migraine with aura consists of reversible focal neurologic symptoms that develop gradually and persist for up to 60 minutes. Auras precede the headache and often include visual disturbances. Studies have shown that radiologic testing in the setting of classic migraine with aura has a low likelihood of significant findings with a negative neurologic examination. Furthermore, comprehensive reviews in the literature have demonstrated that approximately 50–70% of migraineurs have improvement of headaches during pregnancy; however, migraines, often with aura, occasionally present for the first time during pregnancy. Pregnant women who have preexisting migraine symptoms may present with symptoms that are more concerning for an acute intracranial process. Therefore, the onset of new or concerning neurologic symptoms during pregnancy warrants a prompt and complete evaluation. When indicated, CT and MRI scans can be used safely during pregnancy. In general, CT scan is used more commonly when rapid diagnosis is necessary; in less acute situations, MRI scan often is preferred.

The described patient has a history of migraine with aura and exhibits neurologic symptoms with negative neurologic findings on physical examination. However, her symptom course and duration are unlike migraines in that they are abrupt in onset and the neurologic symptoms persisted beyond 60 minutes. Advanced neuroimaging should be obtained for all patients with sudden-onset severe headache, rapidly increasing headache frequency, or neurologic deficits. Additional red flag symptoms that are concerning for nonmigraine headaches include thunderclap headache, new-onset headache, nausea or vomiting, and headaches that differ from baseline. A noncontrast CT scan of the head should be the initial study of choice for this patient. Despite her early-pregnancy status, a CT scan of the head carries minimal fetal radiation exposure and should not be withheld because she is pregnant. Contrast should be avoided unless absolutely necessary.

Because MRI involves no radiation exposure, it is safe to use in pregnancy. It is frequently the preferred imaging modality because of its sensitivity for detecting edema and vascular lesions and its ability to evaluate the posterior fossa. An MRI with arteriography (also called magnetic resonance angiography) may be warranted if cerebral venous thrombosis is a consideration. However, CT scan is more widely available and more useful in evaluating for an acute bleed. An MRI scan should be considered for a patient who has already undergone CT imaging with negative results or who has persistent symptoms.

Reassurance would not be the best course of action for the described patient. Although pain is no longer her primary concern, expectant management would not exclude more worrisome etiologies of her symptoms.

The described patient's elevated white blood cell count is most likely due to her pregnancy, and she has no other signs or symptoms concerning for meningitis, such as fever or neck stiffness. Given the maximal intensity of her headache, a subarachnoid hemorrhage also is a reasonable consideration. A lumbar puncture for cerebrospinal fluid analysis is indicated when there is a clinical suspicion for an infectious etiology or subarachnoid hemorrhage. However, lumbar puncture would not be the most appropriate next step in this patient's evaluation. Her short duration of symptoms would not allow for sufficient development of xanthochromia in the cerebrospinal fluid, and a head CT should be performed first. A negative CT scan of the head performed within 6 hours of headache onset is sufficient to exclude a subarachnoid hemorrhage.

Loder E. Clinical therapeutics. Triptan therapy in migraine. N Engl J Med 2010;363:63–70.

Neurological disorders. In: Cunningham FG, Leveno KJ, Bloom SL, Hauth JC, Rouse DJ, Spong CY, editors. Williams Obstetrics. 24th ed. New York (NY): McGraw-Hill Medical; 2014. p. 1187–203.

Psychiatric disorders. In: Cunningham FG, Leveno KJ, Bloom SL, Hauth JC, Rouse DJ, Spong CY, editors. Williams obstetrics. 24th ed. New York (NY): McGraw Hill Medical; 2014. p. 1204–13.

Sadovsky R, Dodick D. Identifying migraine in primary care settings. Am J Med 2005;118(suppl):11S–17S.

Schoen JC, Campbell RL, Sadosty AT. Headache in pregnancy: an approach to emergency department evaluation and management. West J Emerg Med 2015;16:291–301.

19

Contraception and hypertension

A 37-year-old woman visits your office for her annual well-woman examination. She is using a combination hormonal oral contraceptive pill (OCP) with 35 micrograms of ethinyl estradiol. She is very happy with her OCP because it has controlled her heavy menses and provided contraception. She has used depot medroxyprogesterone acetate in the past but stopped using it because of weight gain. She is not planning to become pregnant in the next several years. A review of her medical history reveals a new diagnosis of hypertension in the past year, which is well controlled on a low-dose diuretic. Her blood pressure today is 120/70 mm Hg, and her examination is normal. Your recommendation for a contraceptive method is

(A) lower-dose combination OCP
(B) vaginal ring
* (C) progestin-only contraception
(D) copper intrauterine device (IUD)
(E) continuation of her current method

Many women of childbearing age will develop chronic medical conditions such as hypertension. Women with such conditions are at an increased risk of morbidity if an unintended pregnancy occurs (Box 19-1), so they have a great need for effective contraception. Women who have been diagnosed with hypertension are at a small but increased risk of adverse cardiac events such as myocardial infarction and stroke. Even well-controlled hypertension is a contraindication to estrogen-containing methods of contraception. There may be a place for careful monitoring of women with well-controlled hypertension who are nonsmokers and younger than 35 years. The Centers for Disease Control and Prevention (CDC) Medical Eligibility Criteria classify combination hormonal OCPs as category 3 (Box 19-2) for women who have been diagnosed with hypertension, even if blood pressure is well controlled; therefore, use of a combination OCP usually is not recommended unless other, more appropriate, methods are not available or acceptable. There is no evidence that a lower dose of ethinyl estradiol confers a lower risk of adverse events. Thus, continued use of the described patient's combination OCP or a lower-dose combination OCP would not be the best birth control method for her.

The vaginal ring provides a lower daily estrogen dose than many combination OCPs. The ring can be used continuously, by placing a new ring immediately upon removal of the last ring, if the woman wishes to suppress the expected withdrawal bleed. Data are lacking on the safety of the vaginal ring in women with hypertension, and the ring should be considered to have a similar risk profile to combination OCPs. The CDC Medical Eligibility Criteria classify the vaginal ring as category 3 for women with well-controlled hypertension, such as the described patient; therefore, the vaginal ring is not her best contraceptive choice.

The copper IUD is a long-acting reversible method of contraception that has few medical contraindications (including uterine infections, severe thrombocytopenia, and cervical and endometrial cancer). The CDC Medical Eligibility Criteria classify the copper IUD as category 1 for women with well-controlled hypertension. Studies have shown high rates of patient satisfaction and continuation with use of the copper IUD, but a common adverse effect is heavy menstrual bleeding. Because this method may lead to resumption of this patient's heavy menses, the copper IUD is not the best contraceptive choice for her. Other nonhormonal methods, such as condoms and diaphragms, are not as effective as other available methods, so they should not be recommended as a first-line contraceptive choice.

There are multiple progestin-only options for contraception that are classified as category 1 for well-controlled or mildly elevated blood pressure, defined as a systolic blood pressure of 140–159 mm Hg or diastolic blood pressure of 90–99 mm Hg. Levonorgestrel IUDs and the contraceptive implant have high rates of patient satisfaction and continuation with very low failure rates (less than 1%). Neither method has been associated with weight gain, which is one of this patient's concerns. In addition to contraception, levonorgestrel IUDs have high rates of oligomenorrhea and amenorrhea. For a woman with a history of heavy menstrual bleeding, such as this patient, levonorgestrel IUD use can diminish menstrual flow and provide excellent long-term contraception.

If the described patient prefers oral contraception, there is one formulation of progestin-only pills in the United States that contains norethindrone. Depot

BOX 19-1

Conditions Associated With Increased Risk of Adverse Health Events as a Result of Unintended Pregnancy

- Breast cancer
- Complicated valvular heart disease
- Diabetes: insulin-dependent; with nephropathy/retinopathy/neuropathy or other vascular disease; or greater than 20 years in duration
- Endometrial or ovarian cancer
- Epilepsy
- Hypertension (systolic blood pressure greater than 160 mm Hg or diastolic blood pressure greater than 100 mm Hg)
- History of bariatric surgery within the past 2 years
- HIV and AIDS
- Ischemic heart disease
- Malignant gestational trophoblastic disease
- Malignant liver tumors (hepatoma) and hepatocellular carcinoma of the liver
- Peripartum cardiomyopathy
- Schistosomiasis with fibrosis of the liver
- Severe (decompensated) cirrhosis
- Sickle cell disease
- Solid organ transplantation within the past 2 years
- Stroke
- Systemic lupus erythematosus
- Thrombogenic mutations
- Tuberculosis

Abbreviations: AIDS, acquired immunodeficiency syndrome; HIV, human immunodeficiency virus.

Centers for Disease Control and Prevention. U.S. Medical Eligibility Criteria for Contraceptive Use, 2010. MMWR 2010;59(No. RR-4):6.

BOX 19-2

Categories of Medical Eligibility Criteria for Contraceptive Use

1 = A condition for which there is no restriction for the use of the contraceptive method

2 = A condition for which the advantages of using the method generally outweigh the theoretical or proven risks

3 = A condition for which the theoretical or proven risks usually outweigh the advantages of using the method

4 = A condition that represents an unacceptable health risk if the contraceptive method is used.

Centers for Disease Control and Prevention. U.S. Medical Eligibility Criteria for Contraceptive Use, 2010. MMWR 2010;59(No. RR-4):3.

medroxyprogesterone acetate injections also are an option, with the highest amenorrhea rate (approximately 50%) of the progestin-only methods, although these injections are associated with weight gain, as this patient experienced. Any of these methods can be recommended to the described patient, who desires highly effective contraception and menstrual control.

Centers for Disease Control and Prevention. U.S. Medical Eligibility Criteria (US MEC) for contraceptive use, 2010. MMWR Morb Mortal Wkly Rep 2010;59:1–85.

Mancia G, Fagard R, Narkiewicz K, Redon J, Zanchetti A, Bohm M, et al. 2013 ESH/ESC guidelines for the management of arterial hypertension: the task force for the management of arterial hypertension of the European Society of Hypertension (ESH) and of the European Society of Cardiology (ESC). Eur Heart J 2013;34(28):2159–219.

20

Cervical insufficiency

A 23-year-old woman, gravida 3, para 2, comes to your office for a routine prenatal visit at 20 weeks of gestation. She has a history of two previous preterm births, both at 30 weeks of gestation. She currently is receiving weekly 17α-hydroxyprogesterone caproate injections. On transvaginal ultrasonography, her cervix measures 20 mm. The most appropriate next step in management is

(A) repeat transvaginal ultrasonography in 1 week
* (B) cervical cerclage
(C) vaginal progesterone gel
(D) strict bed rest

In the United States, the rate of preterm birth (birth before 37 completed weeks of gestation) is approximately 11.4%. In 2012, this equated to 450,000 infants that were born prematurely. Approximately one third of infant deaths are due to prematurity. Preterm birth is the leading cause of long-term neurologic disabilities in children and also is associated with increased risks of morbidity and mortality throughout childhood. The annual cost associated with premature birth in the United States is $26 billion.

A patient's personal history of spontaneous preterm birth is the most predictive risk factor for subsequent preterm birth; it doubles the risk. Other risk factors for preterm birth include tobacco use, multiple gestations, uterine anomalies, and a short interpregnancy interval.

A woman with a history of a spontaneous preterm birth should be offered progesterone supplementation to reduce the risk of recurrent spontaneous preterm birth. Typically, the progesterone offered is 17α-hydroxyprogesterone caproate. Furthermore, women who have a history of preterm birth before 34 weeks of gestation should undergo serial cervical length screenings starting at 16 weeks and continuing until 24 weeks of gestation. If a shortened cervical length (less than 25 mm) is noted during this time, cervical cerclage placement should be offered. Cerclage has been proven to significantly decrease the rate of premature birth and perinatal mortality in such cases.

Cervical cerclage with the transvaginal approach is by far the most common method of cerclage placement. The two most common transvaginal cerclage methods are the McDonald and Shirodkar procedures. In the McDonald procedure, a purse-string suture is placed circumferentially at the cervicovaginal junction. The Shirodkar procedure involves dissecting the bladder and rectum from the vesicocervical mucosa in order to place the stitch as far cephalad as possible.

Transabdominal cerclage may be carried out by means of laparotomy or laparoscopy. This procedure generally is reserved for patients who have anatomic limitations (eg, patients with prior trachelectomy) or who have previously had a transvaginal cervical cerclage followed by a second-trimester pregnancy loss. If a transabdominal cerclage is performed, the stitch may be left in place between pregnancies. These patients would have to undergo cesarean delivery because the cerclage is not meant to be removed.

Repeat ultrasonography in 1 week may be an option for a woman who does not consent to cerclage placement. If the cervical shortening worsens further, she then may agree to have a cerclage placed. However, the obstetrician–gynecologist or other health care provider should be clear that when a significantly shortened cervix (less than 25 mm) is appreciated before 24 weeks of gestation, the woman should be offered a cerclage because further cervical shortening may lead to a preterm birth.

Although 17α-hydroxyprogesterone caproate is the preferred progesterone supplementation, vaginal progesterone gel may be offered to women who refuse injections or who have limited access. Given that the described patient is already receiving 17α-hydroxyprogesterone caproate, adding another progestational agent is not recommended. Progesterone suppositories are indicated for an asymptomatic woman with a singleton gestation with no history of preterm birth and an asymptomatic shortened cervical length (less than 20 mm). Two trials have demonstrated a lower risk of preterm birth and a decrease in composite neonatal morbidity and mortality for women with no history of preterm birth and an asymptomatic shortened cervical length.

Although bed rest often is prescribed as the first intervention to reduce the risk of preterm birth, no evidence is available to support such a management plan. Furthermore, bed rest during pregnancy increases the risk of venous thromboembolic events and adds substantially increased costs to the health care system, a result of lost hours at work and costs of hospitalization. In women with a history of preterm birth and shortened cervical length in a subsequent pregnancy, bed rest has not been demonstrated to reduce the recurrence risk of preterm birth.

Berghella V, Rafael TJ, Szychowski JM, Rust OA, Owen J. Cerclage for short cervix on ultrasonography in women with singleton gestations and previous preterm birth: a meta-analysis. Obstet Gynecol 2011;117:663–71.

Cerclage for the management of cervical insufficiency. Practice Bulletin No. 142. American College of Obstetricians and Gynecologists. Obstet Gynecol 2014;123:372–9.

Hamilton BE, Martin JA, Osterman MJ, Curtin SC, Matthews TJ. Births: Final Data for 2014. Natl Vital Stat Rep 2015;64:1–64.

Prediction and prevention of preterm birth. Practice Bulletin No. 130. American College of Obstetricians and Gynecologists. Obstet Gynecol 2012;120:964–73.

Sosa CG, Althabe F, Belizán JM, Bergel E. Bed rest in singleton pregnancies for preventing preterm birth. Cochrane Database of Systematic Reviews 2015, Issue 3. Art. No.: CD003581. DOI: 10.1002/14651858.CD003581.pub3.

21

Therapy to reduce the risk of colon cancer

A 47-year-old woman comes to your office for a well-woman examination. Her father was diagnosed with colorectal cancer at age 69 years, but her family history is otherwise negative. She asks about the use of aspirin to reduce her risk of colorectal cancer. You recall a recent journal article that suggested reduction in the risk of colorectal cancer after long-term, low-dose aspirin use. In that large prospective trial of low-dose aspirin, after 15 years of follow-up, 98.7% of women who used aspirin did not develop colorectal cancer compared with 98.9% of women who did not use aspirin and did not develop colorectal cancer. The calculation

$$\frac{100}{98.9 - 98.7}$$ is called

(A) relative risk reduction
* (B) number needed to treat (NNT)
(C) absolute risk reduction
(D) hazard ratio
(E) odds ratio

The NNT represents the theoretical number of patients who would need to receive a given treatment or intervention in order for one of those patients to benefit from the intervention. It is a useful measure of effectiveness and one that is readily understood by patients and clinicians. Interventions that require a low NNT usually are seen as preferable to those with a high NNT. A related figure is the number needed to harm (NNH), which is an indicator of the relative safety of the intervention. A high NNH is associated with greater safety. In instances where the intervention carries some risk (eg, gastrointestinal bleeding with nonsteroidal antiinflammatory drug use), then the NNT should be lower than the NNH. The calculation for NNT is simply 100 over the difference between event rates (exposure group versus control group).

The NNT is useful in a global sense but does not take into account the specifics about any individual patient. A patient will not know from the NNT what her likelihood of improvement would be with no treatment. In direct patient care, additional measures of effectiveness will be necessary for informed decision making.

Absolute risk reduction is not a ratio but instead a straightforward quantity by which some outcome is reduced. In the example used in this study, the absolute risk reduction is 0.2% (ie, 98.9–98.7%). The relative risk reduction is calculated by dividing the absolute risk reduction by the baseline rate of the event in question. For example, if an event occurs in 20% of a control population, and with medication (the exposure), the event occurs in 12%, then the relative risk reduction is calculated thus: 8% (the absolute risk reduction) divided by 20% (control incidence), giving a relative risk reduction of 0.4 or 40%. Therefore, the relative risk is 0.6 or 60%. Relative risk is a measure of the effect of the exposure being studied. It is simply a ratio of the percentage of exposed people who experience the outcome divided by the percentage of controls that experience the outcome. In the example given, it is 0.6 or 12% divided by 20%.

Odds is the ratio of probability of some event happening over the probability of the event not happening. An odds ratio is the odds of some outcome in one group (eg, cases) divided by the odds of that outcome in the other group (eg, controls). Odds ratios typically are used in case–control studies, whereas relative risk is used more often in cohort and randomized controlled studies. Odds ratios and relative risks frequently are mistaken for one another because there are similarities in how they are calculated. In comparisons where the outcome is common, the odds ratio frequently overstates the magnitude of the effect. With relatively rare events, the odds ratio and relative risk are numerically close to each other.

A hazard ratio typically is found in studies related to survival or other time-to-event outcomes. It is more complex to calculate and can be confusing to interpret. The key difference is that hazard ratios examine differences in an outcome at a specific point in time and not necessarily at the endpoint of a study. For example, if a trial uses disease resolution as the endpoint, the hazard ratio communicates the relative likelihood of disease resolution in the treated group at any given time before this endpoint. A hazard ratio of less than 1 demonstrates that the event of interest is happening more slowly in the exposed (treatment) group than in the control group.

Cook NR, Lee IM, Zhang SM, Moorthy MV, Buring JE. Alternate-day, low-dose aspirin and cancer risk: long-term observational follow-up of a randomized trial. Ann Intern Med 2013;159:77–85.

Grimes DA, Schulz KF. Making sense of odds and odds ratios. Obstet Gynecol 2008;111:423–6.

Spruance SL, Reid JE, Grace M, Samore M. Hazard ratio in clinical trials. Antimicrob Agents Chemother 2004;48:2787–92.

22

Polycystic ovary syndrome

A 23-year-old nulligravid woman comes to your office for her annual well-woman examination. She reports irregular menses that occur every 35–45 days and a moderate flow without any significant cramping. She regularly plucks hair from her chin, upper lip, and chest. She is not sexually active. Her body mass index (BMI) (calculated as weight in kilograms divided by height in meters squared [kg/m^2]) is 31, and her blood pressure is 138/88 mm Hg. Your examination is significant for moderate acne and unremarkable breast and pelvic findings. Laboratory values include normal levels of thyroid-stimulating hormone, prolactin, and early-morning 17α-hydroxyprogesterone, as well as a normal fasting lipid panel. Her glucose level is 106 mg/dL fasting and 145 mg/dL 2 hours after a 75-g glucose load. You counsel her that the most appropriate intervention to decrease her risk of developing diabetes mellitus is

* (A) low-calorie diet and exercise
(B) metformin hydrochloride
(C) oral contraceptive pills
(D) bariatric surgery

Polycystic ovary syndrome (PCOS) is a constellation of disorders that includes hyperandrogenism, ovulatory dysfunction, and polycystic ovaries. Clinical manifestations of PCOS include menstrual irregularities, infertility, hirsutism, and acne. The condition is associated with metabolic disorders, including diabetes mellitus, and cardiovascular disease. Various criteria have been proposed to make the clinical diagnosis of PCOS. A widely accepted method of diagnosing PCOS is by means of the Rotterdam criteria, with PCOS being diagnosed if two of three criteria are present—androgen excess, ovulatory dysfunction, and polycystic ovaries—assuming exclusion of other endocrine disorders (Appendix C). If a patient meets clinical criteria for ovulatory dysfunction and androgen excess, neither biochemical androgen measurements nor ultrasonographic assessment of the ovaries are necessary. The Endocrine Society Clinical Practice Guideline recommends that all women who are being evaluated for PCOS be screened for thyroid-stimulating hormone level, serum prolactin level, and early-morning serum 17α-hydroxyprogesterone level to rule out thyroid disease, prolactin excess, and nonclassic congenital adrenal hyperplasia. Certain clinical conditions may warrant additional endocrine evaluation, such as primary ovarian insufficiency, hypothalamic amenorrhea, acromegaly, androgen-secreting tumor, or Cushing syndrome.

The described patient meets the criteria for PCOS based on features of ovulatory dysfunction and clinical hyperandrogenism. Insulin resistance often is noted in women who are diagnosed with PCOS, as seen in this patient, but it is not included in the diagnostic criteria for PCOS. Nonetheless, PCOS is associated with a fivefold to 10-fold increased risk of developing type 2 diabetes mellitus. Among women with PCOS in the United States, 30–35% have glucose intolerance and 3–10% have type 2 diabetes. Women with PCOS also have been described to be at increased risk of gestational diabetes, hypertensive disorders of pregnancy, metabolic syndrome, nonalcoholic fatty liver disease, nonalcoholic steatohepatitis, and sleep apnea, in addition to the long-term metabolic sequelae of type 2 diabetes and cardiovascular disease. Chronic anovulation and obesity among women with PCOS place them at increased risk of endometrial cancer. All patients with PCOS should be screened for cardiovascular disease risk factors, including cigarette smoking, impaired glucose tolerance–type 2 diabetes, hypertension, dyslipidemia, obstructive sleep apnea, and obesity.

Obesity is a comorbidity that often is found in patients with PCOS and that may amplify the effects of the disorder, but it also is not a diagnostic criterion. Because obesity makes such a substantial contribution to the metabolic and endocrine abnormalities in PCOS, counseling regarding weight loss is an important part of the management of patients with PCOS. Weight loss can lower circulating androgen levels and allow spontaneous return of ovulation and regular menstruation. It also improves pregnancy rates, decreases hirsutism, and improves glucose and lipid levels.

In patients with impaired glucose tolerance, such as the described patient, lifestyle modification with diet and exercise reduces risk of type 2 diabetes by 58% compared with a 31% decrease with metformin. A low-calorie diet and exercise are recommended lifestyle modifications for overweight and obese women with PCOS and have proven benefits for metabolic and reproductive function. As little as 5% weight loss can improve metabolic abnormalities associated with PCOS. Although no large randomized studies have been carried out of exercise among patients with PCOS, exercise with or without diet has been found to improve weight loss and to decrease risk of diabetes and cardiovascular disease in the general population. Getting 30 minutes a day of moderate-to-vigorous physical activity can effectively reduce the risk of metabolic syndrome and diabetes.

Metformin can delay the development of diabetes; however, recent studies suggest little benefit to the addition of metformin to lifestyle modifications alone. Similarly, although studies have shown weight reduction in patients with PCOS who are treated with metformin, the medication does not increase weight loss in patients who use diet and exercise programs. Diet and exercise, not metformin, constitute first-line therapy for overweight and obese women with PCOS. Metformin is recommended in patients with impaired glucose tolerance or type 2 diabetes who fail lifestyle modification or for patients with menstrual irregularities who cannot take hormonal contraceptives. Metformin is not recommended as first-line treatment of cutaneous manifestations of PCOS, pregnancy complications, or obesity. Adverse effects of metformin include a risk of lactic acidosis in women with diabetes and poor renal function and gastrointestinal symptoms of diarrhea, nausea, vomiting, bloating, flatulence, and anorexia. These effects can be ameliorated by starting at small doses and then gradually increasing them or by using sustained release preparations.

Combination hormonal contraceptives (in the form of a pill, ring, or patch) are recommended for treatment of menstrual irregularities and hirsutism associated with PCOS but not specifically for reduction of diabetes or cardiovascular risk. The effect of hormonal contraceptives on carbohydrate metabolism in patients with PCOS is debated, but the American Diabetes Association and the Centers for Disease Control and Prevention have concluded that hormonal contraceptives are not contraindicated in women who have been diagnosed with diabetes without vascular complications.

Morbidly obese women with PCOS who undergo weight loss surgery experience near normalization of reproductive and metabolic abnormalities. Bariatric surgery typically is indicated in patients who are morbidly obese with a BMI of greater than 40, a BMI of greater than 35 with a serious comorbidity, or a BMI of greater than 30 with uncontrolled type 2 diabetes or metabolic syndrome. Surgery is not the best option for this patient. Even in patients who are offered bariatric surgery, lifestyle modification should be recommended, or even required, before surgery.

Knowler WC, Barrett-Connor E, Fowler SE, Hamman RF, Lachin JM, Walker EA, et al. Reduction in the incidence of type 2 diabetes with lifestyle intervention or metformin. Diabetes Prevention Program Research Group. N Engl J Med 2002;346:393–403.

Legro RS, Arslanian SA, Ehrmann DA, Hoeger KM, Murad MH, Pasquali R, et al. Diagnosis and treatment of polycystic ovary syndrome: an Endocrine Society clinical practice guideline. Endocrine Society. J Clin Endocrinol Metab 2013;98:4565–92.

Lim RB. Bariatric operations for management of obesity: indications and preoperative preparation. In: Post TW, editors. Uptodate. Waltham (MA): UpToDate; 2016.

Polycystic ovary syndrome. ACOG Practice Bulletin No. 108. American College of Obstetricians and Gynecologists. Obstet Gynecol 2009;114:936–49.

23

Thrombophilic disorder associated with recurrent pregnancy loss

A 24-year-old woman, gravida 4, para 1, comes to your office for a prepregnancy visit. Her obstetric history is significant for three consecutive first-trimester pregnancy losses followed by a preterm delivery at 28 weeks of gestation. Upon review of her records from 4 months ago, you notice that she tested positive for lupus anticoagulant with normal levels of anticardiolipin immunoglobulin G (IgG) and anti-β_2-glycoprotein I. In addition, she has had a normal hysterosalpingography, and she and her husband have normal karyotypes. The test that you should order now to establish the diagnosis of antiphospholipid syndrome (APS) is

(A) anticardiolipin IgG
(B) immunoglobulin A
* (C) lupus anticoagulant
(D) anti-β_2-glycoprotein I

Antiphospholipid syndrome is an immune disorder that has been associated with obstetric and medical morbidity, including thrombosis, recurrent miscarriage, fetal loss, fetal growth restriction, preeclampsia, and preterm delivery. For a diagnosis of APS, women must meet laboratory criteria (Box 23-1) as well as clinical criteria (Box 23-2).

The described patient has already met the clinical criteria for APS because she had three first-trimester pregnancy losses. This patient, however, has not yet met the laboratory criteria to confirm APS. To do so would require two positive test results from the same test (lupus anticoagulant, anti-β_2-glycoprotein, or anticardiolipin antibodies) at least 12 weeks apart. Laboratory

BOX 23-1

Laboratory Criteria for the Diagnosis of Antiphospholipid Syndrome

- Lupus anticoagulant present in plasma, on two or more occasions at least 12 weeks apart. It is interpreted as either present or absent. Testing for lupus anticoagulant is ideally performed before the patient is treated with anticoagulants, or
- Anticardiolipin antibody of IgG and/or IgM isotype in serum or plasma, present in medium or high titer (ie, greater than 40 GPL or MPL, or greater than the 99th percentile), on two or more occasions, at least 12 weeks apart, or
- Anti-β_2-glycoprotein I of IgG and/or IgM isotype in serum or plasma (in titer greater than 99th percentile for a normal population as defined by the laboratory performing the test), present on two or more occasions, at least 12 weeks apart.

Abbreviations: GPL, IgG phospholipid; IgG, immunoglobulin G; IgM, immunoglobulin M; MPL, IgM phospholipid.

Modified from Miyakis S, Lockshin MD, Atsumi T, Branch DW, Brey RL, Cervera R, et al. International consensus statement on an update of the classification criteria for definite antiphospholipid syndrome (APS). J Throm Haemost 2006;4;295–306. Copyright 2006, with permission of John Wiley and Sons.

BOX 23-2

Clinical Criteria for Diagnosis of Antiphospholipid Syndrome

- Vascular thrombosis
  One or more clinical episodes of arterial, venous, or small vessel thrombosis, in any tissue or organ, or
- Pregnancy morbidity
  - One or more unexplained deaths of a morphologically normal fetus at or beyond the 10th week of gestation, with normal fetal morphology documented by ultrasound or by direct examination of the fetus, or
  - One or more premature births of a morphologically normal neonate before the 34th week of gestation because of eclampsia or severe preeclampsia, or features consistent with placental insufficiency, or
  - Three or more unexplained consecutive spontaneous pregnancy losses before the 10th week of pregnancy, with maternal anatomic or hormonal abnormalities and paternal and maternal chromosomal causes excluded.

Modified from Miyakis S, Lockshin MD, Atsumi T, Branch DW, Brey RL, Cervera R, et al. International consensus statement on an update of the classification criteria for definite antiphospholipid syndrome (APS). J Throm Haemost 2006;4;295–306. Copyright 2006, with permission of John Wiley and Sons.

testing includes assessment of specified levels of circulating antibodies, specifically lupus anticoagulant, anti-β_2-glycoprotein I, and anticardiolipin antibodies. Because transient positive test results can occur, a positive laboratory finding requires confirmation 12 weeks after the initial test. This patient already had a positive test result for lupus anticoagulant 4 months ago, so it is necessary to confirm that it still is present in order to meet laboratory criteria for diagnosis of APS.

Lupus anticoagulant is a misnomer; it does not indicate that an individual has systemic lupus erythematosus; rather, lupus anticoagulant is associated with thrombosis and is assessed indirectly, usually by a clotting assay (eg, dilute Russell viper venom time or lupus anticoagulant-sensitive activated partial thromboplastin time). Because of a number of factors, such as clotting factor deficiencies, clotting time can be prolonged with these assays, so the next step would be to add normal plasma to the sample. In a patient with lupus anticoagulant, the clotting time remains prolonged because lupus anticoagulant functions to inhibit clotting. In these cases, a second confirmatory test involving phospholipids is recommended.

Enzyme-linked immunosorbent assays are used to detect the presence of anticardiolipin antibodies IgG (designated in international standard units of GPL) or immunoglobulin M (designated as MPL). To enable diagnosis, titers must be greater than 40 units of GPL or MPL twice, 12 weeks apart (ie, 99th percentile). Similarly, anti-β_2-glycoprotein I antibodies are detected using enzyme-linked immunosorbent assays and also have to be greater than the (laboratory-specific) 99th percentile for IgG (designated in international standard units of SGU) or immunoglobulin M (designated as SMU). Immunoglobulin A is of uncertain clinical significance and is not sufficient for diagnosis of APS.

If the described patient with recurrent pregnancy loss eventually is diagnosed with APS, she may benefit from prophylactic heparin and low-dose aspirin; this treatment may decrease her risk of subsequent pregnancy loss. Patients with APS are at increased risk of thrombotic events as their pregnancies advance and throughout the postpartum period. Pregnant patients with APS and a history of thrombotic events should receive prophylactic anticoagulation with heparin throughout pregnancy and through 6 weeks postpartum to minimize the risk of maternal thromboembolism. Pregnant patients without a history of thrombotic events also may benefit from anticoagulation, though the optimal treatment has not been well studied.

Antiphospholipid syndrome. Practice Bulletin No. 132. American College of Obstetricians and Gynecologists. Obstet Gynecol 2012;120:1514–21.

Empson M, Lassere M, Craig JC, Scott JR. Recurrent pregnancy loss with antiphospholipid antibody: a systematic review of therapeutic trials. Obstet Gynecol 2002;99:135–44.

Kearon C, Akl EA, Ornelas J, Blaivas A, Jimenez D, Bounameaux H, et al. Antithrombotic Therapy for VTE Disease: CHEST Guideline and Expert Panel Report. Chest 2016;149:315–52.

24

Pregnancy of unknown location

A 30-year-old woman, gravida 4, para 0, comes to your office and reports vaginal spotting, left lower quadrant pain, and a positive home pregnancy test result. Her last menstrual period was 5 weeks ago. She has a history of two prior pregnancy losses and most recently underwent methotrexate therapy for an ectopic pregnancy. She has been trying to become pregnant for the past year and is extremely anxious about the current pregnancy. Her blood pressure is 120/82 mm Hg and heart rate is 85 beats per minute. Abdominal examination is benign. Pelvic examination is nontender and reveals no masses. On transvaginal ultrasonography, she has an empty uterus with a 2-cm endometrial stripe, normal ovaries bilaterally, with no adnexal masses or free fluid. Laboratory studies demonstrate an initial serum β-hCG level of 647 mIU/mL and Rh-positive blood type. Repeat β-hCG level in 48 hours is 873 mIU/mL. The most appropriate next step in her management is to

* (A) repeat test of β-hCG level in 48 hours
(B) obtain a progesterone level
(C) repeat ultrasonography in 1 week
(D) check serum aspartate aminotransferase, creatinine, and hemoglobin levels

Ectopic pregnancy accounts for 2% of pregnancies and 6–10% of pregnancy-related deaths, and it remains the leading cause of maternal mortality in the first trimester. Approximately 18% of emergency department visits in the United States are women in early pregnancy who have abdominal pain, vaginal bleeding, or both. The diagnosis of ectopic pregnancy relies on serial β-hCG levels in conjunction with transvaginal ultrasonography. A *normal increase in β-hCG levels* traditionally is defined as a minimum 53% increase in 48 hours and is seen in 99% of normal pregnancies. However, 1% of normal intrauterine pregnancies demonstrate a slower increase in β-hCG levels. The diagnosis of pregnancy of unknown location poses a significant clinical challenge, and diagnostic algorithms that exist in clinical practice are not error proof. Although 71% of ectopic pregnancies will exhibit an abnormal increase or decrease in β-hCG levels, 21% of women with ectopic pregnancies will demonstrate a β-hCG increase suggestive of a normal intrauterine pregnancy, and 8% will demonstrate a decrease in β-hCG suggestive of a spontaneous miscarriage. An error in management can result in false reassurance given to a woman who has an ectopic pregnancy; a potential interruption of a desired intrauterine pregnancy; or exposure of an early, potentially viable intrauterine pregnancy to methotrexate.

The described patient has slowly increasing β-hCG levels. Although her β-hCG level did not meet the 53% rise in 48 hours as seen in 99% of patients, her β-hCG levels did increase by 35%, as observed in 1% of normal pregnancies. Given the highly desired pregnancy, hemodynamic stability, and benign physical examination, obtaining an additional data point would be prudent. Thus, a repeat test of her β-hCG levels in another 48 hours is the most appropriate course of action at this time. Serial β-hCG levels can inform clinical management; however, a single measurement is nondiagnostic for pregnancy location or viability. Progesterone levels of less than 5 ng/mL have a specificity of 100% in confirming a nonviable pregnancy, and levels greater than 20 ng/mL are highly correlated with viable pregnancies. The main utility of serum progesterone is to identify whether a pregnancy is normal or failing, but these levels do not clearly delineate the location of the pregnancy. Progesterone levels between 5 ng/mL and 20 ng/mL are considered equivocal, and most ectopic pregnancies demonstrate progesterone levels between 10 ng/mL and 20 ng/mL. Given the limited clinical utility of progesterone level, obtaining a progesterone level would not be the most appropriate course of action for this patient.

Repeat ultrasonography in 1 week is a reasonable option. In general, repeat ultrasonography 2–7 days after initial evaluation may locate a pregnancy that was not identified on initial presentation and will successfully identify 90% of ectopic pregnancies at or beyond 6 weeks of gestation. However, this is not the best course of action for the described patient, who has a history of a prior ectopic pregnancy along with unilateral symptoms and a high level of anxiety. Delay in her diagnosis could lead to avoidable rupture of an ectopic pregnancy. Even with a low-normal increase in her β-hCG levels, her β-hCG would be expected to be above the discriminatory zone well before 1 week. Assessment of a patient's serum aspartate aminotransferase, creatinine, and hemoglobin levels would be appropriate if a need to administer methotrexate was anticipated. Such an assessment may be warranted for this patient later. However, intervention with methotrexate at this point would be inappropriate and could potentially expose an early viable intrauterine pregnancy to the medication's teratogenic effects.

Barnhart KT. Early pregnancy failure: beware of the pitfalls of management. Fertil Steril 2012;98;1061–5.

Barnhart KT. Clinical practice. Ectopic pregnancy. N Engl J Med 2009;361:379–87

Medical management of ectopic pregnancy. ACOG Practice Bulletin No. 94. American College of Obstetricians and Gynecologists. Obstet Gynecol 2008;111:1479–85.

Medical treatment of ectopic pregnancy: a committee opinion. Practice Committee of the American Society for Reproductive Medicine. Fertil Steril 2013;100:638–44.

Seeber BE. What serial hCG can tell you, and cannot tell you, about an early pregnancy. Fertil Steril 2012;98:1074–77.

Senapati S, Barnhart KT. Biomarkers for ectopic pregnancy and pregnancy of unknown location. Fertil Steril 2013;99:1107–16.

25

Complex and benign masses in reproductive-aged women

A 27-year-old nulligravid woman comes to your office for emergency department follow-up. She was seen over the weekend for self-resolving right pelvic pain and underwent transvaginal ultrasonography that revealed a 5.6-cm cyst (Fig. 25-1; see color plate). No free fluid was seen in the pelvis, and color flow was present in both ovaries. In the emergency department, her white blood cell count was 5.2×10^9 per liter, her hemoglobin level was 13.5 g/dL, and her β-hCG level was less than 2 international units/L. She feels well today but is very nervous about what the adnexal mass means, since her friend currently is undergoing chemotherapy for ovarian cancer. Your next step in management should be

(A) CA 125 level testing
(B) pelvic computed tomography scan
* (C) follow-up pelvic ultrasonography
(D) diagnostic laparoscopy
(E) no further follow-up

Adnexal masses, whether noted on physical examination or ultrasonography for gynecologic or other indications, are a common clinical dilemma in office gynecology practice. Women in the United States have a 5–10% lifetime risk of undergoing surgery for a suspected ovarian neoplasm. Of women who undergo surgical management, approximately 13–21% will receive a diagnosis of ovarian cancer. However, most masses are benign and do not require surgical management. Thus, the clinician's job is to use risk factors such as age, family history, and imaging findings to help exclude malignancy and facilitate conservative management. Although the differential diagnosis for an adnexal mass is quite broad and involves gynecologic and nongynecologic sources (Box 25-1), age is of extreme importance in determining the risk of malignancy from a gynecologic source. The median age at diagnosis of ovarian cancer is age 63 years. In menstruating women, functional cysts are the most likely etiology, even when septations are noted. In postmenopausal women, benign neoplasms such as cystadenomas are the most common findings, although the risk of malignancy is much higher relative to the risk for premenopausal women.

Follow-up pelvic ultrasonography is the most appropriate next step in management for this young patient. Although she may be worried about ovarian cancer, her most likely diagnosis is a functional cyst that will resolve spontaneously. Her fears about malignancy are understandable but unlikely. Certain genetic factors, such as *BRCA1* or *BRCA2* gene mutation and Lynch syndrome, have well-known and relatively sizable risk elevations. Other factors that are more common in reproductive-aged women and that also can increase risk of ovarian malignancy include nulliparity, primary infertility, and endometriosis. The only known primary prevention strategy that preserves fertility is the use of oral contraceptives, which has been shown to result in a 40–90% decrease of ovarian cancer risk in users, depending on length of use.

Given the size of the described cyst, the patient is at risk of torsion and cyst rupture. She does need to be counseled regarding concerning symptoms and when she should

BOX 25-1

Differential Diagnosis of Adnexal Mass

Gynecologic
- Benign
  - Functional cyst
  - Leiomyomata
  - Endometrioma
  - Tuboovarian abscess
  - Ectopic pregnancy
  - Mature teratoma
  - Serous cystadenoma
  - Mucinous cystadenoma
  - Breast cancer
  - Hydrosalpinx
- Malignant
  - Germ cell tumor
  - Sex-cord or stromal tumor
  - Epithelial carcinoma

Nongynecologic
- Benign
  - Diverticular abscess
  - Appendiceal abscess or mucocele
  - Nerve sheath tumors
  - Ureteral diverticulum
  - Pelvic kidney
  - Paratubal cysts
  - Bladder diverticulum
- Malignant
  - Gastrointestinal cancer
  - Retroperitoneal sarcomas
  - Metastases

Reprinted from Management of adnexal masses. ACOG Practice Bulletin No. 83. American College of Obstetricians and Gynecologists. Obstet Gynecol 2007;110:201–14.

present again for care. Any evidence of torsion on history or imaging (similar findings but no flow to the affected ovary) may suggest the need for diagnostic laparoscopy. In the absence of new symptoms, she should have repeat imaging within 1 year to ensure resolution of her cyst. The recommendations for exact timing of follow-up are not entirely clear, with many obstetrician–gynecologists and other health care providers routinely repeating imaging in 3–6 months. However, a consensus statement from the Society of Radiologists in Ultrasound suggests that, in a low-risk patient such as the one described, follow-up within 1 year is appropriate. The most likely finding on follow-up ultrasonography is resolution of her cyst.

A woman's lifetime risk of developing ovarian cancer is approximately 1 in 70. Although there are excellent 5-year survival rates for women in whom stage 1 ovarian cancer is diagnosed (more than 90% survival), most women are not diagnosed until later stages, when 5-year survival is approximately 30–55%. Unlike the screening available for cervical cancer through cytology and human papillomavirus testing, ovarian cancer does not yet have an ideal screening test. Although the CA 125 level is elevated in patients with nonmucinous epithelial tumors, it has not been proven beneficial as a screening test, especially in low-risk women.

An alternate form of imaging is not needed at this time for the described patient. Transvaginal ultrasonography is the imaging modality of choice in initial evaluation of an adnexal mass, given its availability, patient tolerability, and cost-effectiveness. Ultrasonography is useful in describing the size and consistency of adnexal masses (cystic, solid, or mixed), whether they are unilateral or bilateral, the presence or absence of septations, mural nodules or excrescences, and the existence of free fluid or ascites. Several of these findings (ie, excrescences, mural nodules, and ascites) increase concern for malignancy. Numerous scoring systems have been developed to help determine malignancy risk. The most consistent predictive findings for a nonmalignant etiology include smooth walls, thin or no septations, and no solid components. Even in postmenopausal patients, the rate of malignancy in women with unilocular, thin-walled, sonolucent cysts with smooth, regular borders is less than 1%. Computed tomography and magnetic resonance imaging scans also are used to evaluate pelvic structures, but their sensitivity and specificity do not exceed ultrasonography to the degree needed to recommend them routinely. A computed tomography scan generally is used when malignancy is suspected to evaluate for the presence of abdominal metastases, such as omental caking, enlarged periaortic lymph nodes, hepatic metastases, or kidney obstruction. There is no role for such imaging in this low-risk, uncomplicated patient with reassuring ultrasonography and benign findings.

Levine D, Brown DL, Andreotti RF, Benacerraf B, Benson CB, Brewster WR, et al. Management of asymptomatic ovarian and other adnexal cysts imaged at US: Society of Radiologists in Ultrasound Consensus Conference Statement. Radiology 2010;256:943–54.

Management of adnexal masses. ACOG Practice Bulletin No. 83. American College of Obstetricians and Gynecologists. Obstet Gynecol 2007;110:201–14.

Reade CJ, Riva JJ, Busse JW, Goldsmith CH, Elit L. Risks and benefits of screening asymptomatic women for ovarian cancer: a systematic review and meta-analysis. Gynecol Oncol 2013;130:674–81.

26

Suppressive herpes simplex virus therapy

A 28-year-old woman has a history of genital herpes simplex virus (HSV) type 2 (HSV-2) infection since age 21 years and is in a new relationship. Over the past 3 years, she had only two recurrent outbreaks of lesions that resolved within 1 week without any treatment. She tells you that her new partner has no history of genital herpes. She wants to know if there is a way to decrease her new partner's risk of acquiring HSV-2 if the couple becomes sexually active. In addition to using condoms, the most appropriate risk-reduction strategy is to use oral medication

* (A) daily for her
(B) daily for her partner
(C) during outbreaks for her
(D) daily for both partners

Genital herpes simplex virus type 1 (HSV-1) and HSV-2 cause common sexually transmitted infections that can be chronic and lifelong. The virus can be shed and transmitted by asymptomatic individuals who are unaware that they have an infection (ie, asymptomatic individuals or individuals with subclinical shedding). The clinical diagnosis of genital herpes virus infection should be confirmed with virologic testing of genital lesions. Viral cell culture is very specific but has an overall sensitivity of only 50%. The polymerase chain reaction test for HSV DNA is much more sensitive and allows differentiation between HSV-1 and HSV-2. Direct fluorescent antibody testing also provides a rapid and sensitive type-specific methodology. Serologic testing is not useful for diagnosis of active genital ulcers unless confirmed with virologic testing. The prevalence of seropositivity for HSV-1 in adults in the United States is 60–70% and is consistent with past oral or genital infection. Seropositivity for HSV-2 has a prevalence of 10–20% and is much more consistent with anogenital infection.

Systemic antiviral drugs are used to treat the first episode of herpes simplex infection and recurrent infections. Acyclovir, valacyclovir, and famciclovir are the antiviral agents of choice. Therapy of 7–10 days for initial infection and 3–5 days for recurrent outbreaks reduce time to healing and viral shedding. Among patients who have frequent recurrences, daily suppressive therapy reduces the frequency of genital herpes recurrence by up to 80%. Suppressive versus episodic treatment (initiation of treatment within 1 day of lesion onset or during the prodrome) also has been shown to improve quality of life.

Indications for chronic, daily suppressive therapy include reducing the risk of occurrence of the following four concerns: 1) the frequency of recurrent outbreaks, 2) viral shedding and recurrent lesions after 36 weeks of gestation in pregnant women, 3) clinical disease in immunocompromised individuals, and 4) transmission to an uninfected partner. Suppressive therapy for infected patients reduced transmission to a discordant, uninfected partner by approximately 50% (1.9% versus 3.6%) in a placebo-controlled trial that randomized patients to valacyclovir once daily versus placebo. This effect was most likely a result of a decrease in asymptomatic viral shedding from 11% of days to only 3% of days during the study. No evidence has been found that treating the uninfected partner with daily suppressive therapy reduces the chances of infection or seroconversion, so suppressive therapy is indicated only for the infected sexual partner.

Transmission of HSV is most likely to occur during asymptomatic viral shedding. This likelihood explains why antiviral treatment is ineffective in reducing transmission to a seronegative partner when administered only during recurrent outbreaks. Hence, episodic treatment is not recommended as a strategy to reduce transmission in discordant couples. Therefore, patients need to understand the importance of safe sexual practices. Even though HSV can be spread by direct contact to skin or mucous membranes, consistent condom usage has been shown to significantly reduce transmission.

Corey L, Wald A, Patel R, Sacks SL, Tyring SK, Warren T, et al. Once-daily valacyclovir to reduce the risk of transmission of genital herpes. Valacyclovir HSV Transmission Study Group. N Engl J Med 2004;350:11–20.

Hollier LM, Wendel GD. Third trimester antiviral prophylaxis for preventing maternal genital herpes simplex virus (HSV) recurrences and neonatal infection. Cochrane Database of Systematic Reviews 2008, Issue 1. Art. No.: CD004946. DOI: 10.1002/14651858.CD004946.pub2.

LeFevre ML. Behavioral counseling interventions to prevent sexually transmitted infections: U.S. Preventive Services Task Force recommendation statement. U.S. Preventive Services Task Force. Ann Intern Med 2014;161:894–901.

Wald A, Langenberg AG, Krantz E, Douglas JM Jr, Handsfield HH, DiCarlo RP, et al. The relationship between condom use and herpes simplex virus acquisition. Ann Intern Med 2005;143:707–13.

Workowski KA, Bolan GA. Sexually transmitted diseases treatment guidelines, 2015. Centers for Disease Control and Prevention [published erratum appears in MMWR Recomm Rep 2015;64:924]. MMWR Recomm Rep 2015;64:1–137.

27

Hymenal variants

A 14-year-old adolescent girl has regular menses that last for 4 days and are associated with mild dysmenorrhea that is relieved with ibuprofen. Although she usually can insert a tampon after a few tries, tampon removal is challenging and sometimes painful. She has never been sexually active. Physical examination reveals a 4-mm longitudinal band of hymenal tissue extending from 6 o'clock to 12 o'clock. The best next step in management is to perform

* (A) office excision
(B) pelvic ultrasonography
(C) pelvic magnetic resonance imaging
(D) operating room excision

The lower portion of the vagina is formed from growth of the urogenital sinus at the caudal end of the paramesonephric (müllerian) ducts in the absence of androgens. Congenital anomalies of the lower vagina occur as the result of incomplete degeneration of cells of the vaginal plate. The hymenal membrane develops from the proliferation of the sinovaginal bulbs and typically becomes perforate before birth. Incomplete perforation of the hymen is the most common congenital anomaly of the female reproductive tract. Commonly observed variants of hymenal presentation include annular, septate, crescentic, cribriform, and microperforate patterns (Fig. 27-1, Fig. 27-2, and Fig. 27-3). An annular hymen is observed most commonly in children younger than 3 years, after which time the hymen forms a crescentic shape along the posterior half of the vestibule. The prepubertal hymen is thin, translucent, and can be exquisitely tender. Normal alterations in hymenal architecture may include ridges at 6 o'clock and 12 o'clock, as well as midline tags.

Variations in hymenal anatomy are common, and girls with semiperforate anomalies, as in the described patient, are most likely to present at or around the time of menarche. Incomplete hymenal canalization frequently is amenable to correction in the office depending on the maturity of the patient and the amount of excision required. The septate hymen is particularly easy to transect in the office under local anesthesia. Thus, in most cases, excision under anesthesia in the operating room would pose unnecessary risk and cost.

Imperforate hymen is the most common of the obstructive genital anomalies, with an incidence of approximately 1 in 1,000. Imperforate hymen generally is detected in infancy secondary to mucocolpos, which presents as a vaginal bulge. Pubertal patients with undiscovered imperforate hymen present with acute, cyclic abdominal or back pain and primary amenorrhea. On examination, a bulging hymen is present, and an abdominal–pelvic mass resulting from hematocolpos and hematometra may be appreciated with complete outlet obstruction. Surgical repair of an imperforate hymen ideally is performed after thelarche and before menarche and is best performed in the operating room with adequate lighting and anesthesia.

The best option for this patient with hymenal variant is transection in the office. Because her minor anomaly is derived from a defect of vaginal plate canalization, imaging studies, such as magnetic resonance imaging, are not indicated to evaluate the upper genital tract in this patient with normal menses and small hymenal septum.

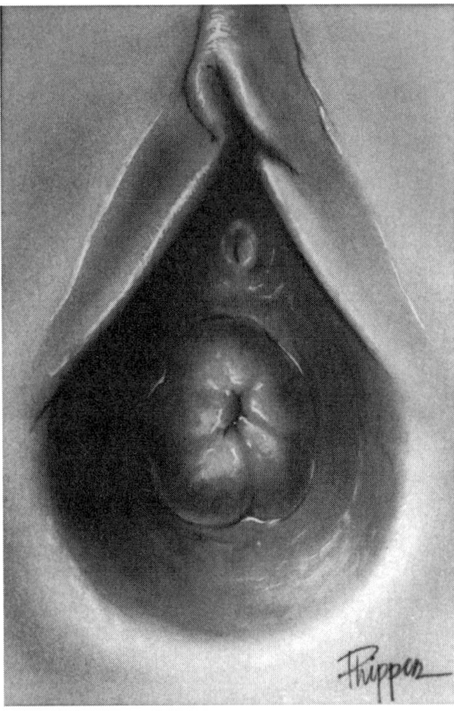

FIGURE 27-1. Fimbriated hymen. (Reprinted from Pokorny SF. Configuration of the prepubertal hymen. Am J Obstet Gynecol 1987;157:950–6. Copyright 1987, with permission of Elsevier.)

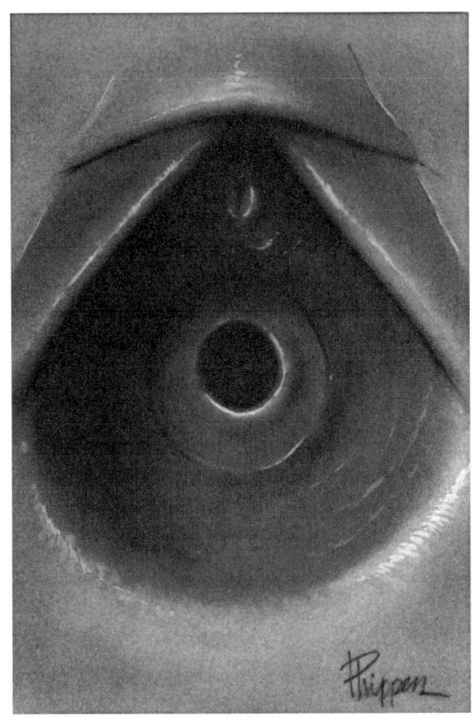

FIGURE 27-2. Circumferential hymen. (Reprinted from Pokorny SF. Configuration of the prepubertal hymen. Am J Obstet Gynecol 1987;157:950–6. Copyright 1987, with permission of Elsevier.)

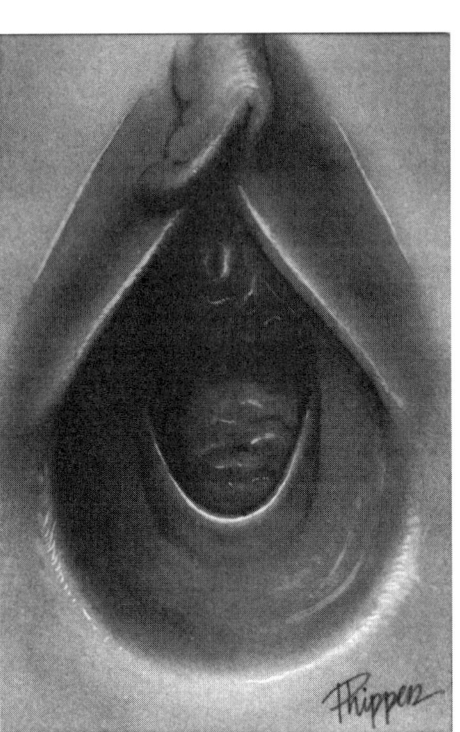

FIGURE 27-3. Posterior rim hymen. (Reprinted from Pokorny SF. Configuration of the prepubertal hymen. Am J Obstet Gynecol 1987;157:950–6. Copyright 1987, with permission of Elsevier.)

Berenson AB, Chacko MR, Wiemann CM, Mishaw CO, Friedrich WN, Grady JJ. A case-control study of anatomic changes resulting from sexual abuse. Am J Obstet Gynecol 2000;182:820–31; discussion 831–4.

Berenson AB. Normal anogenital anatomy. Child Abuse Negl 1998; 22:589–96; discussion 597–603.

Berkoff MC, Zolotor AJ, Makoroff KL, Thackeray JD, Shapiro RA, Runyan DK. Has this prepubertal girl been sexually abused? JAMA 2008;300:2779–92.

Current evaluation of amenorrhea. Practice Committee of the American Society for Reproductive Medicine. Fertil Steril 2006;86:S148–55.

Emans SJ. Office evaluation of the child and adolescent. In: Emans SJ, Laufer MR, editors. Emans, Laufer, Goldstein's pediatric & adolescent gynecology. 6th ed. Philadelphia (PA): Wolters Kluwer Lippincott Williams & Wilkins; 2012. p. 1–20.

Miller RJ, Breech LL. Surgical correction of vaginal anomalies. Clin Obstet Gynecol 2008;51:223–36.

Pokorny SF. Configuration of the prepubertal hymen. Am J Obstet Gynecol 1987;157:950–6.

28

Diet and blood pressure

A 53-year-old woman with chronic hypertension and obesity comes to your office for her annual gynecologic examination. She drinks a glass of wine most nights with dinner and is a nonsmoker. You are concerned about the long-term effects of her chronic hypertension and advise her that the lifestyle modification with the potential for the largest decrease in her blood pressure is

* (A) weight loss
(B) the Dietary Approaches to Stop Hypertension (DASH) diet
(C) reducing dietary sodium
(D) increasing dietary fiber
(E) decreasing wine consumption

Elevated blood pressure, or hypertension, is increasingly common in the United States, affecting approximately one in three adults and contributing to more deaths than any other preventable risk factor. These high rates of hypertension are partially a result of the aging of the population as well as the growing obesity epidemic, with almost two thirds of U.S. adults classified as overweight or obese. Obesity contributes to high blood pressure by direct effects on the heart, as well as through metabolic changes that impair renal function. A body mass index (calculated as weight in kilograms divided by height in meters squared [kg/m^2]) greater than 30 increases the risk of developing hypertension sixfold. This is a significant public health concern, given the overlapping risks between high blood pressure and obesity and their associations with coronary heart disease, heart failure, stroke, and kidney failure.

In otherwise healthy adults, blood pressure is categorized as normal; prehypertension; hypertension, stage 1; and hypertension, stage 2 (Table 28-1). Slightly lower cutoffs are used to define hypertension in adults with comorbidities such as diabetes and chronic kidney disease. The diagnosis is not made until measurements are elevated on two separate occasions taken at least 1 week apart and confirmed outside the clinical setting.

Given the profound personal and public health effects of hypertension, much research has gone into determining the most effective ways to prevent and manage high blood pressure and the associated complications. Lifestyle modifications are recommended as the first-line treatment for hypertension. These include the DASH diet, weight loss, and exercise—all of which have shown beneficial effects on blood pressure in the short term. However, the lifestyle modification that decreases blood pressure the most is weight loss, which is what should be recommended to the described patient.

The DASH diet was developed to prevent hypertension and lower blood pressure by increasing intake of minerals and nutrients that can lower blood pressure, such as potassium, calcium, magnesium, fiber, and protein and by decreasing fat and sodium intake. Despite initial promise and reassuring immediate outcomes, data have been mixed regarding long-term outcomes of the DASH diet alone on sustained blood pressure control. Thus, although the DASH diet may be beneficial in the short term, it is not as effective as weight loss in maintaining blood pressure control.

Numerous recommendations have been made regarding the importance of decreasing sodium intake. The American Heart Association has proposed a general

TABLE 28-1. Classification of Hypertension

Category	Systolic Blood Pressure (mm Hg)		Diastolic Blood Pressure (mm Hg)
Normal	less than 120	and	less than 80
Prehypertension	120–139	or	80–89
Hypertension			
Stage 1	140–159	or	90–99
Stage 2	equal to or greater than 160	or	equal to or greater than 100

population measure to decrease sodium intake to less than 1,500 mg/d by the year 2020. Small blood pressure decreases have been observed in short-term trials of hypertensive and normotensive volunteers eating a low-sodium diet. However, a recent review by the Institute of Medicine was less conclusive about target diet sodium levels, given discrepancies across numerous observational and environmental studies. Thus, more recent recommendations suggest a modified approach to sodium intake based on individual characteristics as opposed to a population level approach.

Colorectal cancer is the second most common neoplasm in women. A low-fiber diet (along with consumption of highly processed food and excess red meat) has been partially implicated for the high rates of colorectal cancer in the United States relative to other developed countries with different dietary patterns. Increasing dietary fiber intake is part of the DASH diet and has been shown to have a beneficial effect on colorectal cancer risk. However, increased fiber intake alone has not been clearly associated with decreased blood pressure and is therefore not the best choice for the described patient.

Alcohol consumption at moderate levels (not more than one beverage per day) has been shown to have a positive effect on hypertension. Excess alcohol consumption is associated with increased blood pressure. The described patient is already drinking a glass of wine most evenings, so she is likely getting some blood pressure benefit. Decreasing her wine intake is not likely to be beneficial for her blood pressure control.

Durko L, Malecka-Panas E. Lifestyle modifications and colorectal cancer. Curr Colorectal Cancer Rep 2014;10:45–54.

Forman JP, Stampfer MJ, Curhan GC. Diet and lifestyle risk factors associated with incident hypertension in women. JAMA 2009;302:401–11.

Hinderliter AL, Sherwood A, Craighead LW, Lin PH, Watkins L, Babyak MA, et al. The long-term effects of lifestyle change on blood pressure: one-year follow-up of the ENCORE study. Am J Hypertens 2014;27:734–41.

James PA, Oparil S, Carter BL, Cushman WC, Dennison-Himmelfarb C, Handler J, et al. 2014 evidence-based guideline for the management of high blood pressure in adults: report from the panel members appointed to the Eighth Joint National Committee (JNC 8) [published erratum appears in JAMA 2014;311:1809]. JAMA 2014;311:507–20.

Stolarz-Skrzypek K, Staessen JA. Reducing salt intake for prevention of cardiovascular disease--times are changing. Adv Chronic Kidney Dis 2015;22:108–15.

29

Meaningful use

In order to be considered an eligible professional through the Medicaid Electronic Health Records (EHR) Incentive Program, the proportion of the obstetrician–gynecologist's private practice patient volume covered by Medicaid must be at least

(A) 10%
(B) 20%
* (C) 30%
(D) 40%
(E) 50%

The Centers for Medicare and Medicaid Services developed a series of incentive programs to encourage health care providers and hospitals to increase implementation and effective use of EHRs in the care of patients. The introduction of the Medicaid EHR Incentive Program in 2011 allowed eligible professionals to receive financial incentives for submitting data showing that they had achieved specific measures.

Physicians, dentists, podiatrists, optometrists, and chiropractors are eligible for incentives under Medicare. Medicaid incentives are provided to physicians, nurse practitioners, certified nurse–midwives, dentists, and some physician assistants (ie, those who work in a federally qualified health care center or those who run a rural health care center). Physicians and other health care providers who are based in a hospital, such as emergency medicine physicians, are not eligible (as individuals or practices) for this program because they are under the umbrella of the hospital incentives.

Eligible professionals as Medicaid providers are defined primarily by the volume of their patients who are covered by Medicaid. Most health care providers, including obstetrician–gynecologists, must document that 30% of their patient volume is covered by Medicaid for eligibility. The measures primarily are meant to target the most vulnerable patient populations; therefore, pediatricians are required to have only a 20% Medicaid patient volume in order to be eligible. Health care providers who work at a federally qualified health care center or a rural health care center are eligible if 30% of their patient volume is attributable to needy individuals, even if those individuals do not use Medicaid.

Professionals who are eligible for the Medicare as well as the Medicaid program must choose one and may switch only once after beginning to submit data. In general, choosing the Medicaid program maximizes incentives for most health care providers.

A hospital is eligible for Medicaid incentives if it has a minimum of 10% Medicaid volume or if it is registered as a children's hospital. Unlike eligible professionals, hospitals can register for the Medicare and the Medicaid incentive programs.

Meaningful use incentives have been released in stages, beginning with stage 1 in 2011. The initial stage required eligible professionals to document in the EHR the three core clinical quality measures for patients older than 18 years: 1) the percentage of patients with a diagnosis of hypertension who had at least one office visit with blood pressure measurement, 2) tobacco use with cessation counseling, and 3) weight screening with follow-up. There were two alternative core clinical quality measures for children—1) immunization status and 2) weight assessment with counseling—and one alternate core clinical quality measure for adults (influenza immunization status for adults 50 years and older). There were many additional clinical quality measures, three of which required submission to receive the incentive payment. A number of these clinical quality measures were specifically relevant to obstetrics and gynecology, such as the percentage of pregnant women screened for human immunodeficiency virus (HIV) in the first or second trimester of pregnancy and the percentage of Rh-negative women who received Rh immune globulin at 26–30 weeks of gestation.

As each stage has been rolled out, the requirements have increased in breadth and depth, including the ability to share information with other EHR systems. The incentives were highest for those who enrolled immediately and decreased with later enrollment. In 2015, eligible professionals and hospitals began to face penalties for failing to demonstrate meaningful use as an eligible Medicare provider. A hardship exemption is available and may be granted to those who, for example, have poor Internet connectivity or a lack of face-to-face patient interactions.

Centers for Medicare & Medicaid Services. Medicare and Medicaid EHR incentive program basics. Baltimore (MD): CMS; 2016. Available at: https://www.cms.gov/regulations-and-guidance/legislation/ehrincentiveprograms/basics.html. Retrieved September 13, 2016.

Centers for Medicare & Medicaid Services (CMS), HHS. Medicare and Medicaid programs; electronic health record incentive program—stage 3 and modifications to meaningful use in 2015 through 2017. Final rules with comment period. Fed Regist 2015;80:62761–955.

30

Full disclosure of medical errors

A 41-year-old woman comes to your office for a 2-week postoperative visit after an uncomplicated vaginal hysterectomy. She has been feeling well but does report some increased vaginal discharge and odor since the surgery. Your pelvic examination shows an intact vaginal cuff with a well-healing vaginal epithelium and a retained vaginal sponge. In addition to immediate removal of the retained sponge, the best next course of action is to

* (A) disclose the medical error to the patient
(B) review sponge count documentation
(C) apologize for the medical error
(D) contact the hospital's risk management department
(E) admit fault

Medical errors and adverse patient outcomes are inevitable in health care. Despite the potentially catastrophic effects of preventable or unavoidable harm on the patient and the obstetrician–gynecologist or other health care provider involved, surveys among health care workers suggest that most feel underprepared and unsupported when faced with the task of disclosing an adverse event. Several national organizations, including the Joint Commission, the American Medical Association, and the Institute of Medicine, have mandated that hospitals develop event reporting systems. These reporting systems ultimately raise the standards for patient safety at local and national levels. Nonetheless, barriers to complete disclosure still exist, such as lack of training, fear of retribution for reporting an adverse event, a culture of blame, and fear of litigation. In order to minimize these barriers, many organizations have adopted a just culture in which clinicians are able to disclose an adverse event without fear of blame, shame, or humiliation while maintaining individual accountability and responsibility.

A variety of programs have been developed to educate physicians about disclosure. Examples include the consensus statement, *When Things Go Wrong: Responding to Adverse Events*, published by the Harvard Hospitals, as well as the Colorado 3 Rs Program, which highlights the core principles of recognizing, responding to, and resolving unanticipated medical events. Basic principles surrounding timely and accurate disclosure of an adverse event emphasize five key components—Who, What, When, Where, and How:

1. "Who" determines the obstetrician–gynecologists or other health care providers who will be involved with and present for the disclosure. Ideally, the team should include a senior physician (ie, attending physician) as well as another member of the health care team, if possible.
2. "What" addresses the content of the disclosure, which should be complete but must include only factual and confirmed information, which is best obtained from a postevent debriefing session.
3. "When" highlights the importance of timely disclosure, which ideally should occur as soon as possible after the event, with opportunities for continued updates for the patient and family as additional information becomes available.
4. "Where" establishes the location of the disclosure, which optimally takes place in a quiet, confidential location that is comfortable for the patient.
5. "How" incorporates critical principles of maintaining dignity and respect for the patient and her family.

The most appropriate course of action for the described scenario is to immediately disclose the medical error to the patient, adhering to the known facts. It is a physician's ethical obligation to disclose medical errors to the patient even if all the details of the incident are not known. In addition, it is the physician's responsibility to protect the patient against further harm by providing necessary medical care and mitigation of any ongoing injury. After the immediate disclosure, it would be appropriate to reassure the patient that she will be provided with additional information as it becomes available. Studies have demonstrated that patients want and expect timely and complete disclosure. In addition, patients are more likely to pursue legal action if they feel that disclosure was lacking, dishonest, or incomplete.

Reviewing the documentation from the operating room sponge count is important from a hospital root cause analysis standpoint. However, this would not be the appropriate next step because it does not address the immediate need to disclose the event to the patient. Acknowledgment of the patient's pain or suffering is always encouraged because it reflects sympathy on the part of the obstetrician–gynecologist or other health care provider. This is in contrast to taking accountability for the suffering through an apology. The question of whether to apologize to a patient after a medical error often is controversial. On one hand, a disclosure without an apology could be perceived as somewhat impersonal to a patient; however, apologies can be admissible in court as evidence. Generally, it is recommended that obstetrician–gynecologists and other health care providers familiarize themselves with local apology laws in their states and consult with risk management to determine if and when an apology is appropriate. Immediately following disclosure, consultation with risk management would be a recommended next step.

Although assuming fault and taking complete ownership for the error demonstrate integrity on the part of the surgeon, it would be most prudent to notify the patient that you will conduct a root cause analysis to determine how and when the error took place. Patients not only appreciate the fact that an investigation is taking place but are often most concerned with how the error will be prevented in the future. Furthermore, assigning or accepting fault may not be productive and could result in unnecessary anger or resentment on the part of the patient.

Disclosure and discussion of adverse events. Committee Opinion No. 520. American College of Obstetricians and Gynecologists. Obstet Gynecol 2012;119:686–9.

Massachusetts Coalition for the Prevention of Medical Errors. When things go wrong: responding to adverse events. A consensus statement of the Harvard Hospital, Burlington (MA): MCPME; 2006. Available at http://www.macoalition.org/documents/respondingToAdverseEvents.pdf. Retrieved June 16, 2016.

Pelt JL, Faldmo LP. Physician error and disclosure. Clin Obstet Gynecol 2008;51:700–8.

Quinn RE, Eichler MC. The 3Rs program: the Colorado experience. Clin Obstet Gynecol 2008;51:709–18.

31

Human papillomavirus testing

A 26-year-old woman visits your office for her annual well-woman examination. She reports no health issues and is happy with her oral contraceptive. She has no significant past medical or gynecologic history; her last cervical cytologic screening 3 years ago was normal. She has heard about primary human papillomavirus (HPV) screening and wonders if she is a candidate for such screening. For this patient, primary screening for HPV without cytology could lead to

(A) undetected cervical intraepithelial neoplasia (CIN) 1
(B) undetected CIN 2 or CIN 3
(C) undetected cervical cancer
* (D) unnecessary colposcopy

The incidence of cervical cancer in the United States has decreased more than 50% in the past 30 years because of widespread cervical cytologic screening. In 2011, a total of 12,109 U.S. women received a cervical cancer diagnosis, and 4,092 women died from the disease. The U.S. mortality rate for cervical cancer is now less than 2 per 100,000 women. As new technologies for cervical cancer screening have become available, the recommendations for screening and results interpretation have evolved (Fig. 31-1).

Infection with an oncogenic strain of HPV is a necessary but insufficient factor for the development of squamous cervical dysplasia and carcinoma. Infection with HPV is most prevalent among females in their teenage years and 20s and most often is a transient infection. Persistent infection, associated with factors such as immunodeficiency and smoking, is related to the development of dysplasia and progression to cancer. Given that HPV-related dysplasia takes about 3–7 years to progress, this provides multiple opportunities for detection and intervention.

Several tests have been approved by the U.S. Food and Drug Administration for the detection of cervical HPV DNA. Most of them test for 13–14 of the most common oncogenic (high-risk) HPV genotypes in the sampled cervical cells. Such HPV testing is initially used in one of two ways:

1. Determining the need for colposcopy in women with an atypical squamous cells of undetermined significance cytology result ("reflex testing")
2. As an adjunct to cytology for screening in women aged 30–65 years ("cotesting"). Three randomized trials have shown that cotesting is superior to cytology alone for

> women aged 30–65 years. Current recommendations for women in this age group state that cotesting with cytology and HPV testing every 5 years is preferred, although screening with cytology alone every 3 years is acceptable.

Testing for HPV, either alone or in combination with cervical cytology, is more sensitive than cytology alone in detecting dysplasia. The ongoing HPV FOCAL Study, a trial including more than 18,000 women aged 25–65 years, assesses several cytology triage strategies after initial HPV testing compared with initial cytology screening with HPV triage. Baseline testing in this trial showed greater sensitivity for CIN 2 with initial HPV testing compared with initial cytology. In 2015, the U.S. Food and Drug Administration approved the first test intended to be used for primary HPV testing for women older than 25 years. The Addressing the Need for Advanced HPV Diagnostics trial evaluated this test and found that HPV primary testing detected significantly more cases of CIN 3 or greater in women older than 25 years than either cytology alone or cotesting. Primary HPV testing did require significantly more colposcopies, though the number of colposcopies required to detect a single case of CIN 3 or greater was the same as the cotesting strategy. Limitations of the study include only 3 years of follow-up and CIN 3, not cervical cancer, as an endpoint.

The 2015 interim guidelines from the Society of Gynecologic Oncology and the American Society for Colposcopy and Cervical Pathology were based on a review of the recent evidence. The guidelines suggest primary HPV testing as an option for women starting at age 25 years; the consensus is that primary HPV testing is superior to cytology alone and no worse than cotesting at the same screening intervals (every 3 years). Primary HPV testing may even be better for women aged 25–29 years, but it does have a higher risk of unnecessary colposcopy. Strategies that include HPV testing increase the number of positive test results and colposcopies performed, and long-term outcomes are uncertain. Future studies should include comparative effectiveness studies along with direct cost comparisons of primary HPV testing with cytology and cotesting. Future studies also must address the optimum intervals for primary HPV testing and use cervical cancer as an additional outcome.

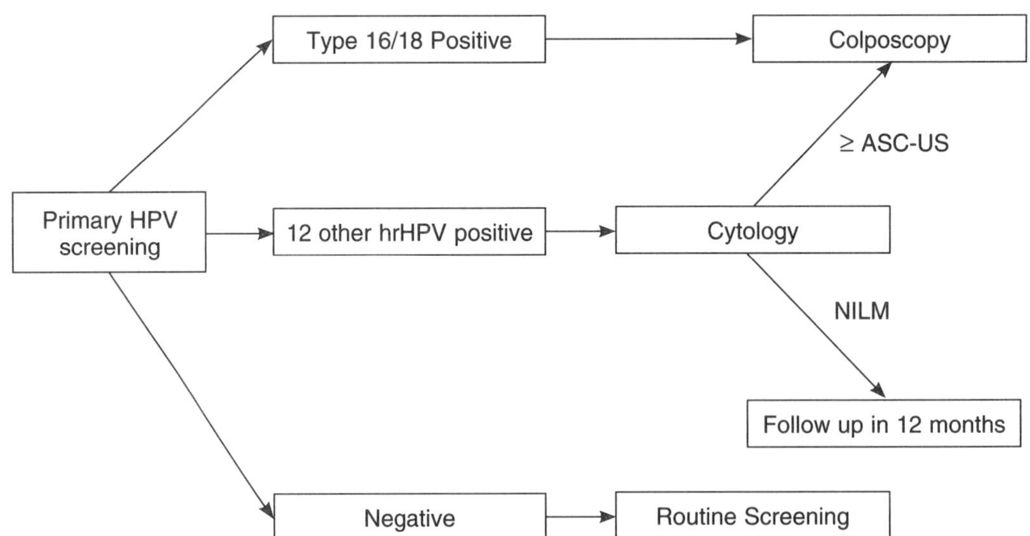

FIGURE 31-1. Primary human papillomavirus (HPV) screening algorithm. Abbreviations: ASC-US, atypical squamous cells of undetermined significance; HPV, human papillomavirus; hrHPV, high-risk human papillomavirus; NILM, negative for intraepithelial lesion or malignancy. (Huh WK, Ault KA, Chelmow D, Davey DD, Goulart RA, Garcia FA, et al. Use of primary high-risk human papillomavirus testing for cervical cancer screening: interim clinical guidance. Gynecol Onc 2015;136:178–82.)

Cervical cancer screening and prevention. Practice Bulletin No. 157. American College of Obstetricians and Gynecologists. Obstet Gynecol 2016;127:e1–20.

Huh WK, Ault KA, Chelmow D, Davey DD, Goulart RA, Garcia FA, et al. Use of primary high-risk human papillomavirus testing for cervical cancer screening: interim clinical guidance. Gynecol Onc 2015;136:178–82.

Katki HA, Kinney WK, Fetterman B, Lorey T, Poitras NE, Cheung L, et al. Cervical cancer risk for women undergoing concurrent testing for human papillomavirus and cervical cytology: a population-based study in routine clinical practice [published erratum appears in Lancet Oncol 2011;12:722]. Lancet Oncol 2011;12:663–72.

Ogilvie GS, Krajden M, van Niekerk DJ, Martin RE, Ehlen TG, Ceballos K, et al. Primary cervical cancer screening with HPV testing compared with liquid-based cytology: results of round 1 of a randomised controlled trial—the HPV FOCAL Study. Br J Cancer 2012;107:1917–24.

Screening for cervical cancer. Practice Bulletin No. 131. American College of Obstetricians and Gynecologists. Obstet Gynecol 2012;120:1222–38.

Wright TC, Stoler MH, Behrens CM, Sharma A, Zhang G, Wright TL. Primary cervical cancer screening with human papillomavirus: end of study results from the ATHENA study using HPV as the first-line screening test. Gynecol Onc 2015;136:189–97.

32

In vitro fertilization and pregnancy outcome

A healthy 26-year-old nulligravid woman is planning to undergo her first in vitro fertilization (IVF) cycle because of unexplained infertility. She is aware of the increased risk of multifetal gestation but asks you if there are other risks associated with IVF. You counsel her that when IVF pregnancies are compared with pregnancies in the general population, the fetal disorder with the largest increase in risk is

(A) autosomal recessive disorder
(B) imprinting disorder
* (C) congenital cardiac defect
(D) Down syndrome

In vitro fertilization has made pregnancy possible for many infertile couples worldwide, but it is not without risks. The most well-known risk of IVF is multifetal gestation. Compared with the general population, IVF is associated with a 30-fold increase in the incidence of twins. Most of these twin gestations are dizygotic, but IVF also raises the incidence of monozygotic twins. In general, the incidence of monozygotic twins is constant at approximately 4 per 1,000 in the population, regardless of race, age, parity, and other demographic factors. However, in a pregnancy achieved through IVF, monozygotic twinning is increased twofold in conventional IVF cycles and is probably even further increased in IVF with intracytoplasmic sperm injection. Retrospective studies have confirmed that certain adverse obstetric outcomes are more prevalent in pregnancies associated with assisted reproductive technologies. Such adverse outcomes include increased rates of preterm delivery, intrauterine growth restriction, and perinatal mortality.

An increased incidence of congenital cardiac defects has been reported in offspring of women who achieved pregnancy through IVF. Compared with a baseline risk of 0.3–1.2%, the risk of congenital cardiac defects is reported to be 1.1–3.3% in pregnancies achieved by IVF, making it the most common disorder in the IVF population compared with the general obstetric population. Most reported anomalies are atrial and ventricular septal defects. The exact cause of this small increase in risk is unknown. It may in part be attributable to the increased incidence of monochorionic twins, a population known to be at increased risk of cardiac anomalies. It also is uncertain if the etiology is due to the number of embryos transferred, twinning process, or underlying infertility. The American Institute of Ultrasound in Medicine and the American Heart Association list a pregnancy achieved by IVF as an indication for fetal echocardiography.

Although uncommon, imprinting disorders have been reported to occur more frequently in pregnancies achieved by IVF. Imprinting is an epigenetic phenomenon in which one of the two alleles of a subset of genes is expressed differently than its parental origin. An example of an imprinting disorder associated with IVF is Beckwith–Wiedemann syndrome. Case series suggest an increased risk of imprinting disorders in pregnancies achieved by IVF. However, because these disorders are so rare (1 in 100,000 to 1 in 300,000), it would be difficult, if not impossible, to definitively confirm an increased risk in prospective studies.

The baseline risk of Down syndrome or other aneuploidies is not increased by IVF pregnancy. However, several studies have noted that there may be a slight increase in sex chromosome abnormalities, specifically in births after intracytoplasmic sperm injection. Risks of Down syndrome include advanced maternal age, history of having a child with Down syndrome, and either parent carrying a balanced robertsonian translocation.

Autosomal recessive disorders are not associated with IVF. Autosomal recessive disorders require the affected person to inherit the deleterious gene mutation from each parent. Examples of autosomal recessive disorders include sickle cell disease, cystic fibrosis, and Tay–Sachs disease.

AIUM practice guideline for the performance of fetal echocardiography. American Institute of Ultrasound in Medicine. J Ultrasound Med 2013;32:1067–82.

Donofrio MT, Moon-Grady AJ, Hornberger LK, Copel JA, Sklansky MS, Abuhamad A, et al. Diagnosis and treatment of fetal cardiac disease: a scientific statement from the American Heart Association. American Heart Association Adults With Congenital Heart Disease Joint Committee of the Council on Cardiovascular Disease in the Young and Council on Clinical Cardiology, Council on Cardiovascular Surgery and Anesthesia, and Council on Cardiovascular and Stroke Nursing [published erratum appears in Circulation 2014;129:e512]. Circulation 2014;129:2183–242.

Multiple gestation associated with infertility therapy: an American Society for Reproductive Medicine Practice Committee opinion. American Society for Reproductive Medicine. Fertil Steril 2012;97:825–34.

Perinatal risks associated with assisted reproductive technology. ACOG Committee Opinion No. 324. American College of Obstetricians and Gynecologists. Obstet Gynecol 2005;106:1143–6.

33

Recurrent pregnancy loss

A 33-year-old woman, gravida 3, para 0, comes to your office with vaginal spotting. Her last menstrual period was 7 weeks ago, and she had a positive home pregnancy test 2 weeks ago. Her past two pregnancies (with the same partner) resulted in spontaneous miscarriages at 6 weeks of gestation. Her ultrasonographic examination from today's visit is shown in Figure 33-1 (see color plate). The crown–rump length is 9 mm. The most appropriate intervention to offer her in this clinical situation is

(A) repeat ultrasonography in 1 week
(B) expectant management
* (C) uterine evacuation and karyotyping of products of conception
(D) parental karyotyping
(E) human chorionic gonadotropin level

The ultrasonographic image shown in Figure 33-1 (see color plate) demonstrates a nonviable embryo based on absence of cardiac activity (ie, no evidence of Doppler flow in the fetus), this patient's third such occurrence. Because the ultrasonographic findings are definitive, repeat ultrasonography in 1 week is unnecessary and gives the patient a false sense of hope. When ultrasonographic evidence of demise is established (ie, no cardiac activity in an embryo of 7 mm or more), there is no benefit to measuring serum pregnancy hormones, such as human chorionic gonadotropin or progesterone. Expectant management in this case would be reasonable if determining the etiology was unimportant. However, karyotyping of spontaneously expelled products of conception is usually unsuccessful.

The definition of recurrent pregnancy loss differs among expert organizations. Most patients with recurrent pregnancy loss have early (ie, first-trimester) losses. Fewer than 5% of women have two consecutive losses, and fewer than 1% have three or more consecutive losses. The American Society for Reproductive Medicine defines *recurrent pregnancy loss* as two or more spontaneous pregnancy losses that do not need to be consecutive. Others define it as three or more losses. Some evaluation after a second pregnancy loss has been shown to be cost-effective.

Approximately one half of spontaneous abortions are attributable to chromosome abnormalities. Documentation of this etiology by karyotyping or array use provides important information to the woman who has suffered a pregnancy loss. Recognizing that no action or inaction on her part contributed to the pregnancy loss provides psychologic benefit. Moreover, the prognosis for successful pregnancy outcomes in subsequent attempts is better if aneuploidy was the explanation for one or more of the losses. Most couples will have a euploid and successful pregnancy after an aneuploid loss. In the event of recurrent euploid pregnancy loss, the prognosis is less favorable.

An etiology for recurrent pregnancy loss can be identified in 50% of couples. A large proportion of explainable causes are genetic. Aneuploidy accounts for approximately one half of all spontaneous abortions. This proportion is even higher in women older than 40 years. Karyotyping of the products of conception is necessary to determine the presence of aneuploidy. In addition, karyotyping the products of conception allows for detection of unbalanced structural rearrangements, which may indicate a parental carrier of a balanced translocation.

A caveat to obtaining a karyotype of the products of conception is that maternal cell contamination frequently leads to unobtainable or erroneous results. Multiple investigators have identified an excess of 46,XX results when karyotyping of the products of conception is performed. However, with sophisticated dissection techniques, or when other molecular approaches are taken, many of these seemingly normal results will be proved to be caused by maternal cell contamination. The clinician should either carefully dissect away maternal decidua from any specimen or use a lab that takes such measures. The presence of aneuploidy in the products of conception provides the etiology of the loss, and further evaluation generally is unwarranted.

Most authorities also recommend karyotyping of the parents, which is a useful measure to identify a balanced carrier. Karyotyping of the products of conception is preferred when possible. In 2–5% of couples with recurrent pregnancy loss, one or both parents will be found to have a structural chromosome rearrangement that may predispose them to unbalanced embryos. Such couples should be referred for genetic counseling to obtain accurate recurrence risk information.

Additional evaluation of couples with recurrent pregnancy loss includes investigation of the presence of antiphospholipid syndrome. This is a relatively rare disorder that is associated with thrombotic predisposition, which is thought to be the mechanism behind its effect on pregnancy. The diagnostic criteria for antiphospholipid syndrome have evolved over time; Box 33-1 delineates the criteria for diagnosis as defined by the International Multidisciplinary Consensus Classification.

BOX 33-1

One of the Following Clinical Criteria AND One of the Laboratory Criteria Are Required for Diagnosis of Antiphospholipid Syndrome*

Clinical criteria

1. Vascular thrombosis
2. Pregnancy morbidity
   a. One or more unexplained deaths of morphologically normal fetus after 10th week of gestation
   b. One or more premature births of a morpho logically normal neonate before the 34th week because of eclampsia, severe pre-eclampsia, or recognized placental insufficiency
   c. Three or more unexplained consecutive spontaneous abortions before the 10th week with evidence of normal karyotype and hormonal state

Laboratory criteria

1. Lupus anticoagulant present on two or more occasions at least 12 weeks apart
2. Anticardiolipin antibody of IgG or IgM in serum or plasma present in medium or high titer (greater than 40 GPL or MPL or greater than 99th percentile) on two or more occasions at least 12 weeks apart
3. Anti-β_2-glycoprotein I antibody of IgG, IgM, or both in serum or plasma (titer greater than 99th percentile) present on two or more occasions at least 12 weeks apart

Abbreviations: GPL, G phospholipid; IgG, immunoglobulin G; IgM, immunoglobulin M; MPL, M phospholipid.

Reprinted from the Practice Committee of the American Society for Reproductive Medicine. Evaluation and treatment of recurrent pregnancy loss: a committee opinion. Practice Committee of the American Society for Reproductive Medicine. Fertil Steril 2012;98:1103–11.

Assessment of the uterine cavity also is recommended frequently, although uterine cavity abnormality is not a common explanation for first-trimester pregnancy loss. Hysterosalpingography, three-dimensional ultrasonography, and magnetic resonance imaging are imaging techniques that can be helpful for this assessment. Other etiologies are less well established. In particular, little to no evidence exists to support the routine incorporation of diagnostic workup for thrombophilias, alloimmune factors, and infectious causes.

Overall, the likelihood for live birth is high for couples with recurrent pregnancy loss, even with a history of four to five miscarriages. Figure 33-2 (see color plate) shows the percentage of women in a large Scandinavian cohort who have had at least one live birth after seeking consultation for recurrent pregnancy loss.

Patients benefit from a reassuring and evidence-based approach to diagnostic workup. Preimplantation genetic screening of embryos has been promoted as a method to reduce the loss rate in couples with recurrent pregnancy loss. Although some centers report success with this approach, no large-scale study has yet demonstrated a generalizable benefit. In addition, preimplantation genetic screening is expensive and its efficacy is questionable. Patients should be made aware of its limitations before considering such an intervention.

Alijotas-Reig J, Garrido-Gimenez C. Current concepts and new trends in the diagnosis and management of recurrent miscarriage. Obstet Gynecol Surv 2013;68:445–66.

Evaluation and treatment of recurrent pregnancy loss: a committee opinion. Practice Committee of the American Society for Reproductive Medicine. Fertil Steril 2012;98:1103–11.

Lund M, Kamper-Jorgensen M, Nielsen HS, Lidegaard O, Andersen AM, Christiansen OB. Prognosis for live birth in women with recurrent miscarriage: what is the best measure of success? Obstet Gynecol 2012;119:37–43.

Murugappan G, Ohno MS, Lathi RB. Cost-effectiveness analysis of preimplantation genetic screening and in vitro fertilization versus expectant management in patients with unexplained recurrent pregnancy loss. Fertil Steril 2015;103:1215–20.

34

Condylomata in a pregnant patient

A 19-year-old woman, gravida 3, para 2, comes to your office at 18 weeks of gestation with genital warts. During your examination, you note that she has multiple 2–3-mm-sized condyloma on her labia majora. She has no visible warts internally on speculum examination. She is very embarrassed by her warts and seeks treatment. Other than cryotherapy, you discuss with her that the best option during pregnancy is

(A) to defer treatment until postpartum
(B) human papillomavirus (HPV) vaccine
* (C) trichloroacetic acid
(D) imiquimod
(E) 5-fluorouracil

Genital warts (condyloma acuminata) are caused by HPV—most commonly, HPV subtypes 6 and 11. The human papillomavirus is transmitted most commonly through close mucosal contact, including sexual intercourse. Perinatal transmission has been described as well, leading to possible laryngeal papillomatosis in the newborn, but the risk is less than 1%. Additionally, young girls can develop genital warts secondary to perinatal transmission years later. More than 100 HPV subtypes have been identified, 30–40 of which are associated with malignancy. The quadrivalent and 9-valent HPV vaccines help protect patients from HPV-related malignancies as well as genital warts. Although the HPV vaccine can be effective in the prevention of genital warts, its use is not indicated for treatment of these lesions. Additionally, it is not recommended during pregnancy because its safety has not been established.

Although there are options for treatment of genital warts during pregnancy, treatment can be deferred until after delivery, especially if significant debulking is required. Deferring treatment until postpartum is not the appropriate choice for the described patient because she desires treatment and does not require extensive debulking. Although this patient does not want cryotherapy, its use is safe in pregnancy. She would benefit most from treatment with trichloroacetic acid, a chemical that results in coagulation of tissue proteins, resulting in destruction of the warts. Trichloroacetic acid has been well studied in pregnancy and is safe to use. It is a good option because it works topically, can be applied easily in the office, and is most effective on smaller, less confluent lesions as observed in this patient. Multiple applications often are required.

Imiquimod treats genital warts by stimulating local cytokine production. Imiquimod has not been studied extensively in pregnancy and, therefore, would not be the best option for this patient. Of note, imiquimod is not indicated for intravaginal use. Podophyllin causes wart necrosis, but its unique mechanism of action as an antimitotic agent makes it unsafe to use in pregnancy. 5-fluorouracil is a pyrimidine antimetabolite and interferes with DNA synthesis. Because of its mechanism of action, it also is contraindicated in pregnancy.

Because the absolute risk of transmission is so low despite the presence of warts, cesarean delivery solely to avoid infant exposure to HPV is not indicated. However, cesarean delivery can be considered if the risk of labor obstruction or bleeding complications secondary to genital warts is significant.

Cervical cancer screening and prevention. Practice Bulletin No. 157. American College of Obstetricians and Gynecologists. Obstet Gynecol 2016;127:e1–20.

Kennedy CM, Boardman LA. New approaches to external genital warts and vulvar intraepithelial neoplasia. Clin Obstet Gynecol 2008;51:518–26.

Lacey CJ, Lowndes CM, Shah KV. Chapter 4: Burden and management of non-cancerous HPV-related conditions: HPV-6/11 disease. Vaccine 2006;24(suppl):S3/35–41.

Workowski KA, Bolan GA. Sexually transmitted diseases treatment guidelines, 2015. Centers for Disease Control and Prevention [published erratum appears in MMWR Recomm Rep 2015;64:924]. MMWR Recomm Rep 2015;64:1–137.

35
Anal incontinence

A 65-year-old woman, gravida 3, para 3, visits your office for her annual well-woman examination. She reports a long history of irritable bowel syndrome with frequent loose stools and rectal urgency. She tells you that over the past 6 months she has had occasional episodes of fecal incontinence. At this point, the incontinence has consisted of mild staining that is not yet bothersome. Her medical history is otherwise unremarkable, and her surgical history is significant for a laparoscopic cholecystectomy. On physical examination, you note perianal staining and dermatitis. Anal wink reflex is positive. Rectal examination reveals no masses or impaction, and she has grossly normal sphincter tone at rest and with voluntary contraction. The best next step for this patient is

* (A) trial of a stool-bulking agent
(B) balloon expulsion test
(C) endoanal ultrasonography
(D) pelvic magnetic resonance imaging (MRI)
(E) anal manometry

Fecal incontinence is the involuntary loss of solid or liquid feces. Anal incontinence also includes the involuntary loss of flatus. Fecal incontinence can affect daily life and may predispose the patient to institutionalization. Many patients do not volunteer these symptoms, making it incumbent on the physician to screen patients with risk factors for fecal incontinence. Box 35-1 shows conditions that may predispose a patient to fecal incontinence.

Concepts based on referral center data suggest that pelvic injury from obstetric trauma is a major risk factor for fecal incontinence in women, with episiotomy and third-degree or fourth-degree lacerations having been associated with anal incontinence. Obstetric injury is associated with early-onset fecal incontinence. However, obstetric trauma may result in pelvic floor injury that is neither clinically recognized at the time of delivery nor symptomatic in the postpartum period. Data from unselected community populations do not confirm obstetric events to be independent risk factors for fecal incontinence. The prevalence of fecal incontinence increases with age; diarrhea and rectal urgency are the strongest risk factors.

BOX 35-1

Factors That Predispose a Patient to Fecal Incontinence

- Anal sphincter weakness of traumatic or nontraumatic etiology
- Neuropathy
- Pelvic floor weakness
- Inflammatory conditions such as radiation proctitis or inflammatory bowel disease
- Central nervous system disorders such as dementia, stroke, or multiple sclerosis
- Irritable bowel syndrome
- Cholecystectomy
- Fecal retention with overflow
- Behavioral disorders

Modified with permission from Macmillan Publishers Ltd: American Journal of Gastroenterology. Wald A, Bharucha AE, Cosman BC, Whitehead WE. ACG clinical guideline: management of benign anorectal disorders. Am J Gastroenterol 2014;109:1141–57;(Quiz)1958.

In community-based epidemiologic studies, advancing age, increased body mass index (calculated as weight in kilograms divided by height in meters squared [kg/m^2]), diarrhea, rectal urgency, cholecystectomy, anal fistula, nonchildbirth anal injury, urinary incontinence, chronic illness, and psychoactive medications all are associated with fecal incontinence. Because semiformed or liquid stools stress pelvic floor continence mechanisms more than formed stools, incontinence for solid stool suggests more severe sphincter weakness than does incontinence for liquid stool.

Physical examination for evaluation of anal incontinence should include a digital anorectal examination to identify rectal masses and to assess anal sphincter tone at rest and during voluntary contraction of the anal sphincter and pelvic floor muscles, as well as change in tone during simulated defecation. Reduced anal resting tone with or without a weak squeeze response are the most common findings in fecal incontinence. Perianal pinprick sensation and the anal wink reflex can evaluate the integrity of the sacral lower motor neuron reflex arc. Further examination findings may include staining by stool or evidence of perianal dermatitis.

For patients with symptoms that are mild or not bothersome as seen in the described patient, conservative measures as needed often suffice and are the best first step. The American College of Gastroenterology recommends the use of education, dietary modification, skin care, and pharmacologic therapy such as limiting fluids, using bulking agents, or using antimotility agents to modify stool delivery and liquidity before diagnostic testing. Antidiarrheal drugs have been shown to improve fecal continence, although they may be associated with adverse effects, such as constipation, abdominal pain, headache, and nausea. Conservative measures, such as verbal instruction on sphincter exercises and hospital-based or home-based biofeedback, have been shown to improve symptoms of fecal incontinence.

In patients who do not respond to conservative measures, additional testing should be pursued. Anorectal manometry, balloon expulsion test, and rectal sensation should be evaluated. Testing should begin with anorectal manometry, with the key parameters being anal sphincter resting and squeeze pressure. Anal sphincter pressures decrease with age. Rectal sensation and balloon expulsion can be evaluated concurrently, with assessment of the patient's sensation of a balloon inflated in the rectum and measurement of manometric changes during expulsion. Rectal sensation may be normal, increased, or decreased in patients with fecal incontinence. Dyssynergia (paradoxical contraction or failure to relax pelvic floor muscles during simulated defecation) or inadequate rectal propulsion indicates a coexisting defecatory disorder. Rectal sensory disturbances and evacuation disorders are potentially amenable to biofeedback. Improvement of defecatory dysfunction, with less stool retained in the rectum, allows such patients to be less prone to leakage. Imaging with endoanal ultrasonography or MRI should be considered in patients with weak pressures if surgery is being considered. Figure 35-1 shows the algorithm for evaluating and managing defecatory disorders. Ultrasonography more clearly visualizes the internal sphincter, whereas MRI better discriminates

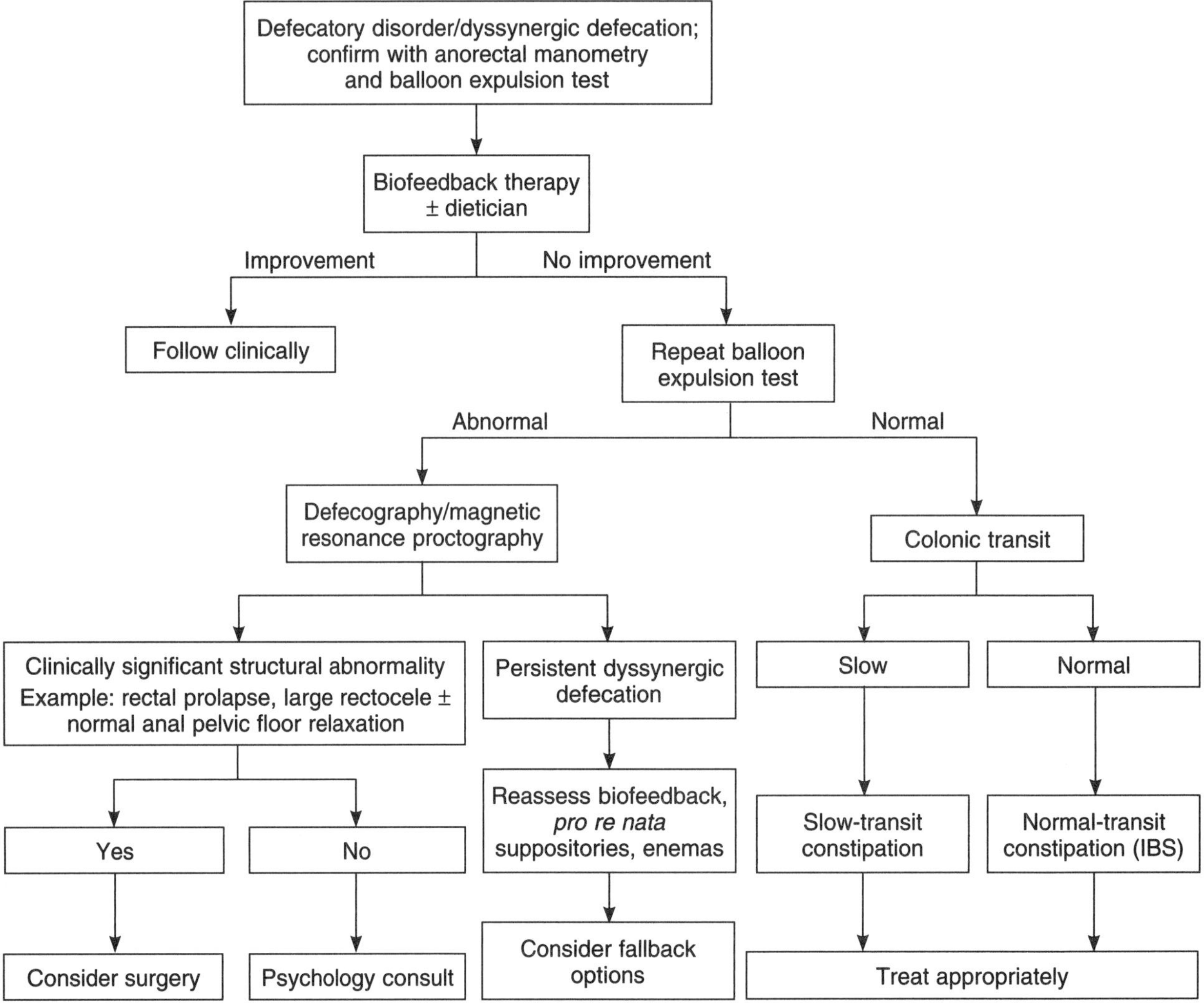

FIGURE 35-1. Suggested algorithm for the evaluation and management of defecatory disorders. Abbreviations: IBS, irritable bowel syndrome; Latin *pro re nata*, as circumstances may require. (Reprinted from Bharucha AE, Dorn SD, Lembo A, Pressman A. American Gastroenterological Association medical position statement on constipation. Gastroenterology 2013;144:211–7. Copyright 2013, with permission from Elsevier.)

between an external anal sphincter tear and a scar and can identify external sphincter atrophy. However, it can be difficult to interpret the clinical significance of anal sphincter injury because even asymptomatic women can have postpartum sphincter defects. Two-dimensional ultrasonography identifies defects in up to one third of women after vaginal delivery, while findings with three-dimensional ultrasonography or MRI show a lower prevalence of approximately 10%.

Pelvic floor rehabilitation techniques are effective and superior to pelvic floor exercises alone in patients with fecal incontinence who do not respond to conservative measures. Sacral nerve stimulation should be considered in patients with fecal incontinence who do not respond to conservative therapy, and anal sphincteroplasty should be considered if there is no response to conservative therapy and an anatomic sphincter defect is present.

Bharucha AE, Fletcher JG, Melton LJ 3rd, Zinsmeister AR. Obstetric trauma, pelvic floor injury and fecal incontinence: a population-based case-control study. Am J Gastroenterol 2012;107:902–11.

LaCross A, Groff M, Smaldone A. Obstetric anal sphincter injury and anal incontinence following vaginal birth: a systematic review and meta-analysis. J Midwifery Womens Health 2015;60:37–47.

Wald A, Bharucha AE, Cosman BC, Whitehead WE. ACG clinical guideline: management of benign anorectal disorders. Am J Gastroenterol 2014;109:1141–57; (Quiz) 1058.

36

Depot medroxyprogesterone acetate and bone density

A 19-year-old nulligravid woman comes to your office with her mother to discuss contraception. She is a competitive gymnast and has been using depot medroxyprogesterone acetate (DMPA) for 2 years, initially for cycle control and now also for contraception. She is satisfied with the amenorrhea and would like to continue DMPA. She has never had a pelvic examination. Her mother is very worried about her bone mineral density (BMD) and has encouraged her to start taking calcium and vitamin D supplements but asks you if she needs to change to a new method. You discuss her options and recommend

(A) insertion of a levonorgestrel intrauterine device (IUD)
* (B) continuation of DMPA
(C) initiation of oral contraceptives (OCs)
(D) insertion of an etonogestrel contraceptive implant
(E) insertion of a copper IUD

For most women, barring any medical concerns, the method of contraception that will have the highest continuation rate is the method she selects for how it fits with her life and her comfort with any adverse effects. Thus, for this patient, continuing DMPA is the best option because it is her preference and it is safe. In 2004, the U.S. Food and Drug Administration added a "black box" warning to DMPA labeling regarding the potential loss of BMD. This warning has concerned many patients and obstetrician–gynecologists and other health care providers regarding DMPA initiation and continuation, limiting access to a very safe and effective form of contraception that is especially appealing to adolescents.

Bone mineral density, which correlates directly with bone strength, is influenced by numerous factors, including gender, age, race, body mass index (calculated as weight in kilograms divided by height in meters squared [kg/m^2]), smoking, alcohol use, physical activity, dietary calcium and vitamin D intake, corticosteroid use, and sex hormones and related changes (eg, pregnancy, breastfeeding, menopause, hormonal contraceptive use). During puberty, BMD accumulation increases up to sixfold in females and then decreases rapidly after menarche. Numerous natural states, such as pregnancy and breastfeeding, result in small (2–8%) and temporary losses in BMD. Similar levels of BMD loss, approximately 5% at 5 years of use, have been seen with DMPA. However, much like other temporary losses, this BMD loss appears to be recoverable after DMPA is discontinued. Although recovery of BMD at the hip and femoral neck appears slower than in the spine, both appear to be recoverable. Although BMD is measured to assess bone health, the clinically meaningful outcome of greatest concern is fractures. No well-designed studies have clearly determined whether use of DMPA results in higher fracture risk. Given these uncertainties, patients should be counseled regarding possible BMD losses that are thought to be recoverable.

Clinicians also can use this discussion as an opportunity to counsel women regarding other ways to improve BMD—such as weight-bearing activity, calcium and vitamin D supplementation, and smoking cessation. Concerns regarding BMD are not a contraindication to initiation of DMPA in otherwise healthy women or a reason for discontinuation in women who are happy with DMPA, even after 2 years of use. There is no need for estrogen supplementation or early dual energy X-ray absorptiometry scanning, especially because this test has not been validated in adolescent populations or for this indication.

Although this patient is a nulligravid adolescent, she has no described contraindications to either the levonorgestrel IUD or the copper IUD. She does report liking the amenorrhea she experiences with DMPA. Although up to one half of women may become amenorrheic with use of a levonorgestrel IUD, it cannot be guaranteed that she will be one of them. She will continue to cycle normally or with slightly heavier periods with a copper IUD.

Oral contraceptives may be an option for this patient. Assuming no absolute contraindications, which are uncommon in women her age, OCs could be initiated safely that day without a pelvic examination. Initiation of OCs the day a patient is seen (quick start) as opposed to waiting until the first Sunday after her menses (conventional start) takes advantage of a woman's current interest and motivation to use contraception. Quick-start regimens are convenient for patients and increase the chance that they will initiate and continue pill use, at least in the short term. However, even if the described patient starts pills the day she is seen, like most women, she probably will experience "typical use" failure rates of 9% as opposed to the "perfect use" failure rate of less than 1%. Thus, continuing DMPA will give her better contraceptive effectiveness.

The etonogestrel contraceptive implant would be a medically appropriate option for the described patient and is recommended by the American College of Obstetricians and Gynecologists and the American Academy of Pediatrics as an ideal method for adolescents and young women. However, this patient currently is amenorrheic and wants to remain that way. With the etonogestrel contraceptive implant, up to a quarter of users have frequent or prolonged bleeding, so this is not the best option for her.

Contraception for adolescents. Committee on Adolescence. Pediatrics 2014;134:e1244–56.

Depot medroxyprogesterone acetate and bone effects. Committee Opinion No. 602. American College of Obstetricians and Gynecologists. Obstet Gynecol 2014;123:1398–402.

Lopez LM, Grimes DA, Schulz KF, Curtis KM, Chen M. Steroidal contraceptives: effect on bone fractures in women. Cochrane Database of Systematic Reviews 2014, Issue 6. Art. No.: CD006033. DOI: 10.1002/14651858.CD006033.pub5.

Mansour D, Korver T, Marintcheva-Petrova M, Fraser IS. The effects of Implanon on menstrual bleeding patterns. Eur J Contracept Reprod Health Care 2008;13(suppl):13–28.

Tepper NK, Curtis KM, Steenland MW, Marchbanks PA. Physical examination prior to initiating hormonal contraception: a systematic review. Contraception 2013;87:650–4.

37

Sonohysterography for postmenopausal bleeding

A 55-year-old woman has been menopausal for 5 years. She has never used postmenopausal hormone therapy and is no longer experiencing vasomotor symptoms. She comes to your office with a history of spotting associated with mild cramping. You perform an office endometrial biopsy, which yields superficial fragments of inactive endometrium. The best next step in management is

* (A) expectant management
(B) transvaginal ultrasonography
(C) sonohysterography
(D) hysteroscopy
(E) repeat endometrial biopsy

The primary goal in the initial management of postmenopausal bleeding is to exclude or diagnose endometrial adenocarcinoma. This can best be accomplished either by endometrial sampling with an office biopsy or by transvaginal ultrasonography to determine the maximal endometrial thickness of the endometrial echo on a long-axis view of the uterus. Even though 90% of cases of endometrial adenocarcinoma are accompanied by postmenopausal bleeding, carcinoma is found in only 1–14% of patients who present with postmenopausal bleeding, depending on age and risk factors. The risk factors for endometrial adenocarcinoma are listed in Box 37-1.

The most common finding to explain postmenopausal bleeding is atrophic endometrial changes. For the described patient, the results of the office biopsy were typical of atrophy and, thus, she should be reassured about the lack of worrisome pathology. Expectant management is the best option, given the negative biopsy. For a number of reasons, however, it is not always possible to perform office endometrial sampling in the postmenopausal patient. It also is very common to obtain inadequate tissue to render a histopathologic diagnosis even if sampling of the endometrial cavity is performed. In either of these situations, a useful tool for the evaluation of postmenopausal bleeding is transvaginal ultrasonography to measure endometrial thickness.

The reliability of endometrial thickness to exclude endometrial adenocarcinoma in women with postmenopausal bleeding has been confirmed in a number of multicenter clinical trials (Table 37-1). Using 4 mm or less as a cut-off, there is a 99.6–100% negative predictive value to exclude adenocarcinoma. A thickness greater than 4 mm is not predictive of any particular pathology but deserves further evaluation. It is important to note that this measurement and its interpretation are useful only in postmenopausal women who have bleeding. The significance of an incidental finding of endometrial thickness greater than 4 mm in postmenopausal women without bleeding has not been established and should not trigger further workup.

It is important to note that the use of endometrial thickness of 4 mm or less is a valuable tool to exclude endometrial adenocarcinoma. However, it does not exclude the presence of other intracavitary pathology, such as

BOX 37-1

Risk Factors for Endometrial Adenocarcinoma

Factors increasing risk
Increasing age
Long-term exposure to unopposed estrogens
Residence in North America or Europe
High concentrations of estrogens postmenopausally
Metabolic syndrome (obesity, diabetes)
Years of menstruation
Nulliparity
History of breast cancer
Long-term use of tamoxifen
HNPCC family syndrome
Hormone-replacement therapy with fewer than 12–14 days of progestogens
First-degree relative with endometrial cancer

Factors decreasing risk
Grand multiparity
Smoking
Oral contraceptive use
Physical activity
Diet of some phytoestrogens

Abbreviation: HNPCC, hereditary nonpolyposis colorectal cancer.

Reprinted from Amant F, Moerman P, Neven P, Timmerman D, Van Limbergen E, Vergote I. Endometrial cancer. Lancet 2005;366:491–505. Copyright 2005, with permission from Elsevier.

TABLE 37-1. Endometrial Thickness and Cancer Findings in Postmenopausal Women With Bleeding

Reference	Endometrial Thickness*	Number of Women	Number of Cases of Cancer	Negative Predictive Value
Karlsson 1995†	≤4 mm	1,168	0	100%
Ferrazzi 1996‡	≤4 mm	930	2	99.8%
	≤5 mm		4	99.6%
Gull 2000§	≤4 mm	163	1	99.4%
Epstein 2001‖	≤5 mm	97	0	100%
Gull 2003¶	≤4 mm	394	0	100%

*Determined by transvaginal ultrasonography.

†Karlsson B, Granberg S, Wikland M, Ylostalo P, Torvid K, Marsal K, et al. Transvaginal ultrasonography of the endometrium in women with postmenopausal bleeding—a Nordic multicenter study. Am J Obstet Gynecol 1995;172:1488–94.

‡Ferrazzi E, Torri V, Trio D, Zannoni E, Filiberto S, Dordoni D. Sonographic endometrial thickness: a useful test to predict atrophy in patients with postmenopausal bleeding. An Italian multicenter study. Ultrasound Obstet Gynecol 1996;7:315–21.

§Gull B, Carlsson S, Karlsson B, Ylostalo P, Milsom I, Granberg S. Transvaginal ultrasonography of the endometrium in women with postmenopausal bleeding: is it always necessary to perform an endometrial biopsy? Am J Obstet Gynecol 2000;182:509–15.

‖Epstein E, Valentin L. Rebleeding and endometrial growth in women with postmenopausal bleeding and endometrial thickness <5 mm managed by dilatation and curettage or ultrasound follow-up: a randomized controlled study. Ultrasound Obstet Gynecol 2001;18:499–504.

¶Gull B, Karlsson B, Milsom I, Granberg S. Can ultrasound replace dilation and curettage? A longitudinal evaluation of postmenopausal bleeding and transvaginal sonographic measurement of the endometrium as predictors of endometrial cancer. Am J Obstet Gynecol 2003;188:401–8.

The role of transvaginal ultrasonography in the evaluation of postmenopausal bleeding. ACOG Committee Opinion No. 440. American College of Obstetricians and Gynecologists. Obstet Gynecol 2009;114:409–11.

endometrial polyps. Therefore, in patients who continue to experience postmenopausal bleeding after endometrial carcinoma has been excluded, further evaluation is warranted. In this circumstance, sonohysterography can be particularly useful to evaluate the endometrial cavity. Indications for sonohysterography are listed in Box 37-2. It is useful to diagnose polyps that then can be removed with hysteroscopy. If the sonohysterography is completely normal, with no polyps or asymmetry of the endometrium, then no further evaluation is necessary. Another option would be to proceed directly to hysteroscopy in either the office or the operating room. Hysteroscopy is the preferred management rather than sonohysterography in patients with persistent bleeding and an endometrial thickness greater than 4 mm, because an explanation for the thickened endometrium will be necessary even if the endometrial cavity appears normal on sonohysterography.

BOX 37-2

Indications for Sonohysterography

- Abnormal uterine bleeding
- Evaluation of uterine cavity
  - Leiomyomas, polyps, synechiae
- Abnormalities present on transvaginal ultrasonography
  - Focal or diffuse endometrial or intracavitary abnormalities
- Congenital anomalies of the uterus
- Infertility
- Recurrent pregnancy loss
- Suboptimal visualization of the endometrium on transvaginal ultrasonography

Sonohysterography. Technology Assessment No. 12. American College of Obstetricians and Gynecologists. Obstet Gynecol 2016;128:e38–42.

Amant F, Moerman P, Neven P, Timmerman D, Van Limbergen E, Vergote I. Endometrial cancer. Lancet 2005;366:491–505.

The role of transvaginal ultrasonography in the evaluation of postmenopausal bleeding. ACOG Committee Opinion No. 440. American College of Obstetricians and Gynecologists. Obstet Gynecol 2009;114:409–11.

Sonohysterography. Technology Assessment in Obstetrics and Gynecology No. 12. American College of Obstetricians and Gynecologists. Obstet Gynecol 2016;128:e38–42.

38

Uterine leiomyoma

You are called to the emergency room to evaluate a 45-year-old woman, gravida 3, para 3, with a history of heavy menstrual bleeding. She reports feeling tired and short of breath when she walks a few blocks. She has not experienced chest pain or dizziness. Her menstrual cycles have become heavier over the past few years, and she is experiencing menstrual bleeding for 7 days each month. Her medical history and surgical history are negative. She smokes one pack of cigarettes a day. Her pulse is 87 beats per minute, and her blood pressure is 117/68 mm Hg. Pelvic examination reveals a small amount of vaginal bleeding and a 14-week-sized mobile uterus. Her hemoglobin level is 7.1 g/dL, and transvaginal ultrasonography shows a solitary 8-cm submucosal leiomyoma and normal-appearing ovaries. After counseling, the patient tells you that she desires a hysterectomy, but she would like to postpone the procedure for a few months. The best initial therapy for this patient is oral iron supplementation plus

(A) depot medroxyprogesterone acetate
(B) combination oral contraceptives (OCs)
(C) levonorgestrel intrauterine device (IUD)
* (D) leuprolide acetate

Women who undergo hysterectomy for treatment of leiomyoma-associated abnormal uterine bleeding have significant improvements in quality of life and mental health scores compared with women treated with medication. Although medical therapy is a reasonable first-line option for women with abnormal bleeding caused by leiomyomas, surgical management in this patient is practical given her age, parity, and significant anemia. Preoperative hormonal manipulation should be considered to minimize perioperative blood loss and correct anemia when feasible. In patients without contraindications to hormonal medications, estrogen-containing OCs or progestin may be considered as a treatment option. However, nearly 60% of women treated with oral medication for heavy menstrual bleeding require hysterectomy within 2 years. This 45-year-old patient smokes and, therefore, is not a candidate for estrogen-containing OCs. Although OCs may decrease blood loss in women with leiomyomas through the development of endometrial atrophy, few studies have evaluated the effects of OCs on anemia in women with leiomyomas. For the described patient, combination OCs are contraindicated because of her smoking habit and age.

Progestational agents are associated with decreased bleeding because of the promotion of endometrial atrophy and may affect uterine size. However, there are no studies that assess the effect of depot medroxyprogesterone acetate on bleeding in women with submucosal leiomyomas and no randomized trials evaluating the effects of this medication on leiomyomas in any location.

The results of a single, small randomized controlled trial to evaluate the effect of the levonorgestrel IUD compared with combination OCs in women with leiomyomas were consistent with a decrease in menstrual blood loss in the levonorgestrel IUD group. Observational studies have found that the use of the levonorgestrel IUD in women with leiomyomas is associated with improvement in hemoglobin and ferritin levels. These studies also suggest an increased rate of IUD expulsion and a greater than 10% incidence of spotting in women with leiomyomas. Uterine volume has been shown to decrease 3 years after levonorgestrel IUD placement without a significant reduction in leiomyoma volume. Studies of the levonorgestrel IUD in women with submucosal leiomyomas are lacking, and the presence of an intracavitary leiomyoma is a contraindication to placement.

Uterine leiomyoma size reduction is greater after the use of gonadotropin-releasing hormone agonists compared with progestins. Leuprolide acetate induces amenorrhea in most women and results in decreased size of a leiomyomatous uterus by as much as 60% after 3 months of use. Women can expect a reduction in anemia and bulk symptoms after injection. Adverse effects of leuprolide acetate include vasomotor symptoms, vaginal dryness, and joint aches. Because of the beneficial effects on leiomyoma symptoms, hemoglobin level, and intraoperative blood loss, leuprolide acetate is approved for preoperative use for women before leiomyoma-related surgery. The use of leuprolide acetate in combination with oral iron supplementation results in greater improvements in hemoglobin concentration than iron supplementation without leuprolide acetate. Studies evaluating the effect that reduction in uterine size after leuprolide acetate has on the route of hysterectomy and incision type have found conflicting results. The reduction in uterine size may positively affect the incision type or route of hysterectomy by increasing the potential for a transverse abdominal incision or a vaginal procedure.

Other potential options for medical management that are not approved by the U.S. Food and Drug Administration for the treatment of leiomyomas may include mifepristone and ulipristal acetate. In small studies, mifepristone use has been associated with decreased bleeding but not decreased leiomyoma size. Ulipristal acetate is a selective progesterone receptor modulator that has been shown to decrease leiomyoma-related bleeding with a shorter treatment-to-amenorrhea interval and fewer adverse effects compared with leuprolide acetate. The use of selective estrogen receptor modulators for the treatment of leiomyomas is not supported in the literature.

Donnez J, Tomaszewski J, Vazquez F, Bouchard P, Lemieszczuk B, Baro F, et al. Ulipristal acetate versus leuprolide acetate for uterine fibroids. PEARL II Study Group. N Engl J Med 2012;366:421–32.

Lethaby A, Vollenhoven B, Sowter M. Efficacy of pre-operative gonadotrophin hormone releasing analogues for women with uterine fibroids undergoing hysterectomy or myomectomy: a systematic review. BJOG 2002;109:1097–108.

Magalhaes J, Aldrighi JM, de Lima GR. Uterine volume and menstrual patterns in users of the levonorgestrel-releasing intrauterine system with idiopathic menorrhagia or menorrhagia due to leiomyomas. Contraception 2007;75:193–8.

Marjoribanks J, Lethaby A, Farquhar C. Surgery versus medical therapy for heavy menstrual bleeding. Cochrane Database of Systematic Reviews 2016, Issue 1. Art. No.: CD003855. DOI: 10.1002/14651858.CD003855.pub3.

Sangkomkamhang US, Lumbiganon P, Laopaiboon M, Mol Ben WJ. Progestogens or progestogen-releasing intrauterine systems for uterine fibroids. Cochrane Database of Systematic Reviews 2013, Issue 2. Art. No.: CD008994. DOI: 10.1002/14651858.CD008994.pub2.

Sayed GH, Zakherah MS, El-Nashar SA, Shaaban MM. A randomized clinical trial of a levonorgestrel-releasing intrauterine system and a low-dose combined oral contraceptive for fibroid-related menorrhagia. Int J Gynaecol Obstet 2011;112:126–30.

Stovall TG, Muneyyirci-Delale O, Summitt RL Jr, Scialli AR. GnRH agonist and iron versus placebo and iron in the anemic patient before surgery for leiomyomas: a randomized controlled trial. Leuprolide Acetate Study Group. Obstet Gynecol 1995;86:65–71.

Tristan M, Orozco LJ, Steed A, Ramírez-Morera A, Stone P. Mifepristone for uterine fibroids. Cochrane Database of Systematic Reviews 2012, Issue 8. Art. No.: CD007687. DOI: 10.1002/14651858.CD007687.pub2.

Vilos GA, Allaire C, Laberge PY, Leyland N, Special Contributors, Vilos AG, et al. The management of uterine leiomyomas. J Obstet Gynaecol Can 2015;37:157–81.

Zapata LB, Whiteman MK, Tepper NK, Jamieson DJ, Marchbanks PA, Curtis KM. Intrauterine device use among women with uterine fibroids: a systematic review. Contraception 2010;82:41–55.

39

Sexually transmitted infection testing

A 32-year-old nulligravid woman comes to your office for her routine annual well-woman examination. She reports regular cycles and has a subdermal contraceptive implant that was placed 2 years ago. Her examination is normal and she has no health issues. During the visit, she tells you that she recently started a new relationship and is discussing the initiation of sex. She asks to be "tested for everything." She has not been sexually active for over 1 year. She states that she has not experienced any vaginal discharge, dysuria, or pelvic pain. You discuss the current recommendations for sexually transmitted infection (STI) screening. The statistical rationale for not routinely screening patients with histories like hers is low

(A) specificity
(B) sensitivity
* (C) positive predictive value (PPV)
(D) negative predictive value (NPV)

Preventive health visits include anticipatory counseling and screening for many conditions. Primary prevention of disease includes treatments and lifestyle modifications geared at prevention of disease. Secondary prevention of disease is detection of the disease state in an early stage, sometimes before the woman recognizes that the disease is present. The obstetrician–gynecologist orders a variety of screening tests on a routine basis. Criteria of a good screening test include the following:

- The disease state must be serious enough to cause a health risk to the woman.
- The disease state must have an effective treatment.
- Treatment is more effective in the asymptomatic state.
- The test should be safe, inexpensive, and readily available.
- The screening test should be accurate and reliable.

The American College of Obstetricians and Gynecologists and the U.S. Preventive Services Task Force agree that women younger than 25 years and women with risk factors (eg, multiple or new sexual partners, inconsistent use of barrier methods of contraception) should be screened for chlamydial infection and gonorrhea. These STIs, if left untreated, have a high risk of causing upper genital tract infections with resulting complications of chronic pelvic pain, infertility, and ectopic pregnancy. Figure 39-1 and Figure 39-2 show rates of reported cases of chlamydial infection and gonorrhea, respectively, by age and sex in the United States.

The ability of a test to identify disease in an affected population is referred to as sensitivity. Specificity is a test's ability to correctly identify individuals without disease (Box 39-1). The populations in question are defined by the criterion standard and are either 100% affected or 0% affected. Sensitivity and specificity are attributes inherent to the test and do not change based on the population examined because the populations are predefined as either all or none. A physician might assume that the best test would be the test with the highest sensitivity. At the extreme, a test that is always positive will have sensitivity of 100% but poor specificity because it will never be negative in the uninfected population. Screening test thresholds seek a balance between sensitivity and specificity. A perfect test (ie, 100% sensitivity and specificity) would identify all patients with disease and would not misidentify any patients without disease. Nucleic acid amplification tests are able to detect even low levels of infectious particles. These tests perform much better than previous testing methodologies (eg, culture, immunoassay, nonamplified testing) and have sensitivities well above 90% and specificities of greater than 99%.

Positive predictive value and NPV are the percentages of test results that correctly identify the presence or absence of disease. Positive predictive value and NPV depend on the frequency of disease in the population. Bayes theorem predicts that for any given test, the PPV is greater if the disease is more common. The curve for specificity of a disease goes up as the prevalence increases (Fig. 39-3). In populations with low prevalence, a positive test result is more likely to be a false-positive result because the disease state is uncommon. Looking at a hypothetical case of two screening populations using the same test (sensitivity 97%, specificity 99%) demonstrates that the PPV is higher in the population with the higher prevalence (88% versus 49.5%) (Box 39-2). Recommendations for screening young women for STIs leverage this phenomenon by identifying the groups at highest risk of having disease, thereby increasing the PPV. It is important for the clinician to recognize the limitations of testing in low-prevalence populations.

Current recommendations for screening asymptomatic women for STIs include screening adolescents and young women or women with risk factors (eg, multiple sexual partners). Sexually transmitted infections are more prevalent in these populations; therefore, the PPV is higher. Routine screening of women at low risk could result in a positive test when no STI is present.

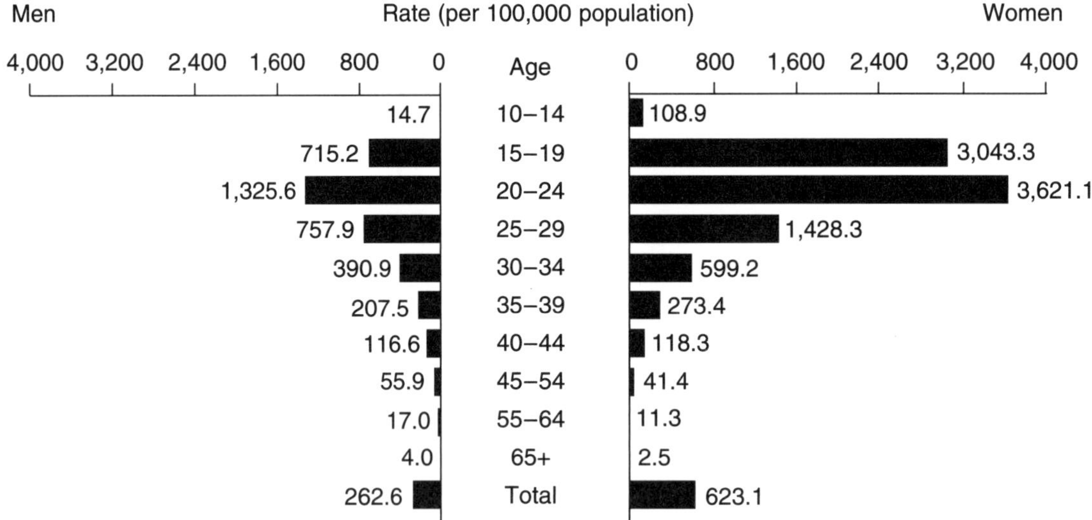

FIGURE 39-1. Rates of reported cases of chlamydial infection, by age and sex, United States, 2013. (Workowski KA, Bolan GA. Sexually transmitted diseases treatment guidelines, 2015. Centers for Disease Control and Prevention [published erratum appears in MMWR Recomm Rep 2015;64:924]. MMWR Recomm Rep 2015;64:1–137.)

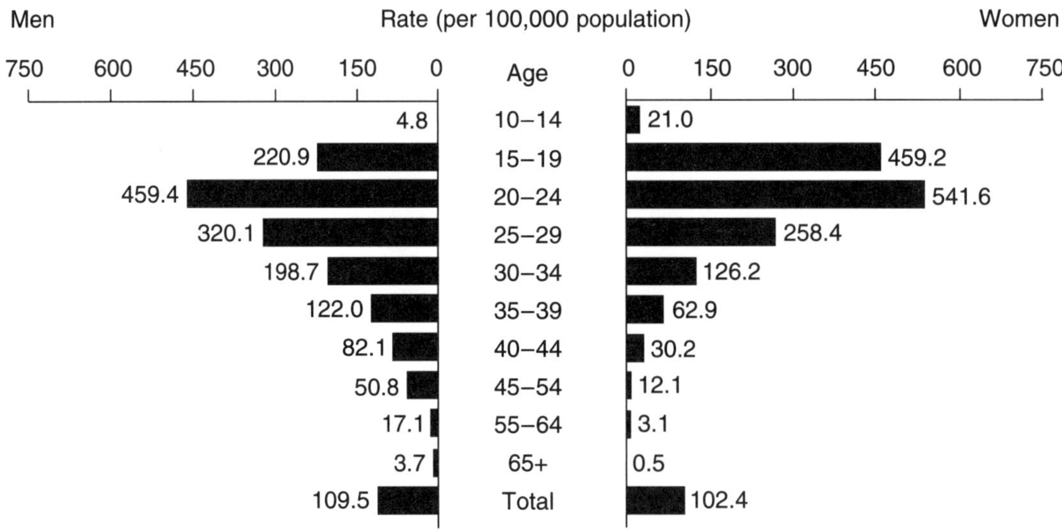

FIGURE 39-2. Rates of reported cases of gonorrhea, by age and sex, United States, 2013. (Workowski KA, Bolan GA. Sexually transmitted diseases treatment guidelines, 2015. Centers for Disease Control and Prevention [published erratum appears in MMWR Recomm Rep 2015;64:924]. MMWR Recomm Rep 2015;64:1–137.)

BOX 39-1

Example of a 2 × 2 Table Illustrating the Relationship Between Test Results and Disease Status Followed by Definitions of Four Common Epidemiologic Terms

	Disease Status	
Test Results	**Present**	**Absent**
+	True positive (TP)	False-positive (FP)
–	False-negative (FN)	True negative (TN)

Sensitivity:

- The proportion of correctly identified individuals with disease among all individuals with disease
- TP/(TP+FN)
- How well the screening test will correctly identify individuals with disease

Specificity:

- The proportion of correctly identified individuals without disease among all individuals without disease
- TN/(TN+FP)
- How well the screening test will correctly identify individuals without disease

Positive predictive value:

- The proportion of individuals with correct positive test results among all individuals in whom the test result was positive
- TP/(TP+FP)
- The probability that, if an individual tests positive, they truly have the disease

Negative predictive value:

- The proportion of individuals with correct negative test results among all individuals in whom the test result was negative.
- TN/(FN+TN)
- The probability that, if a person tests negative, they truly have no disease

Adapted from American College of Obstetricians and Gynecologists. Primary and preventive care. Precis: an update in obstetrics and gynecology. 2nd ed. Washington, DC: ACOG; 1999. p. 10.

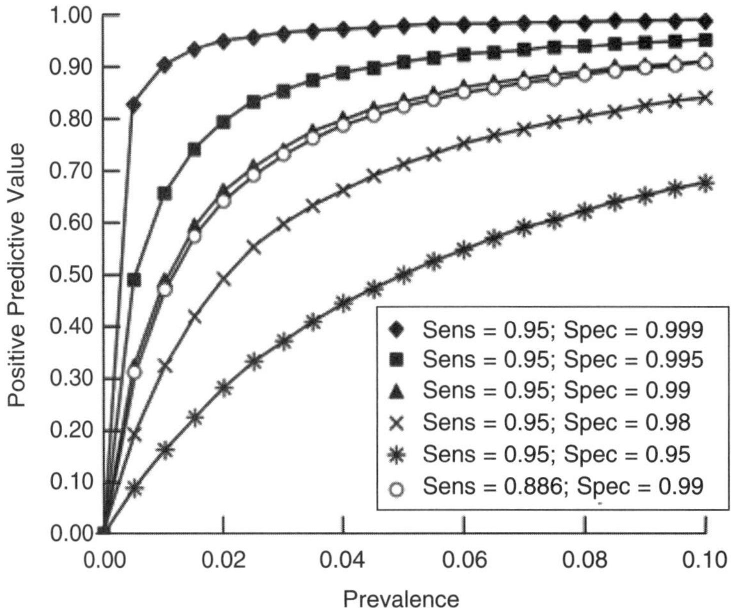

FIGURE 39-3. Calculated positive predictive values for a test with sensitivity of 88.6%–95% and specificity of 95%–99.9% in theoretical populations with disease prevalence of 0.0%–10.0%. (Adapted with permission from BMJ Publishing Group Limited. Zenilman JM, Miller WC, Gaydos C, Rogers SM, Turner CF. LCR testing for gonorrhoea and chlamydia in population surveys and other screenings of low prevalence populations: coping with decreased positive predictive value. Sex Transm Infect 2003;79:94–7.)

BOX 39-2

An Illustration of Test Results in Two Different Populations of 100,000 Individuals With Disease Prevalence of 1% (A) and 7% (B)

A. Population of 100,000 individuals with disease prevalence of 1%

		Disease Status		
		Present	Absent	Total
Test	+	970 (TP)	990 (FP)	1,960
Results	–	30 (FN)	98,010 (TN)	98,040
Total		1,000	99,000	100,000

Sensitivity = TP/(TP+FN) = 970/1,000 = 97%
Specificity = TN/(TN+FP) = 98,010/99,000 = 99%
PPV = TP/(TP+FP) = 970/1,960 = 49.5%
NPV = TN/(TN+FN) = 94,050/94,150 = 99.9%

B. Population of 100,000 individuals with disease prevalence of 7%

		Disease Status		
		Present	Absent	Total
Test	+	6,790 (TP)	930 (FP)	7,720
Results	–	210 (FN)	92,070 (TN)	92,280
Total		7,000	93,000	100,000

Sensitivity = TP/(TP+FN) = 6,790/7,000 = 97%
Specificity = TN/(TN+FP) = 92,070/93,000 = 99%
PPV = TP/(TP+FP) = 6,790/7,720 = 88.0%
NPV = TN/(TN+FN) = 90,250/90,750 = 99.8%

Abbreviations: FN, false-negative; FP, false-positive; NPV, negative predictive value; PPV, positive predictive value; TN, true negative; TP, true positive.

*The same screening test is used in both populations. The screening test has a sensitivity of 97% and a specificity of 99%.

Evans M, Galen R, Britt DW. Principles of screening. Semin Perinatol 2005;29:364–6.

Grimes DA, Schulz KF. Uses and abuses of screening tests [published erratum appears in Lancet 2008;371:1998]. Lancet 2002;359:881–4.

Papp JR, Schachter J, Gaydos CA, Van Der Pol B. Recommendations for the laboratory-based detection of *Chlamydia trachomatis* and *Neisseria gonorrhoeae*—2014. Division of STD Prevention, National Center for HIV/AIDS, Viral Hepatitis, STD, and TB Prevention, CDC. MMWR Recomm Rep 2014;63(RR02):1–19.

40

Pediatric vulvar lichen sclerosus

A healthy 7-year-old girl reports perineal itching and pain as well as dysuria. Her urine culture is negative. She lives with her parents, baby brother, and maternal grandmother, and the family has a low level of concern for the possibility of sexual abuse. Genital examination is significant for normal hymen and vagina and a symmetrical and well-circumscribed perianal and perineal hypopigmentation in a figure-of-eight pattern on her vulva with punctate hemorrhages. The most appropriate initial step is to

(A) obtain vaginal culture
(B) alert child protective services
* (C) prescribe clobetasol propionate ointment
(D) perform a punch biopsy of the affected area
(E) reevaluate after a 2-week period of proper vulvar hygiene

A range of symptoms and physical findings may be encountered in the pediatric patient with a vulvar disorder. The symptoms experienced by the described patient are most consistent with pediatric vulvar lichen sclerosus. Children with lichen sclerosus may present with concerns of vulvar or perineal itching, burning, or localized pain. Discomfort associated with urination and defecation is common. Physical findings of pediatric lichen sclerosus are variable and may not correlate with severity of symptoms, which often leads to misdiagnosis. Classical findings include sharply demarcated white plaques in a figure-of-eight pattern around the labia, perineal body, and anus, with sparing of the vagina and hymen. Frequent scratching can cause small hemorrhages and erosions. The combined effects of the underlying disorder and reactive skin changes can lead to fissures, scarring, and changes in labial architecture.

Lichen sclerosus is a chronic skin disorder with an unclear etiology. Autoimmune, hormonal, genetic, and cell proliferation factors have been considered as potential contributors to the development of this disorder. Associated autoimmune disorders are found commonly in parents or grandparents of girls with lichen sclerosus.

Patients with symptoms respond best to the antiinflammatory properties of high-potency topical corticoid steroid preparations. T-cell modulators such as tacrolimus have been tried without success; thus, the mainstay of medical treatment remains topical steroids such as clobetasol. Clobetasol is applied twice daily for 2–12 weeks with frequent reassessment. The frequency of application is tapered after symptoms abate because rebound may occur with abrupt cessation of steroid use. The relapse rate is high, and long-term surveillance is required for management of symptoms as well as assessment of the labial architecture. If untreated, vulvar lichen sclerosus can result in scarring, architectural distortion, and future sexual dysfunction. A small study of children with lichen sclerosus monitored longitudinally found that symptoms persist past puberty in approximately 75% of patients. In addition to topical corticoid steroid treatment, behavioral modifications such as sitz baths and avoiding irritants are an integral part of treatment and prevention of recurrence.

Although a vulvar biopsy frequently is performed in adults with vulvar skin abnormalities, vulvar lichen sclerosus is associated with typical physical findings in pediatric patients, and a vulvar biopsy is not indicated. For this reason, biopsy may be reserved for children with atypical presentation or poor response to therapy.

Genital infection is a consideration in the differential diagnosis, and pediatric vulvovaginitis is most commonly associated with respiratory and gastrointestinal flora. A culture should be considered in girls with discharge; however, it is not indicated for this patient, and the constellation of symptoms and pattern of hypopigmentation described are classic for lichen sclerosus.

As the initial step in this case, culture would delay diagnosis and therapy. All caretakers of pediatric patients must seriously consider the possibility of abuse when children present with potential evidence of trauma. In this case, the punctate hemorrhages are nonspecific, yet the constellation of findings is consistent with the diagnosis of lichen sclerosus and does not warrant a child protective services investigation at this time. Expectant management is inappropriate in this symptomatic patient with physical findings classic for pediatric lichen sclerosus.

Bercaw-Pratt JL, Boardman LA, Simms-Cendan JS. Clinical recommendation: pediatric lichen sclerosus. North American Society for Pediatric and Adolescent Gynecology. J Pediatr Adolesc Gynecol 2014;27:111–6.

Casey GA, Cooper SM, Powell JJ. Treatment of vulvar lichen sclerosus with topical corticosteroids in children: a study of 72 children. Clin Exp Dermatol 2015;40:289–92.

Smith SD, Fischer G. Childhood onset vulvar lichen sclerosus does not resolve at puberty: a prospective case series. Pediatr Dermatol 2009;26:725–9.

41

Indications for varicella vaccine in nonpregnant patients

A healthy 17-year-old nulligravid female calls your office for advice. Two days ago, she babysat a 4-year-old boy who had a fever. That evening, he developed a generalized, pruritic rash that has now progressed to vesicular lesions (Fig. 41-1; see color plate). The patient cannot recall her vaccination history, nor does she remember having a similar rash. She remains asymptomatic. The best next step in management is

(A) immune globulin
* (B) vaccination
(C) expectant management
(D) oral acyclovir

Varicella infection is caused by the varicella-zoster virus (VZV), which is a member of the herpesvirus group. Primary infection with VZV causes chickenpox, and reactivation of latent infection causes shingles. Varicella is highly contagious and is spread by direct contact, air, or droplets. The incubation period is 14–16 days, and fever and malaise may occur 1–2 days before the onset of a rash. The rash is pruritic and progresses quickly from macules to papules to vesicular lesions, which then crust over.

Varicella vaccination began in the United States in 1995. It is a live, attenuated vaccine and, thus, is contraindicated in pregnant women. It also is contraindicated in individuals who have had a life-threatening allergic reaction to a previous dose of chickenpox vaccine, to gelatin, or to neomycin. Also, people who are moderately or severely ill should not be vaccinated at that time. Individuals with any degree of immune compromise should ask their doctors if vaccination is indicated; it may be safe in some situations of immune compromise. Varicella vaccine is recommended for children in a two-dose series, with the first dose given at age 12–15 months and the second dose at age 4–6 years. Individuals 7 years and older who do not have evidence of varicella immunity also should receive two doses.

For individuals who have no evidence of immunity to varicella (laboratory evidence of immunity, documented history of the disease itself, or documented history of vaccination) and are exposed to the disease, vaccination is recommended, provided that no contraindications exist. Vaccination should be given within 3–5 days of exposure. Vaccination within 3 days of exposure is reported to be more than 90% effective in preventing varicella. When given within 5 days of exposure, vaccination is approximately 70% effective in preventing varicella infection.

Use of varicella immune globulin for postexposure prophylaxis is reserved for individuals in whom vaccination is contraindicated. In these cases, immune globulin should be given to individuals at high risk of severe disease and complications from varicella. Such patients include pregnant women, immunocompromised individuals, neonates of women who have signs and symptoms of varicella around the time of delivery, and premature neonates exposed postnatally. Varicella immune globulin should be given as soon as possible but no later than 10 days after exposure. Information on obtaining varicella immune globulin can be found at the Centers for Disease Control and Prevention website (http://www.cdc.gov/mmwr/preview/mmwrhtml/mm6228a4.htm).

Acyclovir is an antiviral medication that inhibits replication of human herpes viruses, including VZV. It often is used for treatment of severe varicella infection. Acyclovir is not recommended as postexposure prophylaxis.

Expectant management is not appropriate because the described patient has not been vaccinated against VZV, nor has she had the disease. Expectant management would place the adolescent at risk of VZV infection with possible serious complications such as encephalitis and sepsis.

American College of Obstetricians and Gynecologists. Immunization for women. Washington, DC: American College of Obstetricians and Gynecologists; 2016. Available at: http://www.immunizationforwomen.org/. Retrieved June 10, 2016.

FDA approval of an extended period for administering VariZIG for postexposure prophylaxis of varicella. Centers for Disease Control and Prevention. MMWR Morb Mortal Wkly Rep 2012;61:212.

Kimberlin DW, Brady MT, Jackson MA, Long SS, editors. Red book: 2015 report of the committee on infectious diseases. American Academy of Pediatrics. 30th ed. Elk Grove Village (IL): American Academy of Pediatrics; 2015.

Marin M, Guris D, Chaves SS, Schmid S, Seward JF. Prevention of varicella: recommendations of the Advisory Committee on Immunization Practices (ACIP). Advisory Committee on Immunization Practices, Centers for Disease Control and Prevention. MMWR Recomm Rep 2007;56:1–40.

42

Breast cancer screening

A 25-year-old woman of Jewish descent comes to your office. Her mother received a breast cancer diagnosis at age 48 years and was found to carry a *BRCA1* mutation. Your patient recently underwent testing and was found to carry the same mutation. Her mother has encouraged her to start mammography immediately. The most appropriate annual breast surveillance for this patient is

(A) mammography starting at age 30 years
(B) breast magnetic resonance imaging (MRI) starting at age 30 years
(C) breast ultrasonography starting at age 30 years
* (D) magnetic resonance imaging now, adding annual mammography at age 30 years

Women who carry a *BRCA1* or *BRCA2* gene mutation are at significantly increased risk of developing invasive breast cancer. Lifetime risk for *BRCA1* and *BRCA2* mutation carriers originally were reported to be near 75–80% based on studies from breast cancer-affected families, but most newly ascertained patients now benefit from age-specific risk counseling. Updated cumulative risks of breast cancer by age 70 years are 55% for a *BRCA1* mutation carrier and 47% for a *BRCA2* mutation carrier. The age at onset of breast cancer also is notably younger in mutation carriers compared with the general population. For these reasons, breast surveillance is recommended to begin earlier and to be more intensive compared with that in women in the general population.

For women who do not have *BRCA1* or *BRCA2* mutations, breast screening protocols generally specify annual or biennial mammography. The age for initiation of mammography differs among various expert panels, but age 40 years is supported by many professional organizations, including the American College of Obstetricians and Gynecologists. The U.S. Preventive Services Task Force recommendations are for initiation at age 50 years in the absence of other risk factors, such as positive family history.

Table 42-1 demonstrates cumulative breast cancer risk in women with a *BRCA1* or *BRCA2* mutation based on a meta-analysis of several observational studies. Because of the earlier age at onset, breast imaging is recommended beginning at age 25 years. Because of the concern for radiation exposure and the density of normal breast tissue in women in this age category, MRI is the preferred modality. Some women may be unable to undergo MRI because of allergy or other conditions; for these women, ultrasonography should be considered.

The ideal imaging algorithm has not been confirmed in any prospective head-to-head trials. However, consensus panels have agreed upon some combination of MRI and, at a later age, mammography. Such an approach also is supported by statistical models because *BRCA1* and *BRCA2* mutation-bearing women have a risk of breast cancer that rapidly escalates with age compared with noncarriers. Because of biologic properties of breast cancer in women with *BRCA1* or *BRCA2* mutations, prolonged intervals between screenings is undesirable. Many centers use a breast imaging approach that incorporates imaging every 6 months, alternating between mammography and MRI.

Routine ultrasonographic screening for breast malignancies among the average-risk population generally is not recommended. However, ultrasonography serves as a useful adjunct in imaging after suspicious mammography or MRI. In addition, ultrasonography is used for guided biopsies if the lesion is visible or if there is a palpable mass.

After breast cancer has been diagnosed in a *BRCA1* or *BRCA2* mutation carrier, the risk of a second cancer in the contralateral breast is significantly higher than it is in the general population, ranging from 33–40% (compared with 17% in the general population). For this reason, many women with a *BRCA1* or *BRCA2* mutation and newly diagnosed breast cancer choose to undergo bilateral mastectomy.

No randomized controlled trials exist that have examined the sensitivity and specificity of screening algorithms in mutation carriers, but observational studies confirm the additional benefit of combined imaging modalities. Use of mammography plus MRI is associated with detection rates of up to 95% but with specificity lower than either modality alone; MRI plus mammography is reported to have specificity of approximately 75%.

Risk-reducing mastectomy should be discussed with *BRCA1* or *BRCA2* mutation carriers. Such surgery has been shown to lower the risk of breast cancer by 95%. This option precludes the need for further imaging after surgery, frequently can result in excellent cosmetic outcome, and has been shown to reduce anxiety in women

Table 42-1. Cumulative Risks of Developing Breast Cancer in Cancer-Free Women With *BRCA1* or *BRCA2* Mutation by Age

Current Age (Years)	Risk (%) of Developing Breast Cancer at a Later Age				
	30 Years	**40 Years**	**50 Years**	**60 Years**	**70 Years**
BRCA1					
20	1.8	12	29	44	54
30		10	28	44	54
40			20	38	49
50				22	37
60					19
BRCA2					
20	1	7.5	21	35	45
30		6.6	20	35	45
40			15	30	42
50				18	32
60					17

 Chen S, Parmigiani G. Meta-analysis of *BRCA1* and *BRCA2* penetrance. J Clin Oncol 2007;25:1329–33.

who undergo this intervention. The timing of such surgery is dependent on many factors, including desire to breastfeed, age of ascertainment of mutation status, and other demographic factors.

Chen S, Parmigiani G. Meta-analysis of *BRCA1* and *BRCA2* penetrance. J Clin Oncol 2007;25:1329–33.

Hereditary breast and ovarian cancer syndrome. ACOG Practice Bulletin No. 103. American College of Obstetricians and Gynecologists. Obstet Gynecol 2009;113:957–66.

Lowry KP, Lee JM, Kong CY, McMahon PM, Gilmore ME, Cott Chubiz JE, et al. Annual screening strategies in *BRCA1* and *BRCA2* gene mutation carriers: a comparative effectiveness analysis [published erratum appears in Cancer 2012;118:5448]. Cancer 2012;118:2021–30.

Nelson HD, Pappas M, Zakher B, Mitchell JP, Okinaka-Hu L, Fu R. Risk assessment, genetic counseling, and genetic testing for *BRCA*-related cancer in women: a systematic review to update the U.S. Preventive Services Task Force recommendation. Ann Intern Med 2014;160:255–66.

43

Depression in adolescents

A 15-year-old girl presents for a wellness visit. Your nurse indicates that she has screened positive for depression on a self-administered screen filled out in the waiting room. The patient tells you she has felt sad and empty for the past 2 months. Her grades have slipped because she often forgets her homework and cannot concentrate on examinations. She states that she has never tried drugs or alcohol and has never considered hurting herself. Her mother reports that she always looks tired and often snacks late at night. You do not identify any history of recent loss or psychosis. The patient and her mother deny any recent or remote history of manic behavior. Her affect is flat. Her body mass index (calculated as weight in kilograms divided by height in meters squared [kg/m^2]) has increased from 21 last year to 25 at present. The best management is to offer this patient cognitive behavioral therapy and recommend

(A) paroxetine
* (B) fluoxetine
(C) venlafaxine
(D) amitriptyline
(E) St. John's wort

The U.S. Preventive Services Task Force, the National Institute for Health and Care Excellence, the American Academy of Child and Adolescent Psychiatry, and the American Medical Association all recommend routine screening of adolescents for depression. The U.S. Preventive Services Task Force specifies that screening should occur only when there is access to appropriate follow-up and treatment. Up to 80% of adolescents affected by depression do not receive appropriate care. A number of standardized tools can be used for screening, but they should not replace an interview with the patient and, ideally, family members or guardians to confirm the diagnosis.

The described patient exhibits persistent depressed mood, anhedonia, weight gain, insomnia, fatigue, and diminished concentration unexplained by substance use or an underlying medical condition, all of which are criteria indicating a major depressive episode as described in the American Psychiatric Association's *Diagnostic and Statistical Manual of Mental Disorders*, Fifth Edition. Unipolar depression is diagnosed in a patient who has suffered at least one major depressive episode and has no history of a mania or hypomania (see the *Diagnostic and Statistical Manual of Mental Disorders*, Fifth Edition, for the criteria constituting manic and hypomanic episodes). This patient has unipolar major depression.

Treatment of depression can involve pharmacotherapy, psychotherapy, or both. Cognitive behavior therapy, interpersonal psychotherapy, and selective serotonin reuptake inhibitors (SSRIs) have been found to be effective for adolescent depression. Guidelines vary regarding whether to start treatment with psychotherapy, pharmacotherapy, or both. The approach will depend in part on available resources and expertise and in part on input from the patient and her family. Monotherapy with antidepressants does not address the psychosocial context in which depression often occurs, and environmental problems may persist even after mood has stabilized. Psychotherapy to improve coping skills, relationships, and self-esteem can be of particular value during the adolescent years. Some randomized trials suggest that a combination of psychotherapy and pharmacotherapy is better than either alone. However, meta-analyses, including a Cochrane Review, did not find clear evidence of a statistically significant advantage of combined treatment over antidepressant medication. Fluoxetine and cognitive behavioral therapy have been the most widely studied treatments prescribed for adolescents.

Medications that have been used for unipolar major depression include SSRIs, serotonin–norepinephrine reuptake inhibitors, and tricyclic antidepressants (TCAs). As a class, SSRIs have the most evidence for safety and efficacy in adolescents. However, a Cochrane Review of studies of SSRIs in children and adolescents found significant methodologic flaws and risk of bias in all trials. Among the SSRIs, more consistent evidence exists for the efficacy of fluoxetine than for other antidepressants in treating adolescent depression. Most treatment guidelines recommend fluoxetine as first-line medical therapy for adolescents with depression. Therefore, fluoxetine would be the preferred choice for this patient.

Some data show efficacy of sertraline for pediatric unipolar major depression, and the medication often is used as second-line therapy in patients who do not respond to fluoxetine. Escitalopram and citalopram have shown some benefit in pediatric and adolescent depression. Randomized trials of paroxetine, another SSRI, showed no benefit.

Venlafaxine is a serotonin–norepinephrine reuptake inhibitor. It has shown some efficacy in initial treatment of unipolar major depression in adolescents and in treatment-resistant adolescent depression. However, adverse effects are more common in patients treated with venlafaxine, and long-term follow-up outcomes seem better with SSRIs. Therefore, venlafaxine is not the first choice for this patient.

In treatment of adults with depression, TCAs can be effective. Studies in children have not shown benefit. Further, TCAs have an unfavorable adverse effect profile and can be lethal in overdose, which is of particular concern in adolescents at high risk of suicide. Amitriptyline is a TCA and is not the best choice for this patient.

St. John's wort, *Hypericum perforatum*, is a five-petaled yellow flower that has been touted as a natural remedy for depression. Studies in adults have yielded inconsistent results; to date, no good quality data for the use of St. John's wort in children have been published. It is not recommended for pediatric depression. As an herbal product, it is not well standardized or well regulated. Because St. John's wort induces hepatic enzymes, there is significant potential for interaction with prescription medications, including oral contraceptives.

In 2004, the U.S. Food and Drug Administration issued a black box warning on antidepressants indicating that they were associated with an increase in suicidal thinking and behavior in children, adolescents, and young adults. This warning has sparked controversy because of the concern that it will decrease diagnosis and treatment of depression in spite of the known substantial risk of morbidity and mortality posed by untreated depression. Adolescents who screen positive for depression should be assessed for potential to harm self or others. Suicidal ideation is a key predictor of suicide attempts and suicide. Management of depression should include a safety plan that restricts access to lethal means, engages a concerned third party, and develops an emergency communication mechanism.

American Psychiatric Association. Bipolar and related disorders. Diagnostic and statistical manual of mental disorders: DSM-5. 5th ed. Washington, DC: APA; 2013. p. 123–54.

Bonin L, Moreland CS. Overview of treatment for pediatric depression. In: Post TW, editors. Uptodate. Waltham (MA): UpToDate; 2016.

Friedman RA. Antidepressants' black-box warning—10 years later. N Engl J Med 2014;371:1666–8.

Lewandowski RE, Acri MC, Hoagwood KE, Olfson M, Clarke G, Gardner W, et al. Evidence for the management of adolescent depression. Pediatrics 2013;132:e996–1009.

Moreland CS, Bonin L. Pediatric unipolar depression and pharmacotherapy: choosing a medication. In: Post TW, editors. Uptodate. Waltham (MA): UpToDate; 2016.

Stone MB. The FDA warning on antidepressants and suicidality—why the controversy? N Engl J Med 2014;371:1668–71.

44

Thrombophilia

A 36-year-old woman, gravida 4, para 2, at 26 weeks of gestation comes to the emergency department with left leg tenderness. Proximal vein compressive ultrasonography reveals a deep vein thrombosis (DVT). The emergency department physician starts her on anticoagulation and schedules her to see you 2 days later for further evaluation. In addition to factor V Leiden, the thrombophilia that you can confirm in her is

(A) protein C deficiency
(B) protein S deficiency
(C) activated protein C resistance
* (D) prothrombin *G20210A* mutation
(E) antithrombin deficiency

Venous thromboembolism, including DVT and pulmonary embolism, is the leading cause of maternal morbidity in the United States, with an incidence of 1 in 1,600 births. Establishing the etiology in this patient is important for counseling regarding contraception, future pregnancy, and subsequent management of postpartum anticoagulation. The thrombotic potential of pregnancy as a result of decreased anticoagulant activity and fibrinolysis is exacerbated by insulin resistance, hyperlipidemia, hormone-mediated increase in venous capacitance, and venous stasis secondary to compression of the inferior vena cava by the gravid uterus. Physical examination may reveal unilateral swelling with a disparity in calf diameter. A thrombosed vein may be appreciated as a painful, palpable cord. In pregnancy, DVTs tend to be left sided. The D-dimer test is not useful in the diagnosis of DVT in the described patient because D-dimer typically increases in pregnancy. Most often, the diagnosis is based on proximal vein compressive ultrasonography. Wells score has been used in nonpregnant patients to categorize low, moderate, or high risk of DVT, but its use has not been validated in pregnant patients.

All patients with newly diagnosed, unexplained venous thromboembolism should be evaluated for thrombophilias, which can be either inherited or acquired. Inherited thrombophilias include antithrombin, prothrombin *G20210A* mutation, factor V Leiden, protein C deficiency, and protein S deficiency (Appendix D). Prothrombin *G20210A* mutation can be tested regardless of pregnancy, acute thrombosis, or anticoagulation because it involves DNA analysis. Similarly, factor V Leiden mutation can be assessed via DNA analysis at any time. However, because of cost, the initial tests for the factor V Leiden mutation typically are functional assays that detect functional activated protein C resistance. Pregnancy and heparin anticoagulation can result in false-positive test results; therefore, positive test results should prompt confirmatory genetic testing. Protein C, protein S, and antithrombin deficiency can be assessed during pregnancy (although the cutoff values defining protein S deficiency vary by trimester) but cannot be tested during acute thrombosis or while the patient is receiving anticoagulation therapy.

The prevalence of factor V Leiden mutation in Europeans is approximately 5%. It is important to test for all of the aforementioned thrombophilias because the patient may have a low-risk thrombophilia, such as heterozygous factor V Leiden, or a high-risk mutation status, such as homozygous factor V Leiden or prothrombin/factor V Leiden compound heterozygosity. Given her current venous thromboembolism, her risk of recurrent venous thromboembolism in pregnancy would be increased from 10% (heterozygous factor V Leiden) to 17% (homozygous factor V Leiden) to greater than 20% (compound heterozygote).

Once venous thromboembolism is diagnosed in pregnancy, the patient should be started on therapeutic anticoagulation, preferably with low-molecular-weight (LMW) heparin; unfractionated heparin also is acceptable. Therapeutic anticoagulation should be continued for the duration of the pregnancy and, typically, postpartum (Table 44-1). Usually, it is recommended that patients taking LMW heparin convert to unfractionated heparin at approximately 36 weeks of gestation because it can be reversed more readily with protamine sulfate than can LMW heparin and has a shorter half-life. If 24 hours have passed after a patient has taken a therapeutic dose of LMW heparin, regional anesthesia may be administered. Postpartum anticoagulation can be restarted 4–6 hours after a vaginal delivery and 6–12 hours after cesarean delivery. Patients can breastfeed while using these medications.

Table 44-1. Recommended Thromboprophylaxis for Pregnancies Complicated by Inherited Thrombophilias*

Clinical Scenario	Antepartum Management	Postpartum Management
Low-risk thrombophilia† without previous VTE	Surveillance without anticoagulation therapy	Surveillance without anticoagulation therapy or postpartum anticoagulation therapy if the patient has additional risks factors‡
Low-risk thrombophilia with a family history (first-degree relative) of VTE	Surveillance without anticoagulation therapy	Postpartum anticoagulation therapy or intermediate-dose LMWH/UFH
Low-risk thrombophilia† with a single previous episode of VTE—Not receiving long-term anticoagulation therapy	Prophylactic or intermediate-dose LMWH/UFH or surveillance without anticoagulation therapy	Postpartum anticoagulation therapy or intermediate-dose LMWH/UFH
High-risk thrombophilia§ without previous VTE	Surveillance without anticoagulation therapy, or prophylactic LMWH or UFH	Postpartum anticoagulation therapy
High-risk thrombophilia§ with a single previous episode of VTE or an affected first-degree relative—Not receiving long-term anticoagulation therapy	Prophylactic, intermediate-dose, or adjusted-dose LMWH/UFH regimen	Postpartum anticoagulation therapy, or intermediate or adjusted-dose LMWH/UFH for 6 weeks (therapy level should be at least as high as antepartum treatment)
No thrombophilia with previous single episode of VTE associated with transient risk factor that is no longer present—Excludes pregnancy- or estrogen-related risk factor	Surveillance without anticoagulation therapy	Postpartum anticoagulation therapy‖
No thrombophilia with previous single episode of VTE associated with transient risk factor that was pregnancy- or estrogen-related	Prophylactic-dose LMWH or UFH‖	Postpartum anticoagulation therapy
No thrombophilia with previous single episode of VTE without an associated risk factor (idiopathic)—Not receiving long-term anticoagulation therapy	Prophylactic-dose LMWH or UFH‖	Postpartum anticoagulation therapy
Thrombophilia or no thrombophilia with two or more episodes of VTE—Not receiving long-term anticoagulation therapy	Prophylactic or therapeutic-dose LMWH or Prophylactic or therapeutic-dose UFH	Postpartum anticoagulation therapy or Therapeutic-dose LMWH/UFH for 6 weeks
Thrombophilia or no thrombophilia with two or more episodes of VTE—Receiving long-term anticoagulation therapy	Therapeutic-dose LMWH or UFH	Resumption of long-term anticoagulation therapy

Abbreviations: LMWH, low-molecular-weight heparin; UFH, unfractionated heparin; VTE, venous thromboembolism.

*Postpartum treatment levels should be greater or equal to antepartum treatment.

†Low-risk thrombophilia: factor V Leiden heterozygous; prothrombin *G20210A* heterozygous; protein C or protein S deficiency.

‡First-degree relative with a history of a thrombotic episode before age 50 years, or other major thrombotic risk factors (eg, obesity or prolonged immobility).

§High-risk thrombophilia: antithrombin deficiency; double heterozygous for prothrombin *G20210A* mutation and factor V Leiden; factor V Leiden homozygous or prothrombin *G20210A* mutation homozygous.

‖Surveillance without anticoagulation therapy is supported as an alternative approach by some experts.

Inherited thrombophilias in pregnancy. Practice Bulletin No. 138. American College of Obstetricians and Gynecologists. Obstet Gynecol 2013;122:706–17.

Erkens PM, Prins MH. Fixed dose subcutaneous low molecular weight heparins versus adjusted dose unfractionated heparin for venous thromboembolism. Cochrane Database of Systematic Reviews 2010, Issue 9. Art. No.: CD001100. DOI: 10.1002/14651858.CD001100.pub3.

Inherited thrombophilias in pregnancy. Practice Bulletin No. 138. American College of Obstetricians and Gynecologists. Obstet Gynecol 2013;122:706–17.

Kujovich JL. Factor V Leiden thrombophilia. Genet Med 2011;13:1–16.

Prevention of deep vein thrombosis and pulmonary embolism. ACOG Practice Bulletin No. 84. American College of Obstetricians and Gynecologists. Obstet Gynecol 2007;110:429–40.

45

Contraceptive counseling after thrombosis

A 26-year-old woman, gravida 1, para 1, is referred to you by her hematologist for sterilization. She would like to get pregnant again in 2 years, but her hematologist has told her that birth control is not safe for her because of her history of deep vein thrombosis (DVT) in her left leg. During her last pregnancy (delivered 8 months ago), she developed a DVT at 14 weeks of gestation and received anticoagulation therapy during and after her otherwise uncomplicated pregnancy. She reports normal cycles and is otherwise healthy, with a body mass index (calculated as weight in kilograms divided by height in meters squared [kg/m^2]) of 24. She is with a new partner and was diagnosed with chlamydial infection last week but has not yet been treated. She is resistant to injectable contraception (depot medroxyprogesterone acetate) because she fears weight gain and would like to avoid anything that requires a pelvic examination. She has a very busy job and says she is not good at remembering to take medication. The most appropriate birth control method for her is

* (A) contraceptive implant
(B) levonorgestrel intrauterine device (IUD)
(C) progestin-only oral contraceptives (OCs)
(D) surgical sterilization
(E) copper IUD

Pregnancy is known to be a prothrombotic state, with pregnant women having a fourfold to fivefold increased risk of venous thromboembolism relative to their age-matched, nonpregnant counterparts, with risk increasing throughout pregnancy and the postpartum period. In a recent meta-analysis, the pooled incidence of pregnancy-associated venous thromboembolism was 1.4%. Most of these clots occur on the left, likely from compression of the left iliac vein. Pregnancy and the postpartum period offer all three components of the Virchow triad—hypercoagulability, venous stasis, and vascular damage. Thus, pregnancy-related clot risk does not return to baseline until approximately 6 weeks postpartum. Although pregnancy can be managed safely with anticoagulation in women with DVT, this high-risk scenario mandates management by an experienced or specialized obstetrician–gynecologist or other health care provider.

For the described patient, a contraceptive implant is the most appropriate choice, given her medical history and preferences. The device is a 3-year, subdermal, progestin-only (etonogestrel) implant that is inserted into the upper arm. Although estrogen-containing contraception is associated with an approximate doubling of venous thromboembolism risk in the average woman, this is not thought to be the case for progestin-only contraceptives. The estrogen in combination hormonal contraceptives increases hepatic production of serum globulins involved in coagulation (factor VII, factor X, and fibrinogen), thereby increasing clot risk. Although some data suggest variation in thromboembolic risk with different progestins, the main thrombotic effect seen with contraception seems to be from the estrogenic component. Therefore, the Centers for Disease Control and Prevention rates combination hormonal contraception a category 4 in women with a history of DVT who are not taking anticoagulation therapy, meaning that it poses unacceptable health risks and should not be used (Box 45-1). Other women who should not use OCs because of thromboembolic risk include those with an elevated risk of recurrent venous thromboembolism, acute DVT, history of estrogen-associated venous thromboembolism, pregnancy-associated venous thromboembolism,

BOX 45-1

Categories of Medical Eligibility Criteria for Contraceptive Use

1 = A condition for which there is no restriction for the use of the contraceptive method
2 = A condition for which the advantages of using the method generally outweigh the theoretical or proven risks
3 = A condition for which the theoretical or proven risks usually outweigh the advantages of using the method
4 = A condition that represents an unacceptable health risk if the contraceptive method is used

U.S. Medical Eligibility Criteria for Contraceptive Use, 2010. Centers for Disease Control and Prevention. MMWR Recomm Rep 2010;59 (RR-4):1–86.

idiopathic venous thromboembolism, known thrombophilia, active cancer, and history of recurrent venous thromboembolism. The other methods described (ie, implants, levonorgestrel IUDs, and surgical sterilization) are ranked as category 2, except for the copper IUD, which is category 1. For further guidance and a comprehensive set of evidence-based guidelines for contraceptive initiation and continuation, see the Centers for Disease Control and Prevention's *Medical Eligibility Criteria for Contraceptive Use* at http://www.cdc.gov/mmwr/volumes/65/rr/rr6503a1.htm; this information also is available as an app.

Although progestin-only OCs would be safe for the described patient, she is worried about her ability to remember to take medication daily. Progestin-only OCs are very effective if taken at the same time every day, but typical use rates have a failure rate of approximately 9%. The levonorgestrel IUD and the copper IUD are safe in women with a history of thrombosis and share the benefit of having similar perfect-use and typical-use failure rates of less than 1%. Both IUDs must be placed by an obstetrician–gynecologist or other health care provider, but they then require almost no ongoing involvement of the user, which in part explains their high rates of effectiveness. However, this patient prefers a contraceptive method that does not require a pelvic examination. Moreover, she is known to have a chlamydial infection that has not been treated, which would necessitate a delay in IUD placement.

Surgical sterilization is not a reasonable option in a woman who would like to become pregnant again. The American College of Obstetricians and Gynecologists recommends that all patients with a prior DVT in pregnancy should be tested for antiphospholipid antibodies and inherited thrombophilias before becoming pregnant again. Results of this testing can help obstetrician–gynecologists and other health care providers select the most appropriate thromboprophylaxis to maximize fetal and maternal health outcomes.

Meng K, Hu X, Peng X, Zhang Z. Incidence of venous thromboembolism during pregnancy and the puerperium: a systematic review and meta-analysis. J Matern Fetal Neonatal Med 2015;28:245–53.

Thromboembolism in pregnancy. Practice Bulletin No. 123. American College of Obstetricians and Gynecologists. Obstet Gynecol 2011;118:718–29.

Trussell J. Contraceptive failure in the United States. Contraception 2011;83:397–404.

U.S. Medical Eligibility Criteria for Contraceptive Use, 2016. MMWR Recomm Rep 2016;65(RR-3):1–104. DOI: http://dx.doi.org/10.15585/mmwr.rr6503a1.

Vandenbroucke JP, Rosing J, Bloemenkamp KW, Middeldorp S, Helmerhorst FM, Bouma BN, et al. Oral contraceptives and the risk of venous thrombosis. N Engl J Med 2001;344:1527–35.

46

Elder abuse and neglect

An 86-year-old recently widowed woman comes to your office for her annual well-woman examination. She is living independently and has been brought to see you by her son. She is taking multiple medications and is hypertensive despite taking two antihypertensive medications. She has lost 6.8 kg (15 lb) over the past 2 years, and her clothing is soiled and stained. You are worried about her ability to care for herself, but her son tells you that everything is fine and she is just down because of the loss of her husband. The most appropriate next step is to

(A) encourage her to see her primary care physician
(B) assess her financial condition
* (C) report the situation to adult protective services
(D) arrange guardianship

An estimated 1–2 million U.S. citizens older than 65 years have been injured, exploited, or mistreated by someone who is supposed to be caring for them. Elder abuse or neglect is the intentional mistreatment of an elderly person by an individual or facility. This abuse can take many forms (ie, financial, neglect or abandonment, physical, psychological or emotional, sexual). Willful abuse includes infliction of physical or emotional pain and suffering and can include sexual abuse. Financial exploitation has been reported in up to 5% of seniors and includes acts of spending money, forging or forcing the senior's signature, not providing copies of documents, or making poor financial decisions on behalf of the senior.

Populations at increased risk of elder abuse include women older than 75 years; African American women; individuals who have a disability; women with fewer than 12 years of education; and those who have unmarried status, cognitive impairment, a lack of social ties, an annual income of less than $5,000, or nonspousal household members.

Self-neglect is defined as a category of neglect in which the elder may have the capacity to make good decisions for her own sake but does not. A patient who lacks decisional capacity may believe that she is able to take care of herself but is unable to recognize her limitations or even that there is a problem. *Decisional capacity* is defined as the ability of the patient to understand relevant information and the relative situation and consequences or to communicate that decision to caregivers. An elderly woman may be able to make decisions for herself but may lack the ability to carry out or implement those decisions; this is referred to as a lack of executive capacity. If a woman is cognitively impaired, she may not be able to make good decisions for her self-care.

When a patient who is older than 60 years presents for an office visit, the gynecologist has the opportunity to screen for elder abuse. In fact, other than the primary caregivers, the physician may be the only individual with whom such a patient may come into contact. The elderly woman may not be able to recognize that she is being mistreated or may not remember certain circumstances. She also may be reluctant to report mistreatment for fear of being removed from her home or implicating family members. Barriers to clinician recognition include a lack of simple screening tools, time, accurate responses from a cognitively impaired individual, knowledge of risk factors and warning signs, knowledge about what resources are available, or knowledge of the legal requirement in most states to report suspected cases of abuse. Many states have adult protective services in place, and it is important for obstetrician–gynecologists or other health care providers to become familiar with their state's requirements. The obstetrician–gynecologist or other health care provider does not have to ascertain with certainty that mistreatment is occurring but should contact the appropriate authorities to indicate a suspicion of elder abuse. The National Center on Elder Abuse, a division of the Department of Health and Human Services, has resources for obstetrician–gynecologists or other health care providers (http://www.ncea.aoa.gov/resources/). In cases in which the practitioner suspects abuse, the physician has an ethical imperative to report his or her suspicions to government authorities.

The practitioner should be alert to clues that mistreatment is occurring. Poor hygiene or nail care, weight loss, unkempt appearance, missing appliances (eg, glasses, dentures, or hearing aids), or inappropriate attire may be clues of potential neglect. Additional clues may include issues with medication management, inappropriate dosage of medications, or failure to monitor therapy. Patients may be nontherapeutic on medication because they have the medications but do not take them, or they cannot afford them. Physical findings can include pressure ulcers or abrasions, lacerations, bruising, burns, and tearing of skin. Fractures (other than wrist, hip, or vertebrae), particularly spiral fractures, can be signs of ongoing abuse. Malnutrition or dehydration can be a sign of neglect or financial abuse. Financial abuse may be suspected if the patient has a change in the ability to pay for medications, housing, and utilities.

During a patient encounter, the obstetrician–gynecologist or other health care provider should

- interview the patient separately and be aware that family members and caregivers may be abusers
- start with general, open-ended questions and progress to more specific questions
- note inconsistent or frequently changing stories
- observe the patient's reactions to accompanying family members or caregivers
- remain empathetic

Possible cases of elder abuse can be screened using the Elder Abuse Suspicion Index shown in Table 46-1.

Referral to primary care may be appropriate for medical management of chronic medical conditions but does not remove the obstetrician–gynecologist's or other health care provider's responsibility to report cases of possible elder abuse. The obstetrician–gynecologist or other health care provider does not have the responsibility to investigate the financial condition of the patient or to arrange guardianship, but referrals to resources that can make those determinations are the responsibility of the physician.

The practitioner has the ethical and legal imperative to report suspected cases to adult protective services. The prudent clinician also will partner with social workers, nurses, and mental health workers in order to make referrals for at-risk women.

TABLE 46-1. Performing the Elder Abuse Suspicion Index (EASI).

EASI questions 1–5 are asked of the patient; question 6 is answered by the doctor.

All six questions should be queried in the order they appear on this index. A response of "yes" to one or more of questions 2–6 should raise concern about mistreatment.

Within the last six months:

Question			
1) Have you relied on people for any of the following: bathing, dressing, shopping, banking, or meals?	Yes	No	Did not answer
2) Has anyone prevented you from getting food, clothes, medication, glasses, hearing aids or medical care, or from being with people you wanted to be with?	Yes	No	Did not answer
3) Have you been upset because someone talked to you in a way that made you feel shamed or threatened?	Yes	No	Did not answer
4) Has anyone tried to force you to sign papers or to use your money against your will?	Yes	No	Did not answer
5) Has anyone made you afraid, touched you in ways that you did not want, or hurt you physically?	Yes	No	Did not answer
6) **Doctor:** Elder abuse may be associated with findings such as: poor eye contact, withdrawn nature, malnourishment, hygiene issues, cuts, bruises, inappropriate clothing, or medication compliance issues. Did you notice any of these today or in the last 12 months?	Yes	No	Not sure

Yaffe MJ, Wolfson C, Weiss D, Lithwick M. Development and validation of a tool to assist physicians' identification of elder abuse: The Elder Abuse Suspicion Index (EASI). J Elder Abuse Negl 2008;20:276–300. Reprinted by permission of the publisher (Taylor & Francis Ltd, http://www.tandfonline.com).

Acierno R, Hernandez MA, Amstadter AB, Resnick HS, Steve K, Muzzy W, et al. Prevalence and correlates of emotional, physical, sexual, and financial abuse and potential neglect in the United States: the National Elder Mistreatment Study. Am J Public Health. 2010;100:292–7.

Halphen JM, Varas GM, Sadowsky JM. Recognizing and reporting elder abuse and neglect. Geriatrics 2009;64(7):13–8.

Hoover RM, Polson M. Detecting elder abuse and Neglect: Assessment and intervention. Am Fam Physician 2014;89:453–60.

National Center for Elder Abuse. Resources. Available at: http://www.ncea.aoa.gov/resources/. Retrieved June 16, 2016.

Yaffe MJ, Wolfson C, Weiss D, Lithwick M. Development and validation of a tool to improve physicians identification of elder abuse: The Elder Abuse Suspicion Index (EASI). J Elder Abuse Negl 2008;20:276–300.

47

Unintended pregnancy

A 24-year-old woman comes to the emergency department with pelvic pain and irregular bleeding. Her pregnancy test is positive, and ultrasonography confirms an intrauterine gestational sac with a yolk sac but no fetal pole or heartbeat. She is using an oral contraceptive but states that she often starts a new pack of oral contraceptives late. She has had one previous unplanned pregnancy that ended in a miscarriage. On examination, she is not bleeding, her uterus is 6–7 weeks of gestation in size, and her cervix is closed. After discussion of her options, she decides she wants an abortion. The best next step in management is

(A) serum β-hCG level
(B) follow-up ultrasonography
* (C) pregnancy termination
(D) referral to social worker for counseling

Almost one half of U.S. women have experienced an unintended pregnancy, and about one half of unintended pregnancies end in abortion. Counseling of a patient about her options at the time of diagnosis of an unintended pregnancy should be influenced by the patient's desires about pregnancy continuation. When the diagnosis of pregnancy is made early, as with the described patient, it can be unclear if the pregnancy is simply an early intrauterine pregnancy or will become a spontaneous abortion. For a patient who wishes to continue the pregnancy, expectant management and follow-up testing are appropriate to determine viability.

Sometimes a patient is diagnosed with an unintended pregnancy before the location of the gestation can be confirmed. In such cases, ectopic pregnancy is a possibility. In the absence of symptoms, an obstetrician–gynecologist or other health care provider can follow serum β-hCG levels until they reach the discriminatory zone and then perform ultrasonography to locate the pregnancy. If a pregnancy is not desired, another alternative is to perform dilation and curettage to obtain tissue for microscopic pathologic examination. If the tissue examination reveals chorionic villi, then an intrauterine pregnancy is confirmed. Because it has been established that the described patient's pregnancy is intrauterine, there is no need for further β-hCG testing.

New ultrasonographic guidelines have been suggested for how to determine early pregnancy failure. These cutoffs aim for a specificity and positive predictive value of 100% for diagnosis of a nonviable pregnancy. Yet these proposed guidelines do not take into consideration the desirability of the pregnancy. If the patient wants to continue the pregnancy, repeat ultrasonography in 10–14 days would help to determine viability. However, for a patient who does not wish to continue the pregnancy, there is no medical need to establish whether this is a pregnancy loss, and ultrasonography should not be repeated. Because abortion should be performed as early in the pregnancy as possible, there is no need to delay the procedure until viability or loss has been confirmed.

When a patient is faced with an unexpected pregnancy, she may have many feelings and be uncertain as to how to proceed. Options counseling should be performed in a sensitive, unhurried manner and should cover all options for a pregnancy—continuing the pregnancy to term and keeping the baby, continuing the pregnancy and placing the child for adoption, and abortion. Not all patients will be able to make a decision on the day of pregnancy diagnosis. Some patients will need more time to consider the decision, some will consult with family or friends, and some will need more information or even psychologic counseling or spiritual guidance. Social work referral can be helpful to provide guidance about financial resources, as can referral to adoption agencies for more information. Unless the current patient has asked or has demonstrated a clear need for such information, a social work referral is not required.

If the patient is clear that she does not wish to continue with the pregnancy, counseling should shift to management options. A patient in the early first trimester, at 9 weeks of gestation or earlier, can be offered surgical or medical termination (or referral for same). The American College of Obstetricians and Gynecologists has stated that "physicians and other health care providers have the duty to refer patients in a timely manner to other providers if they do not feel that they can in conscience provide the standard reproductive services that patients request." Although an obstetrician–gynecologist or other health care provider is under no legal obligation to provide pregnancy termination, the American College of Obstetricians and Gynecologists' policy holds that obstetrician–gynecologists and other health care providers should not impose their personal beliefs upon their patients, nor should those beliefs be allowed to compromise patient health, access to care (including timely access), or informed consent. The described patient should be either scheduled for pregnancy termination or referred to an obstetrician–gynecologist or other health care provider who offers that service.

American College of Obstetricians and Gynecologists. Abortion policy. College Statement of Policy. Washington, DC: American College of Obstetricians and Gynecologists; 2014. Retrieved June 17, 2016.

Doubilet PM, Benson CB, Bourne T, Blaivas M. Diagnostic criteria for nonviable pregnancy early in the first trimester. N Engl J Med 2013; 369:1443–51.

The limits of conscientious refusal in reproductive medicine. ACOG Committee Opinion No. 385. American College of Obstetricians and Gynecologists. Obstet Gynecol 2007;110:1203–8.

48

Gastroesophageal reflux disease

A 60-year-old obese woman comes to your office with a 12-month history of intermittent, but progressively worsening, nonproductive cough. Her symptoms are most pronounced at night but occur during the day as well, usually after meals. She says she has experienced the sensation of "regurgitating" during these coughing paroxysms, but she reports no dysphagia. She has not experienced fevers, chills, weight loss, gastrointestinal bleeding, or anorexia. She has a 20-pack-per-year history of smoking, although she has recently started a quit-smoking program. Her medical history is otherwise unremarkable. The best next step in this patient's management is

(A) upper endoscopy
(B) barium swallow
* (C) proton pump inhibitor (PPI)
(D) elimination of reflux-triggering foods
(E) promotility agent

Gastroesophageal reflux disease (GERD) is the gastrointestinal condition encountered most commonly by primary care physicians and gastroenterologists in the outpatient setting. In the United States, prevalence rates are as high as 20% in the general population and 6–17% in the elderly. However, a true prevalence is difficult to determine because of the nebulous definition of *GERD* and the fact that prevalence rates are based largely on self-reports of chronic "heartburn." A current definition of *GERD* based on the Montreal classification is "a condition which develops when the reflux of stomach contents causes troublesome symptoms (ie, at least two heartburn episodes per week) and/or complications." Although many cases of GERD can be attributed to lifestyle and environmental factors, additional risk factors include central obesity, trauma, pregnancy, age, and genetic predisposition. New-onset GERD is associated with increasing age, female sex, lower education, gain in body mass index (calculated as weight in kilograms divided by height in meters squared [kg/m^2]), and current or prior tobacco use.

The condition can manifest with a wide array of symptoms that can be either typical or atypical (Appendix E). Typical symptoms of GERD are acid regurgitation and heartburn, which result from the abnormal reflux of gastric contents into the esophagus. However, gastric contents also can enter the oral cavity, larynx, and lungs and result in atypical symptoms, such as chronic cough, halitosis, bronchospasm (asthma), laryngitis, otitis, and chest discomfort. In general, symptoms tend to be more common after meals and often are exacerbated by the patient being in a recumbent position, as in this patient, who has worsening symptoms at night and after meals. A presumptive diagnosis of GERD can be made when a patient has the typical symptoms of heartburn or regurgitation.

Atypical symptoms, such as nausea, bloating, belching, dyspepsia, and epigastric pain, may overlap with typical symptoms but could be suggestive of additional diagnoses, such as achalasia, peptic ulcer disease, gastritis, and gastroparesis. Extraesophageal symptoms, such as chronic cough, asthma, laryngitis, halitosis, and dental erosions, result from microaspiration of refluxate or triggering of the esophagobronchial reflex by the vagal nerve.

The presence of extraesophageal symptoms in isolation should not uniformly be attributed to GERD in the absence of other typical symptoms. A comprehensive history is extremely valuable to facilitate making the correct diagnosis and, thus, allowing for empiric medical therapy. Medical therapy is geared toward acid suppression using antacids, histamine-2 receptor antagonists, or PPIs.

The described patient has typical and atypical symptoms of GERD; thus, empiric medical therapy with a PPI would be the best next course of therapy for her. The use of a PPI has been found to be effective for most patients regardless of age. Although reflux symptoms tend to be chronic, with or without esophagitis, the rate of healing of esophagitis among patients treated with PPIs was 30% greater than the rate of healing among patients treated with histamine-2 receptor antagonists.

Patients may exhibit no symptoms and still have significant findings at the time of endoscopic evaluation. However, upper endoscopy is not required in the presence of typical GERD symptoms. Endoscopic evaluation with biopsies is warranted in the presence of alarm symptoms (ie, dysphagia, bleeding, weight loss, anemia, recurrent vomiting) as well as for screening of patients at high risk of complications. Similarly, routine biopsies of the distal esophagus solely for the diagnosis of GERD are not recommended.

Because of the high prevalence of this condition and the potential for long-term complications, such as erosive esophagitis, peptic stricture, Barrett esophagus, esophageal adenocarcinoma, and pulmonary disease, it is critical that obstetrician–gynecologists and other health care providers have a clear understanding of the current approach to diagnosis and management. A barium swallow would be reserved for more complex evaluations and should not be performed for the routine diagnosis of GERD.

Lifestyle modification, such as weight loss, avoidance of meals 2–3 hours before bedtime, and head-of-bed elevation, often are beneficial for the reduction of reflux symptoms. Additionally, avoidance of fatty or spicy foods also can reduce symptom frequency and severity, but complete elimination of all foods that can trigger reflux is not recommended in the treatment of GERD and would not be the best next therapy for this patient.

Acid suppression therapy remains the mainstay of medical management for GERD. Although most patients affected by this condition typically do not secrete more acid in comparison with controls, reduction of acid does promote healing in the setting of erosive esophagitis. Ideally, the best therapy for GERD would prevent reflux without necessarily altering acid secretion by the use of a promotility agent. There is a lack of evidence to suggest efficacy of promotility agents for the primary treatment of GERD as well as a high rate of adverse effects. As such, routine use of promotility drugs for the treatment of GERD, especially in an elderly patient, should be avoided.

Gastroesophageal reflux disease is a chronic disease that requires long-term management. The optimal criteria for the diagnosis of GERD and for the assessment of extraesophageal symptoms, such as chronic cough, remain unclear. Additionally, the risks and benefits of indefinitely continuing acid suppression therapy and the ideal degree of acid inhibition are important considerations. Prompt diagnosis in conjunction with initiation of empiric therapy can lead to significant improvement in quality of life and avoidance of complications.

Achem SR, DeVault KR. Gastroesophageal reflux disease and the elderly. Gastroenterol Clin N Am 2014;43:147–60.

Badillo R, Francis D. Diagnosis and treatment of gastroesophageal reflux disease. World J Gastrointest Pharmacol Ther 2014;5:108–12.

Hallan A, Bomme M, Hveem K, Moller-Hansen J, Ness-Jensen E. Risk factors on the development of new-onset gastroesophageal reflux symptoms. A population-based prospective cohort study: the HUNT study. Am J Gastroenterol 2015;110:393–400; quiz 401.

Kahrilas P. Gastroesophageal reflux disease: Clinical Practice. N Engl J Med 2008;359:1700–7.

Katz PO, Gerson LB, Vela MF. Guidelines for the diagnosis and management of gastroesophageal reflux disease. Am J Gastroenterol 2013;108:308–28; quiz 329.

49

Dense breast tissue and mammography

A 63-year-old woman, gravida 4, para 4, calls your office after receiving her mammography result in the mail. The report states that she was classified as category 2 using the Breast Imaging Reporting and Data System (BI-RADS) 2 and that she has extremely dense breasts. The report further indicates that she should discuss her results with her physician. She had menarche at age 12 years. Her first child was born when she was age 25 years, and she had a biopsy 8 years ago for fibrocystic disease of the breast. Her maternal grandmother had breast cancer in her 60s. In addition to clinical breast examination and breast self-awareness, you recommend that she receive

* (A) digital mammography
(B) magnetic resonance imaging (MRI) scan
(C) xerography
(D) ultrasonography

Breast cancer is one of the most common types of cancer in women, with a 12% lifetime risk. Well-recognized risk factors for the development of breast cancer include early menarche, low parity, family history, delayed childbirth, and some genetic risk factors. Mammography has been shown to be beneficial in identifying early cancer, and treatment of cancer detected early leads to decreased mortality. For women without risk factors, the American College of Obstetricians and Gynecologists recommends offering screening digital mammography annually starting at age 40 years. Other organizations, including the U.S. Preventive Services Task Force, have published alternative screening schedules. It should be noted that screening mammography implies that the patient is asymptomatic. Symptomatic patients should have a diagnostic procedure that, in addition to mammography, may include ultrasonography or breast biopsy.

Mammography results are commonly reported using the BI-RADS system with risk of underlying malignancy reported using categories 0–6. A woman with an essentially 0% likelihood of malignancy will be reported as BI-RADS 1 or BI-RADS 2. Patients rated as BI-RADS 2, such as the described patient, have normal breast tissue but with the presence of other benign structures (Table 49-1).

Premenopausal women typically have breast tissue that appears denser on mammography. As women age, breast tissue typically becomes less dense; however, a large screening trial showed that almost 50% of women still had dense breasts later in life. Mammography reports also contain a description of the breast composition based on the visual estimate of fibroglandular density. The categories reported are the following:

1. The breasts are almost entirely fatty.
2. There are scattered areas of fibroglandular density.
3. The breasts are heterogeneously dense, which may obscure small masses.
4. The breasts are extremely dense, which lowers the sensitivity of mammography.

Women with heterogeneously or extremely dense breasts are at increased relative risk of breast cancer compared with women who have average breast density. In addition, the ability for mammography to detect cancer is diminished in women with dense breasts (Table 49-2).

Magnetic resonance imaging of the breast has been a cost-effective screening tool for women at very high (greater than 20%) risk of cancer—typically, women with a *BRCA* mutation, a strong family history of breast cancer or ovarian cancer, or a history of chest wall radiation. Women who are at low-to-moderate risk have not been shown to benefit from screening MRI.

Breast ultrasonography of the entire breast has a high false-positive rate and requires specialized personnel that are not widely available, so it is not a good option for screening for this patient. Breast xerography is a technique that enhances fine details such as microcalcifications. The images obtained are not superior to current techniques, and the procedure exposes women to higher radiation levels; therefore, this technique has fallen out of favor.

TABLE 49-1. American College of Radiology Concordance Between Breast Imaging-Reporting Data System (BI-RADS) Assessment Categories and Management Recommendations From the American College of Radiology *BI-RADS Atlas, Breast Imaging-Reporting Data System*

Assessment	Management	Likelihood of Cancer
Category 0: Incomplete—Need additional imaging evaluation, prior mammogram for comparison, or both	Recall for additional imaging, comparison with prior examinations(s), or both	N/A
Category 1: Negative	Routine mammography screening	Essentially 0% likelihood of malignancy
Category 2: Benign	Routine mammography screening	Essentially 0% likelihood of malignancy
Category 3: Probably benign	Short-interval (6-month) follow-up or continued surveillance mammography	>0% but ≤2% likelihood of malignancy
Category 4: Suspicious	Tissue diagnosis	>2% but <95% likelihood of malignancy
Category 4A: *Low* suspicion for malignancy		>2% to ≤10% likelihood of malignancy
Category 4B: *Moderate* suspicion for malignancy		>10% to ≤50% likelihood of malignancy
Category 4C: *High* suspicion for malignancy		>50% to <95% likelihood of malignancy
Category 5: Highly suggestive of malignancy	Tissue diagnosis	≥95% likelihood of malignancy
Category 6: Known biopsy-proven malignancy	Surgical excision when clinically appropriate	N/A

Abbreviation: N/A, not applicable.

Sickles EA, D'Orsi CJ, Bassett LW, Appleton CM, Berg WA, Burnside ES, et al. ACR BI-RADS mammography. ACR BI-RADS mammography. ACR BI-RADS atlas, breast imaging reporting and data system. 5th ed. Reston (VA): American College of Radiology; 2013. p. 13–175.

TABLE 49-2. BI-RADS Breast Density Categories, Demographics, Sensitivity of Cancer Detection, and Breast Cancer Risk

BI-RADS Category	Description	Percentage of Population*	Sensitivity† (%)	Relative Risk of Breast Cancer‡
1	Almost entirely fat	10	88	---
2	Scattered fibroglandular densities	43	82	---
3	Heterogeneously dense	39	69	1.2 (compared with average breast density)
4	Extremely dense	8	62	2.1 (compared with average breast density)

Abbreviation: BI-RADS, Breast Imaging Reporting and Data System.

*Pisano ED, Gatsonis C, Hendrick E, Yaffe M, Baum JK, Acharyya S, et al. Diagnostic performance of digital versus film mammography for breast-cancer screening. Digital Mammographic Imaging Screening Trial (DMIST) Investigators Group [published erratum appears in N Engl J Med 2006;355:1840]. N Engl J Med 2005;353:1773–83.

†Carney PA, Miglioretti DL, Yankaskas BC, Kerlikowske K, Rosenberg R, Rutter CM, et al. Individual and combined effects of age, breast density, and hormone replacement therapy use on the accuracy of screening mammography [published erratum appears in Ann Intern Med 2003;138:771]. Ann Intern Med 2003;138:168–75.

‡Sickles EA. The use of breast imaging to screen women at high risk for cancer. Radiol Clin North Am 2010;48:859–78.

Management of women with dense breasts diagnosed by mammography. Committee Opinion No. 625. American College of Obstetricians and Gynecologists. Obstet Gynecol 2015;125:750–1.

Because of the limitations in mammography in women with dense breasts, many states have enacted specific patient notification laws related to breast density. Currently, no published evidence exists to demonstrate meaningful outcome benefits with supplemental or alternative testing (eg, ultrasonography, MRI) or alternative screening modalities (eg, breast tomosynthesis, thermography) in women without additional risk factors.

Digital breast tomosynthesis. Technology Assessment in Obstetrics and Gynecology No. 9. American College of Obstetricians and Gynecologists. Obstet Gynecol 2013;121:1415–7.

Kaplan SS. Automated whole breast ultrasound. Radiol Clin North Am 2014;52:539–46.

Management of women with dense breasts diagnosed by mammography. Committee Opinion No. 625. American College of Obstetricians and Gynecologists. Obstet Gynecol 2015;125:750–1.

Onega T, Beaber EF, Sprague BL, Barlow WE, Haas JS, Tosteson AN, et al. Breast cancer screening in an era of personalized regimens: a conceptual model and National Cancer Institute initiative for risk-based and preference-based approaches at a population level. Cancer 2014;120:2955–64.

Sickles EA, D'Orsi CJ, Bassett LW, Appleton CM, Berg WA, Burnside ES, et al. ACR BI-RADS Mammography. In: ACR BI-RADS Atlas, Breast Imaging Reporting and Data System. Reston, VA: American College of Radiology; 2013. p. 13–175.

50

Nonhormonal therapy options for vasomotor symptoms

A 50-year-old woman with a history of depression and a diagnosis of stage II ductal carcinoma of the breast has been taking tamoxifen citrate for 12 months. She tells you that her vasomotor symptoms are interfering with her daily activities and that her depression symptoms have returned. She is otherwise healthy. The best pharmacologic option to reduce the bothersome symptoms in this patient is

(A) paroxetine
* (B) venlafaxine
(C) bupropion hydrochloride
(D) sertraline
(E) fluoxetine

At least three quarters of all menopausal women experience vasomotor symptoms, and one third of these women pursue medical relief of these symptoms. Vasomotor symptoms negatively affect quality of life and persist for an average of 7–10 years. As many as 80% of women who take tamoxifen experience hot flushes as an adverse effect of the medication, and genetic polymorphisms in the estrogen receptor gene may make some women more susceptible to tamoxifen-associated hot flushes. Vasomotor symptoms have been associated with persistence of depression symptoms in women with breast cancer.

Estrogen therapy is the most effective treatment for menopausal vasomotor symptoms. Although hormone therapy is associated with a 75% reduction in the frequency of vasomotor symptoms and a marked reduction in their severity, it is contraindicated in most women with a history of breast cancer. Alternative medical therapies for the treatment of vasomotor symptoms include selective serotonin reuptake inhibitors, serotonin–norepinephrine reuptake inhibitors, gabapentin, and clonidine. Approximate reduction in hot flush frequency has been reported in 40–60% of women after nonhormonal pharmacologic therapies (paroxetine, 50%; citalopram, 55%; escitalopram, 30–60%; venlafaxine, 40%).

Paroxetine is the only nonhormonal agent approved by the U.S. Food and Drug Administration for the treatment of hot flushes. Studies of the effects of other selective serotonin reuptake inhibitors (such as sertraline or fluoxetine) on hot flush reduction have been conflicting, with the balance finding no significant reduction in hot flushes. The effect of bupropion on vasomotor symptoms has not been studied. Strong inhibitors of the drug-metabolizing enzyme *CYP2D6*, such as paroxetine, may decrease the conversion of tamoxifen to its active metabolite. Venlafaxine is not a strong inhibitor of this enzyme and, therefore, would offer the better choice for management of vasomotor symptoms in this patient.

Avis NE, Crawford SL, Greendale G, Bromberger JT, Everson-Rose SA, Gold EB, et al. Duration of menopausal vasomotor symptoms over the menopause transition. Study of Women's Health Across the Nation. JAMA Intern Med 2015;175:531–9.

Avis NE, Levine BJ, Case LD, Naftalis EZ, Van Zee KJ. Trajectories of depressive symptoms following breast cancer diagnosis. Cancer Epidemiol Biomarkers Prev 2015;24:1789–95.

Bardia A, Novotny P, Sloan J, Barton D, Loprinzi C. Efficacy of nonestrogenic hot flash therapies among women stratified by breast cancer history and tamoxifen use: a pooled analysis. Menopause 2009;16:477–83.

Bordeleau L, Pritchard KI, Loprinzi CL, Ennis M, Jugovic O, Warr D, et al. Multicenter, randomized, cross-over clinical trial of venlafaxine versus gabapentin for the management of hot flashes in breast cancer survivors. J Clin Oncol 2010;28:5147–52.

Grant MD, Marbella A, Wang AT, Pines E, Hoag J, Bonnell C, et al. Menopausal symptoms: Comparative effectiveness of therapies. Comparative Effectiveness Review No. 147. Rockville (MD): Agency for Healthcare Research and Quality; 2015. Available at: https://effectivehealthcare.ahrq.gov/ehc/products/353/2051/menopause-report-150305.pdf. Retrieved June 15, 2016.

Jin Y, Hayes DF, Li L, Robarge JD, Skaar TC, Philips S, et al. Estrogen receptor genotypes influence hot flash prevalence and composite score before and after tamoxifen therapy. J Clin Oncol 2008;26:5849–54.

Joffe H, Guthrie KA, LaCroix AZ, Reed SD, Ensrud KE, Manson JE, et al. Low-dose estradiol and the serotonin-norepinephrine reuptake inhibitor venlafaxine for vasomotor symptoms: a randomized clinical trial. JAMA Intern Med 2014;174:1058–66.

51

Osteoporosis and low bone mineral density

A 67-year-old white woman had a routine screening dual-energy X-ray absorptiometry (DXA) scan ordered at the time of her well-woman examination. She has no significant past medical or surgical history. She is taking care of her 91-year-old mother, who has limited mobility because of severe kyphosis from compression fractures. She also has a maternal aunt and a cousin with a history of postmenopausal breast cancer. Her recent physical examination was unremarkable. Her weight is 72.6 kg (160 lb) and her height is 1.62 m (64 in.). Her DXA scan reveals the following *T*-scores: spine, –2.3; hip, –1.9; and femoral neck, –2.1. According to the online World Health Organization Fracture Risk Assessment Tool (FRAX), her 10-year probability of major osteoporotic fracture is 12% and her risk of hip fracture is 2.1%. In this patient, the best option at this time to prevent future vertebral fracture is

* (A) raloxifene hydrochloride
(B) bisphosphonate
(C) teriparatide
(D) denosumab

Women disproportionately bear the morbidity and mortality of osteoporosis because their longer life expectancy equates with more years to suffer a major fracture or spinal compression fracture and because of the sudden decrease in estrogen with the onset of menopause. Menopause marks a time of accelerated bone loss, averaging 6–7%, beginning 1 year before through the first 3 years of estrogen deprivation. Morbidity and loss of function with a major fracture represent a significant burden to patients, their families, and society in general. In fact, a woman with a hip fracture after age 80 years has less than a 60% chance of ambulating again without assistance.

Screening and diagnosis of osteoporosis is best accomplished by means of DXA scans of the lumbar spine, total hip, and femoral neck. All major guidelines recommend that screening begin at age 65 years, or earlier if a patient has a major risk factor for osteoporosis, such as the risk factors listed in Box 51-1. An additional way to accurately

BOX 51-1

When to Screen for Bone Mineral Density Before Age 65 Years

Bone density should be screened in postmenopausal women younger than 65 years if any of the following risk factors are noted:

- Medical history of a fragility fracture
- Body weight less than 57.6 kg (127 lb)
- Medical causes of bone loss (medications or diseases)
- Parental history of hip fracture
- Current smoker
- Alcoholism
- Rheumatoid arthritis

Osteoporosis. Practice Bulletin No. 129. American College of Obstetricians and Gynecologists. Obstet Gynecol 2012;120:718–34.

determine if a woman should be screened earlier is to calculate her 10-year risk of a major osteoporotic fracture using the online FRAX tool available at http://www.sheffield.ac.uk/FRAX/. This tool has been validated in multiple cohorts of women across the world. It takes into account not only many of the risk factors in Box 51-1 but also age, race, body mass index, and country of origin. If the calculator predicts a 10-year fracture risk of 9.3% or greater, which is the risk of fracture for a 65-year-old woman with no risk factors, then a DXA scan should be obtained.

The DXA scan provides a *T*-score, which is a measurement that compares current bone mineral density (BMD) with the BMD of a young, healthy cohort of women. A *T*-score of greater than –1.0 is considered to indicate no increased risk of fracture, whereas a score of –2.5 or less defines osteoporosis and usually is the value at which definitive therapy is recommended. A *T*-score of –1.0 to greater than –2.5 is considered to indicate low BMD and to correlate with a slightly increased fracture risk. Low BMD used to be referred to as "osteopenia" but is now more precisely described as low BMD.

Treatment is recommended for patients with a *T*-score of –2.5 or less. Additionally, treatment should be started for women with a FRAX score with a 10-year risk of 3% or greater for a hip fracture or a risk of 20% or greater for a major osteoporotic fracture. An example of the FRAX calculation specific to the described patient is shown in Figure 51-1. It is important to note that when entering data into the FRAX calculation tool, if a *T*-score is used, only the femoral neck value has been validated. It also should be noted that the FRAX calculation does not take into consideration spine BMD, nor does it factor in a patient's individual risk of falls.

The described patient has a *T*-score of –2.1 at the femoral neck and –2.3 at the spine, both of which are above –2.5. Therefore, she does not meet current DXA criteria for treatment of osteoporosis. This is corroborated with a FRAX calculation below the threshold for treatment of 3% for a hip fracture and 20% for a major osteoporotic fracture in the next 10 years. She does, however, have a lower BMD at the spine, a strong family history of severe kyphosis, and several second-degree relatives with a history of postmenopausal breast cancer. She is, therefore, an excellent candidate for 5 years of therapy with raloxifene for the prevention of osteoporotic fractures and reduction of breast cancer risk.

Raloxifene is a selective estrogen receptor modulator that acts as an antiresorptive agent similar to estrogen for BMD. It is approved by the U.S. Food and Drug Administration for the prevention and treatment of osteoporosis, but fracture risk reduction has consistently been proved only for spinal fractures. Raloxifene also has been approved by the U.S. Food and Drug Administration to

Calculation Tool
Please answer the questions below to calculate the ten year probability of fracture with BMD.
Country: US (Caucasian)
Name/ID:
About the risk factors
Questionnaire:
1. Age (between 40 and 90 years) or Date of Birth
Age:
Date of Birth:
67
Y:
M:
D:
2. Sex
Male
Female
3. Weight (kg)
72.57
4. Height (cm)
162.56
5. Previous Fracture
No Yes
6. Parent Fractured Hip
No Yes
7. Current Smoking
No Yes
8. Glucocorticoids
No Yes
9. Rheumatoid arthritis
No Yes
10. Secondary osteoporosis
No Yes
11. Alcohol 3 or more units/day
No Yes
12. Femoral neck BMD (g/cm²)
T-Score
-2.1
Clear
Calculate
BMI: 27.5
The ten year probability of fracture (%)
with BMD
Major osteoporotic
12
Hip Fracture
2.1
Weight Conversion
Pounds kg
160
Convert
Height Conversion
Inches cm
64
Convert
03581044
Individuals with fracture risk assessed since 1st June 2011

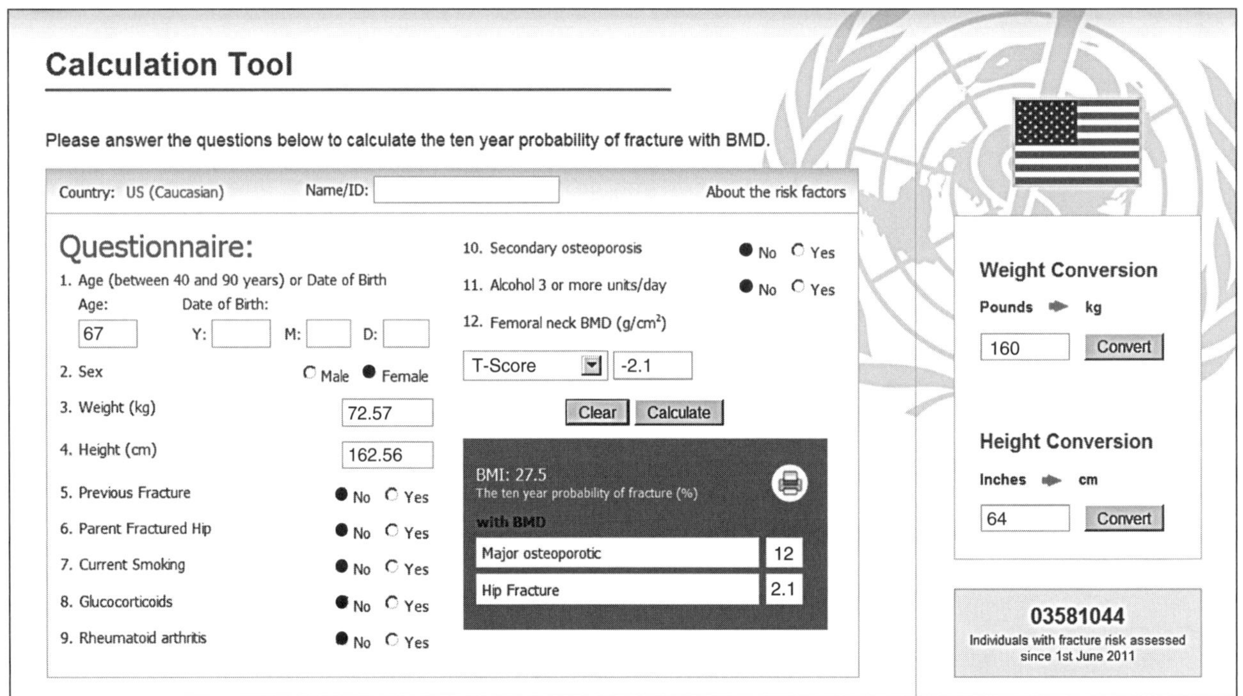

FIGURE 51-1. FRAX calculation tool. Abbreviations: BMD, bone mineral density; BMI, body mass index. FRAX is a sophisticated risk assessment instrument, developed by the University of Sheffield in association with the World Health Organization. It uses risk factors in addition to DXA measurements for improved fracture risk estimation. It is a useful tool to aid clinical decision making about the use of pharmacologic therapies in patients with low bone mass. The International Osteoporosis Foundation supports the maintenance and development of FRAX. Copyright International Osteoporosis Foundation. (Reprinted with permission from the IOF. All rights reserved. WHO Fracture Risk Assessment Tool [FRAX]. Available at: http://www.shef.ac.uk/FRAX/. Retrieved March 7, 2016; June 16, 2016.)

reduce the risk of invasive breast cancer in postmenopausal women. Raloxifene has a similar thromboembolic disease risk to that posed by estrogen, and women may experience an increase or reappearance of vasomotor symptoms.

Bisphosphonates generally are considered to be first-line agents for pharmacologic treatment of osteoporosis, with a proven benefit in fracture risk reduction at the spine and the hip. Patients who have a history of gastrointestinal problems or a history of intolerance to bisphosphonates secondary to gastrointestinal adverse effects are excellent candidates for a parenteral bisphosphonate. Denosumab injection is a good choice for women at very high risk of fracture or who have failed other therapies. Studies have shown a 68% and 40% decrease in fractures at the spine and hip, respectively, with the use of denosumab. Teriparatide injection usually is reserved for patients who have experienced fractures. Because this patient has not been diagnosed with osteoporosis and does not meet FRAX criteria for treatment, raloxifene is the only one of the aforementioned pharmacologic therapies that is indicated for her.

Florence R, Allen S, Benedict L, Compo R, Jensen A, Kalogeropoulou D, et al. Diagnosis and treatment of osteoporosis. 8th ed. Bloomington (MN): Institute for Clinical Systems Improvement; 2013. Available at: https://www.icsi.org/_asset/vnw0c3/Osteo.pdf. Retrieved June 16, 2016.

Management of osteoporosis in postmenopausal women: 2010 position statement of The North American Menopause Society. Menopause 2010;17:25–54; quiz 55–6.

Osteoporosis. Practice Bulletin No. 129. American College of Obstetricians and Gynecologists. Obstet Gynecol 2012;120:718–34.

Screening for osteoporosis: U.S. Preventive Services Task Force Recommendation statement. U.S. Preventive Services Task Force. Ann Intern Med 2011;154:356–64.

WHO Fracture Risk Assessment Tool (FRAX). Available at: http://www.shef.ac.uk/FRAX/. Retrieved March 7, 2016; June 16, 2016.

52

Weight gain associated with contraception

An 18-year-old nulligravid woman is referred to you by her pediatrician for contraceptive counseling. She is newly sexually active and is about to leave for college. She recently worked very hard to lose 4.5 kg (10 lb) and her body mass index (calculated as weight in kilograms divided by height in meters squared [kg/m^2]) is down to 32. She is otherwise healthy but has a severe needle phobia. She has light, predictable menstrual periods and wants a contraceptive method that will maintain little or no bleeding. However, her biggest concern is ensuring that her contraceptive will not cause weight gain. You counsel her that the best birth control method for her is

* (A) levonorgestrel intrauterine device (IUD)
(B) depot medroxyprogesterone acetate (DMPA)
(C) oral contraceptives (OCs)
(D) etonogestrel contraceptive implant
(E) copper IUD

Overweight and obesity is a growing epidemic, with 34% of U.S. adults qualifying as overweight and 35% qualifying as obese. Thus, for many women, additional weight gain from a contraceptive method is not only of personal concern but also of medical concern. Pregnancy is well known to cause weight gain. Despite recent, more conservative recommendations regarding appropriate weight gain in pregnancy from the Institute of Medicine, many women still gain significantly more weight than is recommended and have difficulty with postpartum weight loss. Weight gain often is given as a reason not to initiate a contraceptive method or to discontinue use of one. Thus, offering contraception that will meet a patient's pregnancy prevention goals and also not affect her weight is an important clinical concern.

There is biologic plausibility to the idea that hormonal contraception could cause weight gain. Estrogen could lead to increased fat deposition or mineralocorticoid activity resulting in fluid retention. More androgenic components of hormonal contraception could cause increased muscle mass or increased appetite from anabolic effects. However, numerous well-conducted studies have failed to demonstrate any significant weight gain attributable to contraception, perhaps excluding DMPA. Oral contraceptives are the best studied contraceptive methods, and dozens of randomized trials have not documented any clinically meaningful association between OC use and weight gain. With progestin-only methods, there is less information. However, the levonorgestrel IUD and the etonogestrel contraceptive implant seem to have no significant effect on weight.

There is no consistent finding of clinically significant weight gain in DMPA users. However, there may be specific populations, such as overweight and obese adults and adolescents, with the potential for rapid and significant weight gain. Despite these findings, even among obese adolescents and adult women, most users will not experience significant weight gain. Because minimizing weight gain is of primary concern for this patient, DMPA probably is not the best choice. Although most obese adolescents using DMPA do not gain weight, there can be early and very significant weight gain in those who do. This patient also reports a needle phobia, making DMPA and the etonogestrel contraceptive implant less ideal options for her. Although weight gain is a commonly reported reason for implant discontinuation, the most common reason for removal is irregular bleeding.

For the described patient, the levonorgestrel IUD is the best option because it fits all of her preferences for an ideal contraceptive method. Although she is a nulligravid adolescent, that is not a contraindication to IUD use. The American College of Obstetricians and Gynecologists and the American Academy of Pediatrics have promoted IUDs as a safe and recommended method in this age group. The superior effectiveness and minimal adverse effect profile offered by IUDs make them an ideal choice for many patients. Because perfect use and typical use are almost the same with IUDs, even young women who often have poor pill adherence can expect high contraceptive efficacy. The local effects of levonorgestrel result in a more than 70% decrease in blood loss after the first few months of use. Amenorrhea rates at 1 year and 5 years are 20% and 60%, respectively.

The copper IUD has no association with weight gain and provides highly effective contraception for 10 years. However, this patient desires a contraceptive method that will make her periods lighter or go away. Menstrual blood loss increases on average by 30% in women who use copper IUDs, so this is not a good choice for her. Although OCs will not cause weight gain and could lead to lighter or even less frequent menses with extended cycle use, this patient is an adolescent about to make a major life transition. Numerous studies demonstrate that women often miss pills, with some suggesting an average of four missed pills per cycle. Thus, a levonorgestrel IUD is the best option for her.

Flegal KM, Carroll MD, Ogden CL, Curtin LR. Prevalence and trends in obesity among US adults, 1999-2008. JAMA 2010;303:235–41.

Gallo MF, Grimes DA, Schulz KF, Helmerhorst FM. Combination estrogen-progestin contraceptives and body weight: systematic review of randomized controlled trials. Obstet Gynecol 2004;103:359–73.

Le YC, Rahman M, Berenson AB. Early weight gain predicting later weight gain among depot medroxyprogesterone acetate users. Obstet Gynecol 2009;114:279–84.

Lopez LM, Edelman A, Chen M, Otterness C, Trussell J, Helmerhorst FM. Progestin-only contraceptives: effects on weight. Cochrane Database of Systematic Reviews 2013, Issue 7. Art. No.: CD008815. DOI: 10.1002/14651858.CD008815.pub3.

Vickery Z, Madden T, Zhao Q, Secura GM, Allsworth JE, Peipert JF. Weight change at 12 months in users of three progestin-only contraceptive methods. Contraception 2013;88:503–8.

53
Resistant otitis media

A 32-year-old woman comes to your clinic with ear pain and sudden loss of hearing in the left ear. She has no significant medical history. She has not had an ear infection since childhood. Examination of the ear reveals a bulging, erythematous tympanic membrane. She is afebrile. She has no known drug allergies and is given a prescription for amoxicillin and acetaminophen. Three days later, she returns to the clinic with worsening pain and night sweats. Her temperature is 38.0°C (100.3°F). Examination of the ear reveals continued erythema and bulging of the tympanic membrane without rupture. At this time, the most appropriate treatment for her is

* (A) amoxicillin–clavulanate
(B) vancomycin
(C) sulfamethoxazole–trimethoprim
(D) ciprofloxacin
(E) ibuprofen

Acute otitis media is one of the most common conditions treated with antibiotics. Most cases of acute otitis media affect children aged 6 months to 2 years, although 20% of acute otitis media cases affect adults. Acute otitis media results from eustachian tube dysfunction during an acute upper respiratory tract infection. Fluid accumulates in the narrow part of the eustachian tube, which then becomes infected. *Streptococcus pneumoniae, Haemophilus influenzae*, and *Moraxella catarrhalis* are the most commonly implicated organisms in these infections. Risk factors for acute otitis media include environmental allergies, craniofacial abnormalities, and gastroesophageal reflux. Children with otitis media typically have fever and ear pain, whereas adults may have ear pain, diminished hearing, and sore throat.

Accurate diagnosis of acute otitis media may be difficult. The standard tool used to diagnose otitis media is the pneumatic otoscope. Pneumatic otoscopy allows assessment of tympanic membrane contour, color, and mobility. When a bulging, erythematous tympanic membrane is noted with poor mobility after pneumatic pressure is applied, acute otitis media is diagnosed.

The initial treatment for acute otitis media is amoxicillin. The advantages of amoxicillin include inexpensive cost, acceptable effectiveness rate, and a narrow microbiologic spectrum. Despite amoxicillin being a first-line treatment, the failure rate is 10.5%. If significant symptoms of acute otitis media persist beyond 72 hours, the patient should be reexamined because this signifies resistant otitis media. The appropriate treatment for resistant acute otitis media is amoxicillin–clavulanate. In the described patient, who continued to have acute symptoms and physical examination findings consistent with otitis media despite treatment with amoxicillin, amoxicillin–clavulanate is the most appropriate next step in management. Cefuroxime, ceftriaxone, or clindamycin would be an acceptable alternative treatment for resistant acute otitis media in a patient with a penicillin allergy.

Untreated otitis media in adults may lead to several serious complications. These complications are rare because of the wide availability of antibiotics. If a patient does not improve with treatment, complications still may occur, including mastoiditis, labyrinthitis, and hearing loss. More severe sequelae include meningitis, facial paralysis, and brain abscess.

Vancomycin, sulfamethoxazole–trimethoprim, and ciprofloxacin are not acceptable treatments for acute otitis media because of insufficient microbial coverage. Ibuprofen is a treatment for the pain associated with acute otitis media, but antibiotic therapy is the mainstay of treatment.

Currie C, Berni E, Jenkins-Jones S, Poole C, Ouwens M, Driessen S, et al. Antibiotic treatment failure in four common infections in UK primary care 1991–2012: longitudinal analysis. BMJ 2014:349:g5493.

Harmes KM, Blackwood RA, Burrows HL, Cooke JM, Harrison RV, Passamani PP. Otitis media: diagnosis and treatment [published erratum appears in Am Fam Physician 2014;89:318]. Am Fam Physician 2013;88:435–40.

Hendley JO. Clinical practice. Otitis media. N Engl J Med 2002;347:1169–74.

Leskinen K, Jero J. Acute complications of otitis media in adults. Clin Otolaryngol 2005;30:511–6.

Lieberthal AS, Carroll AE, Chonmaitree T, Ganiats TG, Hoberman A, Jackson MA, et al. The diagnosis and management of acute otitis media [published erratum appears in Pediatrics 2014;133:346]. Pediatrics 2013;131:e964–99.

54

Pelvic organ prolapse

A 75-year-old woman, gravida 3, para 3, comes to your office with a vaginal bulge. She tells you that the bulge is most bothersome when gardening or walking. She reports no urinary problems. She moves her bowels regularly, occasionally with some straining, and she notices the bulge at such moments. She is occasionally sexually active with her husband. She has hypertension that is well controlled with hydrochlorothiazide. On examination, she is 1.63 m (64 in.) tall and weighs 54.4 kg (120 lb). Her pelvic organ prolapse quantification result is shown below and her pelvic floor muscle strength is 4/5.

Aa 2	Ba 3	C –1
Gh 4	Pb 2	Tvl 7
Ap –2	Bp –2	D –5

The best next step for this patient is

(A) reassurance
(B) physical therapy
* (C) pessary
(D) urodynamic testing

Prolapse is the most common indication for hysterectomy in U.S. women 55 years or older; a woman's risk of undergoing prolapse surgery by age 80 years is upwards of 20%. With the advancing age of the U.S. population, the practicing gynecologist can expect to encounter women with prolapse frequently. Nonsurgical management of prolapse can result in significant symptomatic improvement in many patients. There are few well-designed studies of conservative management of pelvic organ prolapse, so most recommendations are based on expert opinion, retrospective studies, or prospective studies that are short term or observational in nature.

The hallmark symptom of pelvic organ prolapse is the awareness of a vaginal bulge or protrusion. This symptom typically is not present until the leading edge of the prolapse is beyond the hymenal ring. The pelvic organ prolapse quantification is used to standardize documentation of examination findings and to assign a stage from 0 (no prolapse) to 4 (complete procidentia). Typically, treatment of prolapse should be focused on alleviating symptoms that are bothersome to the patient rather than on specific physical examination findings. When asymptomatic prolapse is found on examination, as in the described patient, some gynecologists use the opportunity to educate the patient regarding pelvic floor muscle strengthening, but it is important not to give the patient the impression that she has a worrisome condition that necessitates intervention (Box 54-1, Fig. 54-1, and Fig. 54-2).

Pessaries can be fitted in most women with prolapse and should be offered to women with symptomatic prolapse before surgical intervention. Pessaries have been found in short-term studies to result in significant improvement in urinary symptoms and quality of life. The two most popular types of pessaries are the ring pessary with support and the Gellhorn pessary (Fig. 54-3 and Fig. 54-4, respectively). The ring pessary with support is the first-line therapy in most patients, and many patients will be able to remove and reinsert this pessary themselves. Therefore, the best next step for this patient would be to try a ring pessary with support.

If a patient cannot retain a ring pessary with support, a Gellhorn pessary may be the second-line choice. The Gellhorn pessary creates more friction and suction effects within the vagina, which may keep the pessary in place

BOX 54-1

Stages of Pelvic Organ Prolapse

Stages are based on the maximal extent of prolapse relative to the hymen in one or more compartments.

Stage 0: No prolapse; anterior and posterior points are all –3 cm, and C (cervix) or D (posterior fornix) is between –TVL and –(TVL – 2) cm.

Stage I: The criteria for stage 0 are not met, and the most distal prolapse is more than 1 cm above the level of the hymen (less than –1 cm).

Stage II: The most distal prolapse is between 1 cm above and 1 cm below the hymen (at least one post is –1, 0, or +1).

Stage III: The most distal prolapse is more than 1 cm below the hymen but no further than 2 cm less than TVL.

Stage IV: Represents complete procidentia or vault eversion; the most distal prolapse protrudes to at least (TVL – 2) cm.

Pelvic Organ Prolapse Quantification System

Six vaginal sites used in staging prolapse:

Points Aa and Ba anteriorly

Points Ap and Bp posteriorly

Point C for the cervix or vaginal apex

Point D for the posterior fornix (not measured after hysterectomy)

Three additional measurements:

GH — genital hiatus

PB — perineal body

TVL — total vaginal length

Reprinted from Bump RC, Mattiasson A, Bo K, Brubaker LP, DeLancey JO, Klarskov P, et al. The standardization of terminology of female pelvic organ prolapse and pelvic floor dysfunction. Am J Obstet Gynecol 1996;175:10–7. Copyright 1996, with permission from Elsevier.

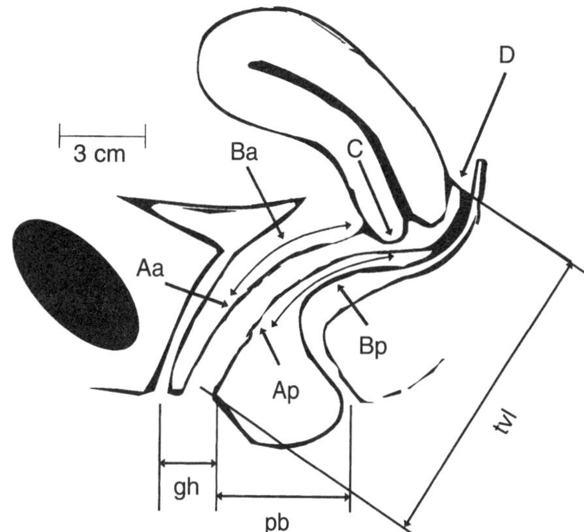

FIGURE 54-1. Six sites (points *Aa, Ba, C, D, Bp,* and *Ap*), genital hiatus (gh), perineal body (*pb*), and total vaginal length *(tvl)* used for pelvic organ support quantitation. (Reprinted from Bump RC, Mattiasson A, Bo K, Brubaker LP, DeLancey JO, Klarskov P, et al. The standardization of terminology of female pelvic organ prolapse and pelvic floor dysfunction. Am J Obstet Gynecol 1996;175:10–7. Copyright 1996, with permission from Elsevier.)

Anterior wall **Aa**	Anterior wall **Ba**	Cervix or cuff **C**
Genital hiatus **gh**	Perineal body **pb**	Total vaginal length **tvl**
Posterior wall **Ap**	Posterior wall **Bp**	Posterior fornix **D**

FIGURE 54-2. Three-by-three grid for recording quantitative description of pelvic organ support. (Reprinted from Bump RC, Mattiasson A, Bo K, Brubaker LP, DeLancey JO, Klarskov P, et al. The standardization of terminology of female pelvic organ prolapse and pelvic floor dysfunction. Am J Obstet Gynecol 1996;175:10–7. Copyright 1996, with permission from Elsevier.)

but also makes it difficult for the patient to insert or remove the device on her own. The Gellhorn pessary is not compatible with intercourse when it is in place and may be difficult for patients to remove before intercourse, so it is not as good a choice for patients who wish to remain sexually active. The PESSRI study, a randomized crossover trial comparing the ring pessary with the Gellhorn pessary, did not find a difference in effectiveness between the two types.

There is no consensus on frequency of follow-up visits to check for pessary-associated abrasions or excoriations. Most patients who use pessaries do not need to use vaginal estrogen or antibiotics regularly. Such medications can be used as needed for discharge or abrasions. Most minor vaginal abrasions can be treated with estrogen cream with or without the pessary in place. Severe ulcerations are only likely in cases of prolonged loss to follow-up. Other problems with pessaries include the unmasking of occult stress incontinence, pessary-related discharge, spontaneous expulsion, or Pap test abnormalities related to inflammation.

Certain factors have been shown to be associated with successful pessary use. Increasing age is associated with greater likelihood of choosing a pessary over surgery, whereas patients with diabetes, occult stress incontinence, and lack of family support are more likely to discontinue pessary use. A study of factors that influence

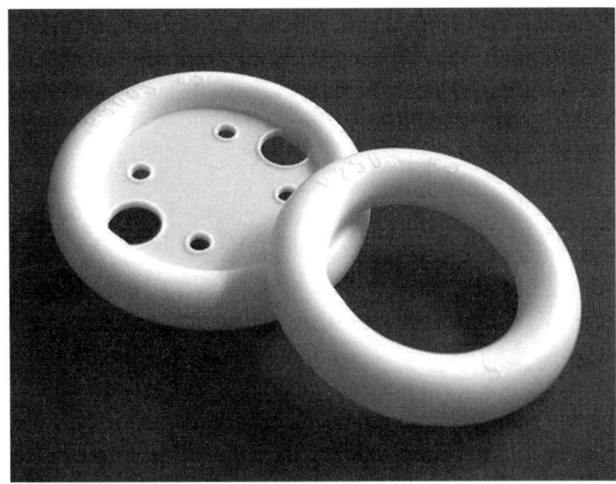

FIGURE 54-3. Plain ring and ring with support. Courtesy Bioteque America Copyright 2012. (Culligan PJ. Nonsurgical management of pelvic organ prolapse. Obstet Gynecol 2012;119:852–60.)

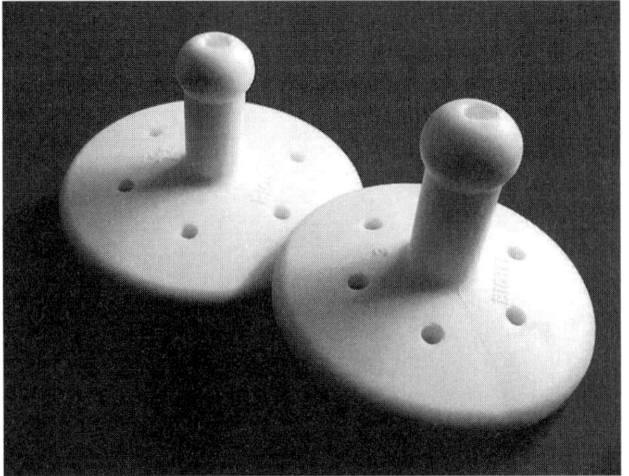

FIGURE 54-4. Gellhorn pessary. Courtesy Bioteque America Copyright 2012. (Culligan PJ. Nonsurgical management of pelvic organ prolapse. Obstet Gynecol 2012;119:852–60.)

long-term pessary use found that age older than 72 years was associated with continued pessary use, whereas prior hysterectomy or prolapse surgery and stress incontinence were associated with discontinuation.

Reassurance alone would not be appropriate for this patient. She reports her prolapse symptoms as "bothersome," and she is seeking help in alleviating those symptoms.

Patients with weak pelvic floor muscles may be able to arrest development of further prolapse with exercise and education. Patients who already possess very strong pelvic floor muscles with good voluntary control are less likely to experience improvement with further exercise. Because this patient already has 4/5 pelvic floor muscle strength, pelvic floor physical therapy is less likely to have a significant effect on her symptoms. Several short-term trials have demonstrated improvement in prolapse symptoms or examination findings with pelvic floor muscle training, but long-term efficacy has not been shown. In addition, evidence shows that patients tend to give up these exercise regimens over time. One study that compared 12 weeks of traditional pelvic floor muscle training with Pilates classes showed significant improvement in both groups and no difference between groups.

The described patient does not have urinary concerns that necessitate urodynamic testing. However, it is important to counsel patients that reduction of prolapse with a pessary may unmask occult stress incontinence. Patients with a positive prolapse-reduced stress test are at increased risk of postoperative stress incontinence after surgical correction of prolapse and benefit from the performance of an incontinence procedure at the time of prolapse repair. This incontinence procedure aids counseling and surgical decision making and is another benefit to offering pessaries for first-line treatment of pelvic organ prolapse.

Culligan PJ. Nonsurgical management of pelvic organ prolapse. Obstet Gynecol 2012;119:852–60.

Friedman S, Sandhu KS, Wang C, Mikhail MS, Banks E. Factors influencing long-term pessary use. Int Urogynecol J 2010;21:673–8.

Ko PC, Lo TS, Tseng LH, Lin YH, Liang CC, Lee SJ. Use of a pessary in treatment of pelvic organ prolapse: quality of life, compliance, and failure at 1-year follow-up. J Minim Invasive Gynecol 2011;18:68–74.

Persu C, Chapple CR, Cauni V, Gutue S, Geavlete P. Pelvic Organ Prolapse Quantification System (POP-Q) — a new era in pelvic prolapse staging. J Med Life 2011;4:75–81.

Wu JM, Matthews CA, Conover MM, Pate V, Jonsson Funk M. Lifetime risk of stress urinary incontinence or pelvic organ prolapse surgery. Obstet Gynecol 2014;123:1201–6.

55

Fetal cardiovascular malformation and inheritance

A 36-year-old woman, gravida 1, comes to your office at 20 weeks of gestation for routine fetal anatomy ultrasonography. She has no health risks and previously declined aneuploidy screening and carrier testing. There is no family history of cardiac disease. On ultrasonography, she is noted to have a male fetus with a ventricular septal defect, overriding aortic root, and pulmonary artery stenosis. Estimated fetal weight is normal for gestational age. No other anomalies are identified. She is counseled about further genetic testing and agrees to undergo amniocentesis. The most likely fetal karyotype is

* (A) 46,XY
(B) 47,XY,+21
(C) 47,XY,+18
(D) 46,XY,del*22q*
(E) 46,XY,del*15q11-13*

This fetus has tetralogy of Fallot, and the most likely fetal karyotype is 46,XY. This is one of the more common forms of congenital heart disease and the most common cyanotic cardiac malformation. The word "tetralogy" indicates that four features make up this syndrome. These features are ventricular septal defect, overriding aorta, pulmonic valve stenosis, and right ventricular hypertrophy. Right ventricular hypertrophy typically is not seen on prenatal ultrasonography, given fetal circulation hemodynamics.

When fetal cardiac malformations are identified, the patient should be advised of the increased risk of chromosomal and other genetic disorders, although most fetuses with isolated cardiac malformations are euploid. Overall, the risk of aneuploidy when cardiac malformations are identified is around 30%. When isolated tetralogy of Fallot is identified, the risk of aneuploidy is approximately 20%. Cardiac outflow (conotruncal) abnormalities also can be associated with genomic microdeletions, especially 22q11 deletions. A microdeletion involving 22q11 (also known as DiGeorge syndrome) is a multiple anomaly syndrome that, in addition to cardiac malformations, also results in problems such as velopharyngeal insufficiency, learning disabilities, and immune deficiency. If a couple chooses to undergo prenatal diagnostic testing as a result of congenital heart disease, it is recommended that genomic microarray be used as first-line testing as opposed to just a karyotype. The additional diagnostic yield for microarray in a large National Institute of Child Health and Human Development trial demonstrated a 6% added detection of genomic abnormalities when there was an otherwise normal karyotype. It is important to counsel patients that chromosomal or genomic abnormalities can have a significant effect on prognosis for the newborn.

Many fetuses with Down syndrome (trisomy 21) will have structural heart malformations. The classic association is atrioventricular septal defect, sometimes called A–V canal, although ventricular septal defects also are common in Down syndrome. The proportion of newborn children with Down syndrome that have a structural heart malformation is approximately 50%.

Fetuses with trisomy 18 almost always have some type of heart defect, most commonly ventricular septal defect. Other cardiac abnormalities associated with trisomy 18 include atrioventricular septal defect and valvular anomalies.

The karyotype result del*15q11-13* is associated with either Prader–Willi syndrome (more common) or Angelman syndrome (less common), depending on which parental chromosome 15 contains the deletion. Approximately 70% of children who are diagnosed with Prader–Willi syndrome have a paternal deletion of this region. These two disorders exemplify the concept of genomic imprinting. Most of these microdeletion disorders occur de novo and are unlikely to recur, but some parental chromosome translocations may predispose a couple to microdeletion syndromes in their offspring. Cardiac abnormalities are not a feature of Prader–Willi syndrome. Prenatally, these fetuses may be found to have reduced fetal movement in the third trimester but otherwise typically do not have structural malformations that would trigger diagnostic testing.

Most structural heart malformations occur sporadically with no family history, but most also are believed to be polygenic, multifactorial, or both. Disorders with this inheritance pattern do carry an increased risk of recurrence to others. For example, siblings of a child with a nonsyndromic structural heart malformation have a 2–3% risk of recurrence, though not necessarily with the same type of malformation. Similarly, if a parent had a structural heart malformation, the risk for the offspring is approximately 2–3%. The risk appears to be higher for certain types of malformations, such as hypoplastic left heart syndrome, presumably as a result of a stronger genetic component.

Suspicion of fetal cardiac malformation is an indication for fetal echocardiography. Consultation with a pediatric cardiologist prenatally can help parents better comprehend the possible course their infant may face. In addition to abnormal fetal ultrasonography and family history, other indications for echocardiography include maternal diabetes mellitus, teratogenic exposures, monochorionic twinning, and in vitro fertilization.

Donnelly JC, Platt LD, Rebarber A, Zachary J, Grobman WA, Wapner RJ. Association of copy number variants with specific ultrasonographically detected fetal anomalies. Obstet Gynecol 2014;124:83–90.

Fahed AC, Gelb BD, Seidman JG, Seidman CE. Genetics of congenital heart disease: the glass half empty [published erratum appears in Circ Res 2013;112:e182]. Circ Res 2013;112:707–20.

Oyen N, Poulsen G, Boyd HA, Wohlfahrt J, Jensen PK, Melbye M. Recurrence of congenital heart defects in families. Circulation 2009;120:295–301.

Peyvandi S, Ingall E, Woyciechowski S, Garbarini J, Mitchell LE, Goldmuntz E. Risk of congenital heart disease in relatives of probands with conotruncal cardiac defects: an evaluation of 1,620 families. Am J Med Genet A 2014;164A:1490–5.

56

Thyroid disease

A 32-year-old woman is referred to your office for prenatal care at 8 weeks of gestation. On review of her laboratory assessment, you notice that she has an abnormally elevated serum thyroid-stimulating hormone (TSH) concentration with normal free thyroxine (T_4) and triiodothyronine (T_3) levels. She is asymptomatic and has a normal heart rate. The most appropriate management is

(A) propylthiouracil
(B) levothyroxine
(C) methimazole
(D) desiccated thyroid
* (E) no treatment

The described patient has subclinical hypothyroidism because she is asymptomatic with an elevated serum TSH and normal serum free T_4 and T_3. This condition may result from administration of thyroid hormone, overproduction of thyroid hormone, delayed recovery of TSH-producing cells after treatment for hyperthyroidism, pregnancy, nonthyroidal illnesses (eg, euthyroid sick syndrome), or medication administration (eg, dopamine, corticosteroids, and possibly dobutamine). The American College of Obstetricians and Gynecologists does not recommend treatment of subclinical hypothyroidism in pregnancy.

Propylthiouracil and methimazole are treatments for hyperthyroidism. Patients with hyperthyroidism have suppressed TSH and elevated serum free T_4. Because this patient does not have hyperthyroidism, treatment with these medications is not indicated. Propylthiouracil and methimazole block organification of iodide, resulting in decreased thyroid hormone synthesis. In addition, propylthiouracil blocks the peripheral conversion of T_4 to T_3.

The risks of not treating a pregnant hyperthyroid woman are that she may experience hyperthyroid symptoms, be at risk to develop cardiac arrhythmias or preeclampsia, have calcium drawn from her bones (resulting in osteoporosis), or experience thyroid storm. Additional risks of untreated hyperthyroidism include preterm delivery, fetal growth restriction, impaired fetal neuropsychologic development, miscarriage, placental abruption, low birth weight, and stillbirth. When possible, it is recommended to treat hyperthyroidism with propylthiouracil in the first trimester and to switch to methimazole in the second trimester. This is suggested in an attempt to balance the risk of hepatotoxicity (seen with propylthiouracil) and methimazole embryopathy (eg, aplasia cutis and esophageal or choanal atresia), although these conditions rarely occur.

Levothyroxine and desiccated thyroid are used for treatment of hypothyroidism. Patients with hypothyroidism have elevated TSH levels and low serum free T_4 levels. Because this patient does not have hypothyroidism, treatment with these medications is not indicated. The aforementioned risks of uncontrolled maternal hypothyroidism during pregnancy are modifiable with thyroid-replacement medications. Thyroid-replacement therapies are safe to use during pregnancy and are essential to normal fetal development in the presence of maternal hypothyroidism.

Typically, women with thyroid disease in pregnancy should have serial thyroid function tests assessed (4 weeks after any change in therapy) to maintain euthyroidism. Fetal growth assessments are indicated in the setting of uncontrolled disease. Table 56-1 shows thyroid function test results in the setting of normal pregnancy and thyroid disease.

TABLE 56-1. Changes in Thyroid Function Test Results in Normal Pregnancy and in Thyroid Disease

Maternal Status	TSH	Free T_4
Pregnancy	Varies by trimester*	No change
Overt hyperthyroidism	Decrease	Increase
Subclinical hyperthyroidism	Decrease	No change
Overt hypothyroidism	Increase	Decrease
Subclinical hypothyroidism	Increase	No change

Abbreviations: T_4, thyroxine; TSH, thyroid-stimulating hormone.

*The level of TSH decreases in early pregnancy because of weak TSH receptor stimulation due to substantial quantities of human chorionic gonadotropin during the first 12 weeks of gestation. After the first trimester, TSH levels return to baseline values.

Thyroid disease in pregnancy. Practice Bulletin No. 148. American College of Obstetricians and Gynecologists. Obstet Gynecol 2015;125:996–1005.

Surks MI, Ortiz E, Daniels GH, Sawin CT, Col NF, Cobin RH, et al. Subclinical thyroid disease: scientific review and guidelines for diagnosis and management. 2004, Issue 2. Art. No.: PMID: 14722150; 291/2/228 [pii]. DOI: 10.1001/JAMA.291.2.228.

Thyroid disease in pregnancy. Practice Bulletin No. 148. American College of Obstetricians and Gynecologists. Obstet Gynecol 2015; 125:996–1005.

57

Vaginal bleeding—foreign object

A 5-year-old girl is brought to your clinic by her mother. The mother reports seeing spots of blood on her daughter's underwear. The child says she has not had any abdominal or pelvic pain, nor does there appear to have been any sexual abuse or inappropriate touching, as far as you can ascertain by taking the patient's history. Her mother has no increased concern about abuse. The patient is otherwise healthy and meets all developmental milestones for a child of her age. She has no signs of thelarche or adrenarche. You place the girl in the frog-leg position on the examination table to examine her. External examination shows Tanner stage I development and normal findings on examination of her external genitalia with no vulvar or urethral excoriations or ulcerations and a normal anus. You attempt a vaginal examination to perform irrigation, but she stops the examination and will not allow you to further examine her; you do not notice any vaginal lacerations or bruising during your limited examination. The best next step in management is

(A) reassurance
(B) urinalysis
(C) wet mount preparation
* (D) examination under anesthesia
(E) consultation with social worker

Vaginal bleeding in a premenarchal girl is always abnormal and must be investigated. Sometimes an etiology will not be identified, but complete evaluation is justified because, although rare, some causes (like ovarian or cervical tumors) can be life threatening, and abuse should always be considered. The causes of vaginal bleeding before puberty fall into four main categories: 1) trauma, 2) vulvovaginitis, 3) endocrine or hormonal (exogenous estrogen exposure or precocious puberty), and 4) anatomic (Box 57-1). This patient, who lacks breast budding, does not have a history or examination consistent with hormonal causes, so the diagnosis most likely will come from a complete physical examination or additional testing. Parental reassurance is premature before a complete physical examination assessing the upper vagina and cervix is performed.

Blood noticed by a child's parents may not be coming from the vagina but instead from the bladder or rectum. Urinary tract infections (UTIs) are common in childhood. Common features of a UTI in a girl older than 2 years include abdominal pain or back pain; dysuria, frequency, or both; and new-onset urinary incontinence. Macroscopic hematuria is a possible but less common symptom. In the described patient, who has no other health concerns, vaginal bleeding is less likely to indicate a UTI. Similarly, because she does not report abdominal pain and her anus appears normal, without evidence of fissures or hemorrhoids, constipation is less likely to be the cause of her bleeding.

BOX 57-1

Differential Diagnosis for Vaginal Bleeding in the Child

- Trauma
  - Accidental
  - Sexual abuse
- Vulvovaginitis
  - Irritation
  - Infectious (eg, *Shigella*, *Streptococcus*, pinworm)
  - Lichen sclerosus
  - Sexually transmitted infections (eg, condylomata)
- Endocrine/hormonal
  - Precocious puberty
  - Hypothyroidism
  - Exogenous estrogen
  - Foreign body
- Anatomic lesions
  - Urethral prolapse
  - Neoplasia (eg, hemangioma, granulosa cell tumor, sarcoma, adenocarcinoma, endodermal sinus tumor, müllerian papilloma)

Adapted from Swaim LS, Zietz B, Qu Z. An uncommon cause of vaginal bleeding in a child. Obstet Gynecol 2008;110:416–20.

Vulvovaginitis is one of the most common gynecologic problems in prepubertal girls. The most common infectious causes associated with bleeding are group A streptococci and *Shigella*; however, most cases are thought to be noninfectious and dermatologic in origin. Vulvovaginitis cases with specific bacterial causes typically have acute onset of a visible discharge. A pediatric patient with vulvovaginal symptoms should undergo a careful vulvar examination for evidence of a dermatologic cause and for vaginal discharge. If the described patient's physical examination is nondiagnostic, the vaginal secretions should be evaluated by microscopy and sent for culture. A wet mount preparation without visible discharge is unlikely to be helpful and does not obviate the need for a thorough physical examination.

Trauma to the vulva and vagina can result from blunt trauma like a straddle injury, penetrating trauma, or sexual abuse. In a child, the hymenal and vaginal tissues are particularly vulnerable to bleeding because of hypoestrogenism, marked vascularity, and lack of protective labial fat pads. A careful history should be obtained, and the physical findings on examination should be consistent with the history. Straddle injuries are more common in the anterior area of the vulva, including the mons, clitoral hood, and anterior aspect of the labia, whereas an injury to the posterior fourchette and hymenal area suggests possible sexual abuse. Genital warts or other sexually transmitted infections resulting from sexual abuse also can cause vaginal bleeding. If sexual abuse is suspected, child protective services should be notified and the child referred to a professional trained in the management of child sexual abuse. In the described patient, unless a thorough physical examination completed later is suggestive of abuse, there is no need for a social work consultation.

A foreign body is a highly likely diagnosis in girls who present with vaginal bleeding but no history of trauma; another accompanying symptom may be a persistent, malodorous discharge. The most common foreign body in young children is toilet paper, although small toys, hair bands, and paper clips also are common. Other etiologies of prepubertal bleeding identified on physical examination include urethral prolapse and lichen sclerosus; much less common is a vaginal polyp or tumor, such as a sarcoma botryoides, which has a peak incidence at age 2–5 years. This tumor can involve the hymen, lower urethra, or anterior vaginal wall, or higher up along the vagina closer to the cervix in older premenarchal girls. Benign polyps also can occur involving the vagina and hymenal area, but they are rare and can be removed with surgical excision. Because the most likely cause of bleeding in the described patient will be found on physical examination, the obstetrician–gynecologist or other health care provider must be able to see the length of the vagina to rule out a foreign body, tumor, or other vaginal trauma, even if it means an examination under anesthesia with vaginoscopy and cultures. Because of her discomfort, postponing the examination until sedation is available is recommended to allow for a thorough examination.

Stricker T, Navratil F, Sennhauser FH. Vaginal foreign bodies. J Paediatr Child Health 2004;40:205–7.

Striegel AM, Myers JB, Sorensen MD, Furness PD, Koyle MA. Vaginal discharge and bleeding in girls younger than 6 years. J Urol 2006;176:2632–5.

Swaim LS, Zietz B, Qu Z. An uncommon cause of vaginal bleeding in a child. Obstet Gynecol 2008;110:416–20.

Vaginitis. ACOG Practice Bulletin No. 72. American College of Obstetricians and Gynecologists. Obstet Gynecol 2006;107:1195–206.

58

Health Insurance Portability and Accountability Act rules

Your office manager discusses with you the recent implementation of software and security upgrades to your network to comply with changes in the Health Insurance Portability and Accountability Act (HIPAA) rules. She informs you of the increased costs associated with these upgrades and the need for ongoing security checks. She states that the new regulations are mandated by the Health Information Technology for Economic and Clinical Health (HITECH) Act. The part of HIPAA that addresses provisions from the HITECH Act is the

(A) Privacy Rule
(B) Technology Rule
(C) Enforcement Rule
* (D) Omnibus Final Rule
(E) Security Rule

Since the original version of HIPAA was passed by Congress in 1996, many revisions and additions have occurred. The Omnibus Final Rule, which addresses the provisions of the HITECH Act, was added in 2009 as part of the American Recovery and Reinvestment Act. This legislation imparts new guidelines for electronic health records (EHRs) and is an attempt to standardize EHR capabilities across the many platforms that are available. In addition, funding was legislated to assist hospitals and practices in incorporating EHRs. Incentives for practices to incorporate such capabilities include monetary rewards for those facilities that made "meaningful use" of EHRs. As an example, electronic prescribing is a feature that is considered meaningful use.

Another section of the HITECH Act addresses data breaches. A data breach in this legislation is defined as "acquisition, access, use, or disclosure of protected health information." Any data breach affecting 500 patients or more must be reported to federal authorities. More than 82% of data breaches reported from 2010 through 2013 were of this magnitude. Most occurred as a result of theft or other overt criminal activity and illicitly acquired electronic hardware, such as laptops or other portable electronic devices.

The Privacy Rule, or the "Standards for Privacy of Individually Identifiable Health Information," is a set of national standards created to ensure there is no misuse of protected health information. The Office of Civil Rights within the Department of Health and Human Services has jurisdiction in cases of violation of these standards.

The Security Rule protects a subset of patient data that is covered by the Privacy Rule. It explicitly addresses any and all electronic methods to create, receive, maintain, or transmit protected health information. It mandates protections that will address the technical and nontechnical safeguards that medical organizations have in place to ensure this security.

There is no explicit Technology Rule; this aspect of electronic health data management is covered under the Security Rule and HITECH Act. However, given that technology plays a central role in successful creation and use of these systems, an understanding of the technologies involved is critical for medical offices and hospitals.

The Enforcement Rule outlines the methods and logistics for how the Department of Health and Human Services can regulate compliance and carry out investigations. Additionally, the rules surrounding civil monetary penalties for violations of HIPAA are delineated in the Enforcement Rule, as are the rules governing procedures and hearings addressing these violations.

Blumenthal D. Implementation of the federal health information technology initiative. N Engl J Med 2011;365:2426–31.

Blumenthal D. Wiring the health system--origins and provisions of a new federal program. N Engl J Med 2011;365:2323–9.

Liu V, Musen MA, Chou T. Data breaches of protected health information in the United States [published erratum appears in JAMA 2015;313:2497]. JAMA 2015;313:1471–3.

59

Breast cancer chemoprevention

A 55-year-old white woman, para 2, asks you about her risk of developing breast cancer. She has no significant medical history and is taking no medications. With the use of the Gail Model Breast Cancer Risk Assessment Tool, you determine that her 5-year risk of developing breast cancer is 3.1% and her lifetime risk is 20.1%. To reduce her risk of breast cancer, the best medical therapy for her is

* (A) raloxifene hydrochloride
(B) anastrozole
(C) leuprolide acetate
(D) tamoxifen citrate
(E) exemestane

The Gail Model Breast Cancer Risk Assessment Tool, available online at www.cancer.gov/bcrisktool, is one of a number of risk assessment tools for breast cancer. Although it is a very easy and rapid tool to use, it only takes into consideration patient age, some reproductive factors, history of breast biopsies without pathologic findings, and contribution of family history, which is limited to first-degree female relatives. Women are considered to be at an elevated risk if they have a 5-year breast cancer risk of 1.67% or greater (which is equivalent to the average risk for a woman at age 60 years) or a lifetime risk of 20% or greater. At a minimum, these women should be offered enhanced screening to include clinical breast examination every 6–12 months, annual mammography, and instruction on breast self-awareness. Other models for breast cancer risk prediction are available. The Claus model is particularly useful in women with at least one female first-degree or second-degree relative who has been diagnosed with breast cancer because it takes into consideration an extended family history; however, the Claus model lacks an online calculator. The Breast Cancer Surveillance Consortium risk calculator includes radiologic breast density.

Screening for breast cancer allows for early detection and has been shown to reduce the mortality odds ratio in screened populations, but it does nothing to prevent breast cancer development. Data are limited to show that behavioral modifications, such as weight loss or eliminating alcohol from the diet, will significantly reduce a woman's lifetime risk of breast cancer. Because the described patient has a 5-year risk of 3.1% for developing breast cancer, she is an excellent candidate for chemoprevention.

Multiple studies have clearly established the role of tamoxifen in the treatment of breast cancer. The 1998 National Surgical Adjuvant Breast and Bowel Project Breast Cancer Prevention P-1 Study demonstrated that tamoxifen reduced the risk of invasive breast cancer by 49% in risk-eligible women. The National Surgical Adjuvant Breast and Bowel Project Study of Tamoxifen and Raloxifene P-2 Trial was the first large trial that did a head-to-head comparison of the effectiveness of the selective estrogen receptor modulators tamoxifen and raloxifene to reduce the risk of breast cancer in women who are at an increased risk. The study demonstrated raloxifene to be as effective as tamoxifen in reducing the risk of invasive breast cancer but with lower risk of thromboembolic disease, endometrial cancer, and need for cataract surgery.

In 2013, the U.S. Preventive Services Task Force (USPSTF) reviewed existing evidence on the effectiveness and adverse effects of tamoxifen and raloxifene for breast cancer chemoprevention. The USPSTF concluded that the net benefit for use over a 5-year course of therapy is moderate to substantial for women who are aged 35 years or older, at increased risk of breast cancer, and at low risk of adverse medication effects (Table 59-1). Tamoxifen and raloxifene have been approved by the U.S. Food and Drug Administration for this indication in postmenopausal women, and tamoxifen has been approved for use in premenopausal women. The USPSTF found the strongest benefit among women with a 5-year risk of breast cancer of 3% or more, but the balance of risks to benefits depended on age, race, medications, and whether the patient had a uterus. Additional benefits were found with the use of tamoxifen in regard to nonvertebral fracture risk reduction and with use of raloxifene for vertebral fracture risk reduction.

The primary risk associated with tamoxifen and raloxifene is thromboembolic disease, including deep vein thrombosis, pulmonary embolism, stroke, or transient ischemic attack. The actual increased risk of thromboembolic disease was 4–7 events per 1,000 women over 5 years of use, with a slightly higher risk with tamoxifen

TABLE 59-1. Medications for Risk Reduction of Primary Breast Cancer in Women: Clinical Summary of U.S. Preventive Services Task Force (USPSTF) Recommendations

Population	Asymptomatic women 35 years or older without a prior diagnosis of breast cancer who are at increased risk of breast cancer	Asymptomatic women aged 35 years or older without a prior diagnosis of breast cancer who are not at increased risk of breast cancer
Recommendation	Engage in shared, informed decision making and offer to prescribe risk-reducing medications, if appropriate. Grade: B	Do not prescribe risk-reducing medications. Grade: D
Risk assessment	Important risk factors for breast cancer include patient age, race and ethnicity, age at menarche, age at first live childbirth, personal history of ductal or lobular carcinoma in situ, number of first-degree relatives with breast cancer, personal history of breast biopsy, body mass index, menopause status or age, breast density, estrogen and progestin use, smoking, alcohol use, physical activity, and diet. Available risk assessment models can accurately estimate the number of breast cancer cases that may arise in certain study populations, but their ability to accurately predict which individual women will (and will not) develop breast cancer is modest.	
Preventive medications	The selective estrogen receptor modulators tamoxifen and raloxifene have been shown to reduce the incidence of invasive breast cancer in postmenopausal women who are at increased risk of the disease. The usual daily doses for tamoxifen and raloxifene are 20 mg and 60 mg, respectively, for 5 years.	
Balance of benefits and harms	There is a moderate net benefit from use of tamoxifen and raloxifene to reduce the incidence of invasive breast cancer in women who are at increased risk of the disease.	The potential harms of tamoxifen and raloxifene outweigh the potential benefits for breast cancer risk reduction in women who are not at increased risk of the disease. Potential harms include thromboembolic events, endometrial cancer, and cataracts.
Other relevant USPSTF recommendations	The USPSTF has made recommendations on risk assessment, genetic counseling, and genetic testing for *BRCA*-related cancer, as well as screening for breast cancer. These recommendations are available at www.uspreventiveservicestaskforce.org.	

Abbreviation: USPSTF, U.S. Preventive Services Task Force.

For a summary of the evidence systematically reviewed in making this recommendation, the full recommendation statement, and supporting documents, please go to www.uspreventiveservicestaskforce.org.

Republished with permission of Annals of Internal Medicine, from Moyer VA. Medications to decrease the risk for breast cancer in women: recommendations from the U.S. Preventive Services Task Force recommendation statement. U.S. Preventive Services Task Force. Ann Intern Med 2013;159:698–708. Copyright 2013, with permission from Elsevier.

compared with raloxifene. The USPSTF defined *low risk* as no personal or family history of thromboembolic disease. It is important to note that tamoxifen, but not raloxifene, increased the risk of endometrial cancer in women with a uterus by approximately 4 cases per 1,000 women. The task force also confirmed that tamoxifen may increase the risk of cataracts, which is more substantial in postmenopausal women, who are already at higher risk based on age.

Considering the increased risk of thromboembolic disease, endometrial neoplasia, and cataracts with the use of tamoxifen, the described patient is best suited for 5 years of therapy with raloxifene. In addition to counseling the patient on the risk of thromboembolic disease, she should be cautioned that she may experience a return of vasomotor symptoms, most commonly when she is first starting raloxifene. Aromatase inhibitors, such as anastrozole or exemestane, have not been approved by the U.S. Food and Drug Administration for breast cancer chemoprevention, and concerns for accelerated loss of bone mineral density probably will limit their use for this indication. Leuprolide has no indication for breast cancer prevention and would have no therapeutic benefit in a woman who is already postmenopausal. It is used for ovarian suppression in premenopausal women who need to take an aromatase inhibitor as part of adjuvant therapy for breast cancer.

Breast cancer risk assessment tool. Available at: http://www.cancer.gov/bcrisktool/. Retrieved June 11, 2016.

Breast Cancer Surveillance Consortium. Introduction. Breast cancer surveillance consortium risk calculator. Bethesda (MD): BCSC; 2016. Available at: https://tools.bcsc-scc.org/bc5yearrisk/intro.htm. Retrieved June 16, 2016.

Claus EB, Risch N, Thompson WD. Autosomal dominant inheritance of early-onset breast cancer. Implications for risk prediction. Cancer 1994;73:643–51.

Fisher B, Costantino JP, Wickerham DL, Redmond CK, Kavanah M, Cronin WM, et al. Tamoxifen for prevention of breast cancer: report of the National Surgical Adjuvant Breast and Bowel Project P-1 Study. J Natl Cancer Inst 1998;90:1371–88.

Moyer VA. Medications to decrease the risk for breast cancer in women: recommendations from the U.S. Preventive Services Task Force recommendation statement. U.S. Preventive Services Task Force. Ann Intern Med 2013;159:698–708.

Vogel VG, Costantino JP, Wickerham DL, Cronin WM, Cecchini RS, Atkins JN, et al. Update of the National Surgical Adjuvant Breast and Bowel Project Study of Tamoxifen and Raloxifene (STAR) P-2 Trial: Preventing breast cancer. National Surgical Adjuvant Breast and Bowel Project. Cancer Prev Res (Phila) 2010;3:696–706.

Vogel VG. The NSABP Study of Tamoxifen and Raloxifene (STAR) trial [published erratum appears in Expert Rev Anticancer Ther 2009;9:388]. Expert Rev Anticancer Ther 2009;9:51–60.

60

Chronic pelvic pain in adolescents

A 13-year-old adolescent girl is referred to you by her family physician because of a 3-month history of pelvic pain. She lives with her mother and stepfather, both of whom are present during the visit. You note that the patient's eye contact is poor and that her mother answers all questions directed to the girl, and her parents are hesitant about her being interviewed by herself. The pain is localized to the lower quadrants and is sharp, nonradiating, and not associated with diet or activity. She has not experienced diarrhea or pain with urination. She has not had a fever, and her weight has remained stable. She denies sexual activity. The most appropriate next step is to

* (A) interview the patient separately
(B) perform pelvic examination
(C) order pelvic ultrasonography
(D) refer to child protective services

Chronic pelvic pain in the adolescent is defined as persistent or recurrent pain that occurs for at least 3 months. The differential diagnosis of chronic pelvic pain in the child and adolescent is broad and includes gynecologic, gastrointestinal, urologic, musculoskeletal, and psychosocial causes. Symptoms that have been associated with organic as opposed to functional causes of chronic pain in children and adolescents include involuntary weight loss, unexplained fever, persistent diarrhea, urinary symptoms, and blood in the stool.

Most abdominopelvic pain in children and adolescents is functional in origin. Somatic symptoms may be the presenting symptom in patients with a history of sexual assault, which must be considered in the differential diagnosis of females of all ages with chronic pain. Although it is frequently appropriate to interview small children in the presence of a parent, a portion of interviews with adolescents should take place in the absence of family members.

Laws regarding confidentiality in adolescent health vary between states, and practitioners should become familiar with local regulations. The issue of confidentiality should be discussed with the patient and her family. Conditional confidentiality, whereby the patient and parents are instructed that information shared between the patient and obstetrician–gynecologist or other health care provider will remain confidential except where required by law, or if the physician determines that the patient may be acting in a way that is unsafe, is recommended for obstetrician–gynecologists or other health care providers of adolescents. Social and psychologic factors strongly influence individual response to pain. Stress, violence in the home, family member or personal substance abuse, and other psychosocial factors may manifest as chronic pelvic pain in the adolescent. The use of specific tools for the determination of risk-taking behavior (eg, the Home, Education/Employment, Activities, Drugs/Dieting, Sexuality, Suicide and Safety assessment) can provide insight into the patient's social situation.

Pelvic examination in a sexually naïve adolescent is rarely warranted as a first step; however, vulvar and rectal examination may yield helpful information. Examination should not take place until the physician builds rapport and trust with the patient.

Pelvic ultrasonography should be reserved for adolescents with chronic pelvic pain who are suspected of having pain with gynecologic etiology, an abnormal physical finding, or suboptimal examination.

A child protective services investigation must be initiated if the physician suspects assault after evaluation. Absolute proof of assault is not required to begin an investigation. Physicians who are unsure may contact local community child advocacy centers for guidance.

The described patient's symptoms and poor eye contact may be due to pain and teenage anxiety unrelated to sexual assault, but the lack of other signs and symptoms and the apparent controlling nature of her parents raise concern for abuse or potential social factors that may contribute to her pain. Alternatively, the behavior of her parents may be the result of anxiety over the cause of her pain as opposed to a desire to prevent the disclosure of accusatory information. To attempt to engage in history taking with the described patient in a calm and supportive environment separate from her parents is the most reasonable option.

Alfven G. One hundred cases of recurrent abdominal pain in children: diagnostic procedures and criteria for a psychosomatic diagnosis [published erratum appears in Acta Paediatr 2003;92:641]. Acta Paediatr 2003;92:43–9.

Di Lorenzo C, Colletti RB, Lehmann HP, Boyle JT, Gerson WT, Hyams JS, et al. Chronic abdominal pain in children: a technical report of the American Academy of Pediatrics and the North American Society for Pediatric Gastroenterology, Hepatology and Nutrition. AAP Subcommittee, NASPGHAN Committee on Chronic Abdominal Pain. J Pediatr Gastroenterol Nutr 2005;40:249–61.

Hewitt GD, Brown RT. Acute and chronic pelvic pain in female adolescents. Med Clin North Am 2000;84:1009–25.

Sacks D, Westwood M. An approach to interviewing adolescents. Paediatr Child Health 2003;8:554–6.

Song AH, Advincula AP. Adolescent chronic pelvic pain. J Pediatr Adolesc Gynecol 2005;18:371–7.

Thrall JS, McCloskey L, Ettner SL, Rothman E, Tighe JE, Emans SJ. Confidentiality and adolescents' use of providers for health information and for pelvic examinations. Arch Pediatr Adolesc Med 2000;154:885–92.

61

Pyelonephritis in pregnancy

A 25-year-old woman, gravida 1, at 26 weeks of gestation presents to the emergency department with fever, dysuria, and back pain. Physical examination is notable for left costovertebral angle tenderness. There is no fundal tenderness noted. Her temperature is 38.6°C (101.5°F), her heart rate is 115 beats per minute, and her blood pressure is 100/55 mm Hg. Cardiovascular examination reveals a holosystolic murmur. Fetal heart tones are present at 165 beats per minute by Doppler ultrasonography. Her complete blood count reveals a white blood cell count of 17 g/dL. Urinalysis is notable for more than 100 white blood cells per high-power field. The patient is admitted to the hospital for intravenous (IV) antibiotics, and after 48 hours of IV ceftriaxone, she demonstrates clinical improvement and is discharged with oral antibiotics. She presents to your office for follow-up and is feeling well. Upon review of her hospital records you note a urine culture that shows 100,000 colony forming units/mL *Escherichia coli*, which is sensitive to her current antibiotic regimen, as well as blood cultures positive for gram-negative rods. The most appropriate next step in management is

(A) repeat blood cultures
(B) broad-spectrum IV antibiotics
* (C) continue current oral antibiotics
(D) echocardiography

Urinary tract infections constitute one of the most common medical complications during pregnancy. These infections can be classified as asymptomatic bacteriuria in which the bacterial growth is limited to the urine, cystitis in which there is an infection of the lower urinary tract, or pyelonephritis, which is an ascending infection that involves the upper urinary tract. The presence of asymptomatic bacteriuria and cystitis is associated with an increased risk of developing an upper urinary tract infection, and up to 40% of pregnant women with untreated lower tract bacteriuria will develop pyelonephritis.

Because of the possible adverse maternal and fetal outcomes that can result from pyelonephritis during pregnancy, routine screening and treatment of lower urinary tract bacteriuria in all pregnant women is recommended by several organizations, including the American College of Obstetricians and Gynecologists, the U.S. Preventive Services Task Force, the Infectious Diseases Society of America, the American Academy of Pediatrics, and the American Academy of Family Physicians.

There are a variety of structural, physiologic, and functional urinary tract changes unique to pregnancy that predispose women to ascending infections, such as pyelonephritis, during pregnancy. Acute pyelonephritis complicates 1–2% of pregnancies and most commonly occurs in the second and third trimesters of pregnancy, when stasis and hydronephrosis are more evident. Additional risk factors for acute pyelonephritis include maternal age, nulliparity, diabetes mellitus, sickle cell anemia, nephrolithiasis, illicit drug use, urinary tract abnormalities, and prior history of pyelonephritis. Pyelonephritis remains one of the most common nonobstetric causes for hospitalization during pregnancy and is the leading cause of septic shock during pregnancy.

Among pregnant women with pyelonephritis, approximately 10–20% are found to have concurrent bacteremia by positive blood cultures. Blood cultures often are obtained in conjunction with urine cultures as part of the diagnostic evaluation of pyelonephritis; however, the necessity of obtaining blood cultures has not been validated. Given their sterile nature, organisms found in the blood are good targets for antimicrobial therapy. However, obtaining blood cultures adds little clinical value when urine culture results are known and can appropriately guide clinical therapy. Research questioning the utility of blood cultures in the management of pyelonephritis in pregnant women has demonstrated successful therapy without the need for blood culture results and susceptibility testing. Treatment decisions were based on a patient's clinical course rather than on blood culture results. Although the described patient had positive blood cultures, her uropathogen probably is the same pathogen found in the blood culture. Given her clinical improvement, repeat blood cultures are not warranted because they would not alter the patient's clinical management.

The pathogens responsible for urinary tract infections during pregnancy are organisms commonly found in the gastrointestinal tract, with *E coli* accounting for up to 80% of cases. Among the remaining cases, *Klebsiella pneumoniae*, coagulase-negative *Staphylococcus, Staphylococcus aureus*, and group B streptococci often are implicated. A diagnosis of pyelonephritis is based on a constellation of clinical findings, including lumbar pain, fever higher than 38°C (100.4°F), and costovertebral angle tenderness in conjunction with laboratory evidence of bacteriuria or pyuria confirmed with subsequent urine culture. Acute pyelonephritis complicating pregnancy requires inpatient hospitalization with IV antibiotics for the initial 24–48 hours, which are continued until the patient is afebrile and shows clinical improvement.

Approximately 75% of patients will have clinical resolution of symptoms within 48 hours, and 95% of patients will see resolution within 72 hours of therapy. After clinical improvement, patients are transitioned to oral antibiotics to complete a 2-week course and require daily antibiotic suppression for the duration of the pregnancy and 6 weeks postpartum. The initial antibiotic therapy is empiric and should then be altered based on urine culture results. Common empiric regimens include ampicillin plus gentamicin or a single-agent cephalosporin such as ceftriaxone. Although some studies have demonstrated a resistance rate to ampicillin close to 50%, no single antibiotic treatment regimen has been shown to be clinically superior to others, and patient treatment plans ultimately should be determined by local antibiograms and susceptibility patterns.

The described patient was treated appropriately with empiric IV antibiotics at the time of her initial presentation, and they were continued until she demonstrated clinical improvement. In addition, her urine culture susceptibility testing reveals an organism that is sensitive to her current antibiotic regimen. Broad-spectrum IV antibiotics are not warranted at this time. Given her ongoing clinical improvement, in conjunction with known susceptibility testing, continuing her current antibiotic regimen is the most appropriate next step in management.

The most significant and feared complication of bacteremia is infective endocarditis. The most common uropathogen implicated in pyelonephritis during pregnancy is *E coli*. However, gram-negative *Enterobacteriaceae* are less likely to cause endocarditis than gram-positive cocci. The described patient has no clinical signs or symptoms concerning for infective endocarditis. Her holosystolic murmur is likely a physiologic flow murmur seen in pregnancy that was exacerbated at the time of her initial presentation. Echocardiography is not indicated at this point in her management.

Dawkins JC, Fletcher HM, Rattray CA, Reid M, Gordon-Strachan G. Acute pyelonephritis in pregnancy: a retrospective descriptive hospital based study. ISRN Obstet Gynecol 2012;519321.

Glaser AP, Schaeffer AM. Urinary tract infection and bacteriuria in pregnancy. Urol Clin N Am 2015;42:547–60.

Gomi H, Goto Y, Laopaiboon M, Usui R, Mori R. Routine blood cultures in the management of pyelonephritis in pregnancy for improving outcomes. Cochrane Database of Systematic 2015, Issue 2. Art. No.: CD009216. DOI: 10.1002/14651858.CD009216.pub2.

Matuszkiewicz-Rowińska J, Małyszko J, Wieliczko M. Urinary tract infections in pregnancy: old and new unresolved diagnostic and therapeutic problems. Arch Med Sci 2015;11:67–7.

62

Urethral lesions

A 65-year-old woman comes to your office for her annual well-woman examination. She has a history of four vaginal deliveries and urinary urge incontinence, for which she takes oxybutynin. During her physical examination, you notice an abnormality (Fig. 62-1; see color plate). The mass is soft on palpation with no evidence of necrosis or groin lymphadenopathy. The patient tells you that she has no dysuria, difficulty urinating, discharge, vaginal bleeding, or pain. The next step in management is

(A) biopsy
(B) estrogen cream
* (C) observation
(D) stop oxybutynin
(E) surgical excision

A urethral caruncle is a benign polypoid lesion at the distal portion of the urethral meatus. It is the most common abnormality of the female urethra and occurs primarily in postmenopausal women. A urethral caruncle appears as a soft pink or red nodule protruding from the urethral meatus on examination. It is differentiated from a urethral prolapse by the degree of urethral eversion; urethral prolapse has mucosa that is circumferentially everted at the meatus, whereas the caruncle has only a segment that is prolapsed, generally on the posterior margin. Symptoms may include light bleeding, dysuria, pain, obstruction to urine flow, and patient awareness of the mass.

It is important to distinguish a caruncle or prolapse, which are benign lesions, from a urethral carcinoma. Signs suggestive of malignancy include a mass larger than 2 cm or increasing size, firmness, induration, ulceration, irregular borders, additional palpable lesions not visible on examination (local extension), or inguinal lymphadenopathy. Biopsy is indicated if the diagnosis is uncertain. The described patient has no signs or symptoms consistent with malignancy, so a biopsy is not required at this time.

For symptomatic patients, the first-line treatment is topical estrogen cream for 2–3 months. A small amount of estrogen cream can be applied to the caruncle once daily for 2 weeks and then twice a week for 2–3 months. Because the described patient lacks symptoms, such as bleeding or dysuria, treatment with estrogen cream is not necessary.

The most common symptoms of urethral caruncle are light bleeding and pain; urinary symptoms are less common. Studies have found an association between urethral instability and detrusor instability, but there does not appear to be a relation between benign urethral lesions and the treatment of incontinence. Thus, there is no need to stop the patient's use of oxybutynin.

If the patient's symptoms are refractory to estrogen, or if the caruncle is large, then biopsy and surgical excision under local or regional anesthesia would be recommended. The traditional procedure is excision of the lesion at its base with reapproximation of the edges with a small (3-0 or 4-0) synthetic absorbable monofilament suture. If the defect is large, the edge of the urethral mucosa is everted onto the adjacent vaginal epithelium to minimize the risk of meatal stenosis, which is the major complication of this procedure. A technique involving suture ligation that can be done in the office without analgesia has been described. Because the described patient is asymptomatic and the caruncle is small, she is not a candidate for surgical excision at this time.

Urethral caruncles and prolapse most often are benign conditions. If the patient is asymptomatic, as this patient is, the conditions should be managed expectantly with observation.

Conces MR, Williamson SR, Montironi R, Lopez-Beltran A, Scarpelli M, Cheng L. Urethral caruncle: clinicopathologic features of 41 cases. Hum Pathol 2012;43:1400–4.

Park DS, Cho TW. Simple solution for urethral caruncle. J Urol 2004;172(5 Pt 1):1884–5.

Schreiner L, Nygaard CC, Anschau F. Urethral prolapse in premenopausal, healthy adult woman. Int Urogynecol J 2013;24:353–4.

63
Zika virus in pregnancy

A 24-year-old nulligravid woman who recently emigrated from Brazil presents for her first prenatal visit. Although she has no history of any significant medical conditions, she does indicate that 6 weeks ago she had a mild flu-like illness with associated joint discomfort and watery eyes. Pelvic examination is consistent with 14 weeks of gestation. A fetal heart rate was detected. At this time, in addition to standard antenatal testing, you recommend

(A) routine care
(B) serial fetal ultrasonography
(C) pregnancy termination
(D) reverse transcription polymerase chain reaction (PCR) testing for Zika virus infection
* (E) immunoglobulin M (IgM) antibody testing for Zika virus infection

Zika virus infections during pregnancy have been associated with birth defects, specifically microcephaly and intracranial calcifications. This flavivirus is spread among humans by infected *Aedes aegypti* mosquitoes and has an incubation period of 3–12 days. Sexual transmission also has been reported. Symptoms are nonspecific and may include fever, rash, arthralgia, and conjunctivitis. Although cases of Guillain-Barré syndrome have occurred with this viral infection, most illnesses are mild, and only approximately 20% of infected individuals exhibit any symptoms. It is unknown whether pregnant women are at increased risk of these infections. Transmission of the virus has been documented in all trimesters. Evidence of the infection has been found in fetal tissue from missed abortions, amniotic fluid, and placentas, as well as in the brains of fetuses with microcephaly and term neonates. At this time, there is no treatment or vaccine available. There is a great deal of epidemiologic uncertainty regarding the incidence of Zika virus infection in pregnant women in endemic areas, the rate of vertical transmission to the fetus, and the rate at which an infected fetus manifests a complication such as microcephaly.

The presence of a serum reverse transcription PCR from a blood sample of a possible infected individual is diagnostic. However, samples must be obtained within 3–7 days of the onset of symptoms. Immunoglobulin M testing and plaque-reduction neutralizing tests can be used after 4 days have elapsed since the onset of the illness. Plaque-reduction neutralizing tests are difficult to interpret because of false-positive test results and cross-reactions with other flavivirus infections, such as dengue, West Nile virus, and yellow fever. Despite the complexity of interpretation, a negative IgM test result obtained 2–12 weeks after travel would suggest that a Zika virus infection did not occur.

Figure 63-1 provides the approach to evaluating women with possible exposure to Zika virus. Use of Zika virus reverse transcription PCR or IgM testing is the first step in evaluating pregnant women. Because the described patient is outside the window for reverse transcription PCR testing, she would undergo IgM testing. Serial fetal ultrasonography every 3–4 weeks is done to detect the manifestations of significant infection, microcephaly, or intracranial calcifications in the fetuses of women with positive or inconclusive testing. However, fetal ultrasonography may not detect these changes until the late second trimester or early third trimester. The described patient has not undergone serologic testing, so serial fetal ultrasonography would not be the appropriate option for her. The Centers for Disease Control and Prevention recommend considering amniocentesis when fetal manifestations are detected or a pregnant woman has received a positive test result for the Zika virus infection. Such testing would provide more insight into the epidemiology of this viral infection and, thus, would not be an appropriate option for this patient without initial serologic testing. In the absence of a known serious manifestation of the infection, and because of the uncertainty of whether the fetus is even infected, pregnancy termination because of a possible Zika virus infection is not indicated. Routine care is not recommended unless the patient prefers it because there is some risk the fetus may be affected.

Because there is no treatment or vaccine available for Zika virus, pregnant women should avoid travel to endemic areas. Pregnant women who live in such areas should protect themselves against mosquito bites by wearing appropriate clothing to protect their skin, using

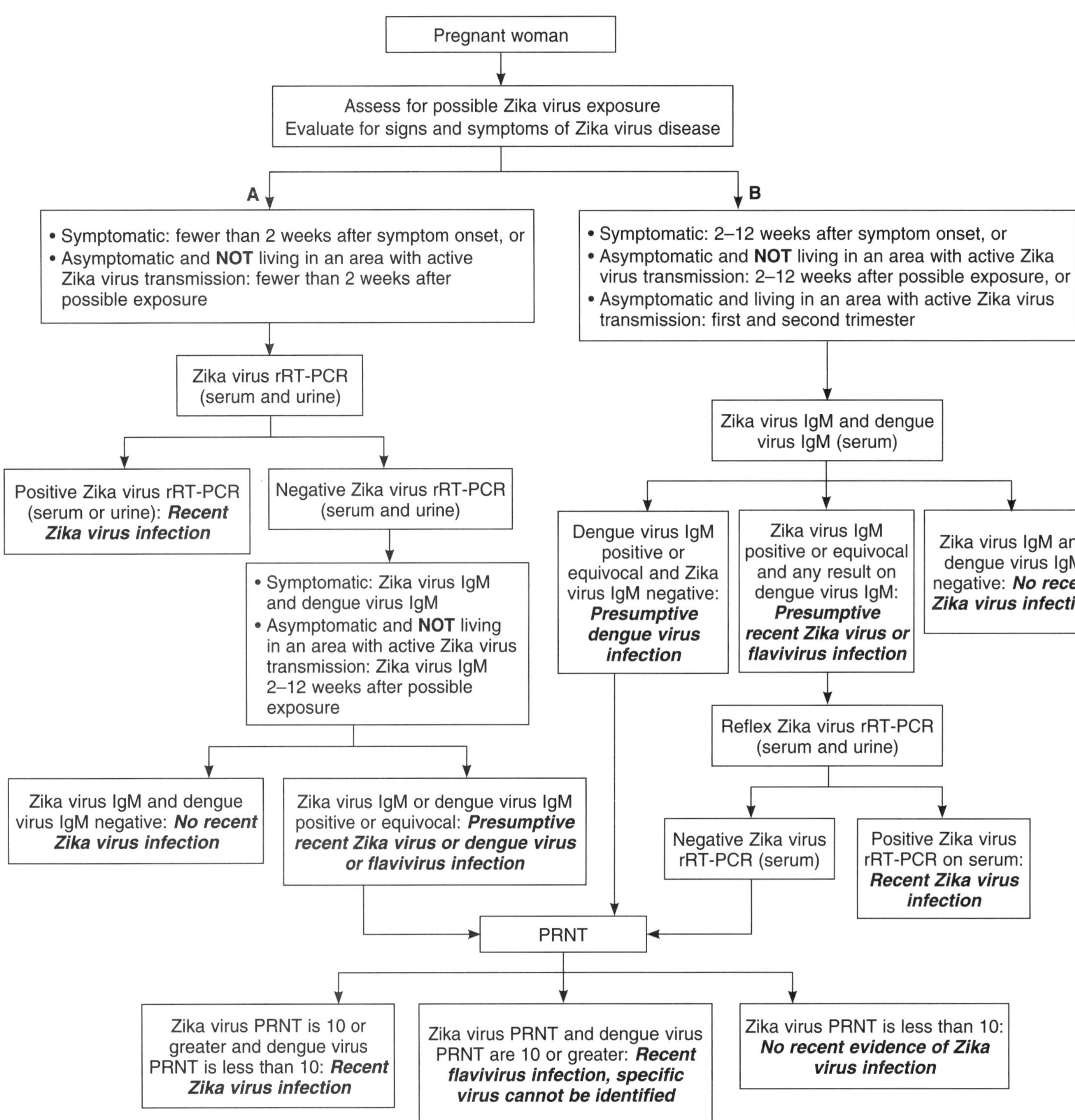

FIGURE 63-1. Updated interim guidance: testing and interpretation recommendations for a pregnant woman with possible exposure to Zika virus. Abbreviations: IgM, immunoglobulin M; PRNT, plaque-reduction neutralization test; rRT-PCR, real-time reverse transcription–polymerase chain reaction. A pregnant woman is considered symptomatic if one or more signs or symptoms (acute onset of fever, rash, arthralgia, or conjunctivitis) consistent with Zika virus disease is reported. A pregnant woman is considered asymptomatic if these symptoms are NOT reported. Testing includes Zika virus rRT-PCR on serum and urine samples, Zika virus and dengue virus IgM, and PRNT on serum samples. PRNT results that indicate recent flavivirus infection should be interpreted in the context of the currently circulating flaviviruses. Refer to the laboratory guidance for updated testing recommendations (http://www.cdc.gov/zika/laboratories/lab-guidance.html). Because of the overlap of symptoms in areas where other viral illness are endemic, evaluate for possible dengue or chikungunya virus infection. Dengue virus IgM antibody testing is recommended only for symptomatic pregnant women. If Zika virus rRT-PCR testing is requested from laboratories without IgM antibody testing capacity or a process to forward specimens to another testing laboratory, storing of additional serum samples is recommended for IgM antibody testing in the event of an rRT-PCR negative result. Possible exposure to Zika virus includes travel to or residence

in an area with active Zika virus transmission (http://wwwnc.cdc.gov/travel/notices/), or sex (vaginal sex [penis-to-vagina sex], anal sex [penis-to-anus sex], oral sex [mouth-to-penis sex or mouth-to-vagina sex], and the sharing of sex toys) without a barrier method to prevent infection (male or female condoms for vaginal or anal sex, male condoms for oral sex [mouth-to-penis], and male condoms cut to create a flat barrier or dental dams for oral sex [mouth-to-vagina]) with a partner who traveled to or lives in an area with active Zika virus transmission. (Petersen EE, Polen KN, Meaney-Delman D, Ellington SR, Oduyebo T, Cohn A, et al. Update: Interim Guidance for Health Care Providers Caring for Women of Reproductive Age with Possible Zika Virus Exposure—United States, 2016. MMWR Morb Mortal Wkly Rep. ePub: 25 March 2016. DOI: http://dx.doi.org/10.15585/mmwr.mm6512e2er.)

Environmental Protection Agency-approved bug spray containing diethyltoluamide, spending as much time as possible in screened-in or air-conditioned areas, and treating clothing with permethrin. When used as directed, diethyltoluamide-containing sprays and permethrin are safe during pregnancy. Because sexual transmission of the virus occurs, men who reside in or who have traveled to an area with active Zika virus transmission and who have a pregnant partner should abstain from sexual activity or consistently and correctly use condoms for the duration of the pregnancy.

Petersen EE, Polen KN, Meaney-Delman D, Ellington, SR, Oduyebo, T, Cohn A, et al. Update: Interim Guidelines for Health Care Providers Caring for Pregnant Women and Women of Reproductive Age with Possible Zika Virus Exposure — United States, 2016. MMWR Morb Mortal Wkly Rep 2016;65:122–127. DOI: http://www.cdc.gov/mmwr/volumes/65/wr/mm6512e2.htm?s_cid=mm6512e2_w.htm.

64

Endometrial thickness in an asymptomatic postmenopausal woman

A 55-year-old menopausal woman is referred to you for a uniform endometrial thickness of 7 mm discovered on ultrasonography. Her past medical history and family history are normal, and she takes no medications. The patient is asymptomatic and reports no bleeding. The most appropriate next step in management is

(A) endometrial biopsy
(B) hysteroscopy
* (C) expectant management
(D) sonohysterography
(E) repeat ultrasonography

The significance of an ultrasonographic finding of a thickened endometrium in an asymptomatic postmenopausal woman has not been determined, and routine endometrial sampling based on this finding alone is not recommended. Results of a decision analysis found that asymptomatic postmenopausal women with an endometrial thickness of less than 11 mm have a similar risk of endometrial cancer compared with postmenopausal women with bleeding and a measurement of less than 4 mm.

The lifetime risk of uterine cancer for women living in the United States is just below 3%. Type I endometrial (endometrioid cell type) cancer accounts for 75% of these cases. Type II endometrial cancer includes clear cell and papillary serous histology and is responsible for 40% of deaths related to uterine cancer. Risk factors for the development of type I endometrial cancer are listed in Appendix F.

Endometrial evaluation is indicated for all women with postmenopausal bleeding who do not take hormone therapy. Ultrasonographic determination of endometrial thickness may be used as part of the evaluation of the endometrium in symptomatic postmenopausal women. An endometrial stripe measurement of 4 mm or less is associated with a negative predictive value of greater than 99% for endometrial cancer in postmenopausal women who experience bleeding. For this reason, the American College of Obstetricians and Gynecologists suggests that endometrial stripe measurement may be a reasonable first test in a postmenopausal woman with bleeding or for the triage of women with insufficient endometrial sampling.

The described patient should undergo endometrial sampling if she has a history of recent bleeding. Endometrial biopsy in the office with a pipelle sampler is highly sensitive for the detection of endometrial cancer in postmenopausal women. Repeat ultrasonography in the absence of bleeding is costly and unlikely to affect management decisions in this case. Hysteroscopy and directed biopsy are recommended in a postmenopausal woman with focal endometrial findings on ultrasonography or in a persistently symptomatic woman who has had negative biopsy and ultrasonography results. Hysteroscopy may be avoided in a postmenopausal woman with negative sonohysterography and tissue sampling. Although sonohysterography may be indicated in a patient with focal findings on ultrasonography or with abnormal or unscheduled vaginal bleeding, this patient is asymptomatic, so sonohysterography is not the best next step. The incidental finding of a 7-mm endometrium in this asymptomatic woman without risk factors for endometrial cancer does not warrant further testing. Expectant management is the most appropriate next step.

Dijkhuizen FP, Mol BW, Brolmann HA, Heintz AP. The accuracy of endometrial sampling in the diagnosis of patients with endometrial carcinoma and hyperplasia: a meta-analysis. Cancer 2000;89:1765–72.

Endometrial cancer. Practice Bulletin No. 149. American College of Obstetricians and Gynecologists. Obstet Gynecol 2015;125:1006–26.

Gupta JK, Chien PF, Voit D, Clark TJ, Khan KS. Ultrasonographic endometrial thickness for diagnosing endometrial pathology in women with postmenopausal bleeding: a meta-analysis. Acta Obstet Gynecol Scand 2002;81:799–816.

The role of transvaginal ultrasonography in the evaluation of postmenopausal bleeding. ACOG Committee Opinion No. 440. American College of Obstetricians and Gynecologists. Obstet Gynecol 2009;114:409–11.

Smith-Bindman R, Weiss E, Feldstein V. How thick is too thick? When endometrial thickness should prompt biopsy in postmenopausal women without vaginal bleeding. Ultrasound Obstet Gynecol 2004;24:558–65.

Tabor A, Watt HC, Wald NJ. Endometrial thickness as a test for endometrial cancer in women with postmenopausal vaginal bleeding. Obstet Gynecol 2002;99:663–70.

65

Prepregnancy counseling

A 33-year-old nulligravid woman, who is a registered nurse, comes to see you for a prepregnancy visit. She states that she is healthy and that she takes no medications other than prenatal vitamins. She is having regular menstrual cycles. She reports that her 40-year-old husband, a former professional athlete, is healthy with the exception of some mild musculoskeletal concerns and is not taking any medications. She has stopped drinking alcohol. Review of her immunization records reveals that she is immune to rubella and varicella. Her test result for syphilis is negative. The infectious disease for which prepregnancy interventions are most likely to improve perinatal outcome is

(A) vaginal group B streptococci (GBS)
(B) herpes simplex virus (HSV)
* (C) human immunodeficiency virus (HIV)
(D) asymptomatic bacteriuria
(E) hepatitis C

The goal of prepregnancy care and counseling is to address health, environmental, and resource issues that may have an adverse effect on pregnancy outcome. Ideally, all women should seek such an evaluation before pregnancy, but about one half of pregnancies are unplanned. Addressing prepregnancy concerns should be part of routine well-woman care throughout the patient's reproductive years.

An effective prepregnancy program addresses health promotion (eg, weight loss), infectious disease (eg, hepatitis, HIV), medical conditions (eg, hypertension), parental exposures (eg, alcohol, lead), nutrition (eg, folate supplementation), and genetic risk factors (family history of genetic disorders). The length of this list may appear burdensome, but interventions before pregnancy are more likely to have a positive effect on the pregnancy than those undertaken after a pregnancy is established.

One aspect of prepregnancy care is identification of infectious disease risk. Many sexually transmitted infections can have an adverse effect on pregnancy, whereas others are less of a problem or can be assessed by appropriate history taking. Other infectious morbidities are limited to those who travel internationally (eg, malaria) or engage in specific behaviors (eg, intravenous drug use).

Since the first appearance of HIV as a public health crisis, HIV diagnosis and screening have undergone significant evolution. There are therapies that can reduce transmission, improve survival, and reduce morbidity. In the prepregnancy setting, identification of HIV infection allows for initiation or alteration of therapies that can reduce the chances of vertical transmission to the fetus or newborn. For these reasons, routine screening for HIV infection is widely endorsed. The American College of Obstetricians and Gynecologists recommends routine screening for females aged 13–64 years. The decision to perform annual screening after an initial negative assessment is based on risk factors; however, it should be considered for all patients. Nearly 20% of individuals who have HIV infection are not aware of their status. Identification of HIV status before pregnancy will give the patient various options with respect to reproduction, including prevention of pregnancy. Other modalities to reduce vertical transmission include taking a maximally suppressive antiretroviral regimen. Although no regimen guarantees prevention of transmission, maintaining a low or undetectable viral load will reduce the likelihood of mother-to-child transmission.

There are no data to support routine screening for hepatitis C before pregnancy. Certain high-risk patients may benefit from screening (eg, intravenous drug users). Antiviral treatment during pregnancy is an active area of research.

Routine screening of pregnant patients at the initial prenatal visit for asymptomatic bacteriuria is advised because, if it is left untreated, it may progress to pyelonephritis in pregnancy and may result in perinatal morbidity. However, prepregnancy testing for asymptomatic bacteriuria is not advised because the likelihood of serious infection in nonpregnant women is very low, and persistent or recurrent bacteriuria is common. Retreatment during pregnancy would thus be necessitated, and overtreatment can lead to antibiotic resistance.

Testing for GBS also is a routine part of prenatal care but is not indicated before pregnancy. No increased risk of early pregnancy complications has been associated with vaginal GBS infections. Therefore, testing should be limited to the 35–37 weeks of gestation window, as recommended by the American College of Obstetricians and Gynecologists and the Centers for Disease Control and Prevention. Similarly, prepregnancy screening for HSV has not been shown to result in better pregnancy outcomes. Treatment during pregnancy of HSV-positive women starting at 36 weeks of gestation, however, can reduce outbreaks at term, as well as perinatal transmission in women known to be infected.

Other elements of effective prepregnancy counseling include dietary interventions, such as initiation of folate supplementation (400 micrograms daily) to reduce fetal neural tube defects and other birth defects. Another area of increasing importance is encouraging obese women to lose weight before pregnancy. Perinatal outcomes are better if a woman has a body mass index (calculated as weight in kilograms divided by height in meters squared [kg/m^2]) of less than 30. Consultation with a nutritionist should be considered for women who would benefit from weight loss before pregnancy.

Routine screening for certain environmental exposures (eg, lead, mercury) generally is not recommended, but some general guidance to reduce these exposures is warranted. Certain fish that contain higher amounts of mercury should be avoided (eg, shark, swordfish, king mackerel, and tilefish). Some skin-lightening creams contain mercury and also should be avoided. Consultation with a toxicologist may be warranted if suspicion for excess mercury exposure is present.

Finally, patients should be advised to stop smoking and avoid alcohol use if they are considering pregnancy. Many women will cease smoking and avoid alcohol use on their own when they become pregnant, but encouragement and positive reinforcement from health care professionals has been shown to increase substance avoidance.

Coonrod DV, Jack BW, Stubblefield PG, Hollier LM, Boggess KA, Cefalo R, et al. The clinical content of preconception care: infectious diseases in preconception care. Am J Obstet Gynecol 2008;199: S296–309.

Humphrey JR, Floyd RL. Preconception health and health care environmental scan: Report on clinical screening tools and interventions. Atlanta (GA): National Center on Birth Defects and Developmental Disabilities Centers for Disease Control and Prevention; 2012. Available at: http://www.cdc.gov/preconception/documents/environmental-scan-report.pdf. Retrieved June 11, 2016.

Routine human immunodeficiency virus screening. Committee Opinion No. 596. American College of Obstetricians and Gynecologists. Obstet Gynecol 2014;123:1137–9.

Sathyanarayana S, Focareta J, Dailey T, Buchanan S. Environmental exposures: how to counsel preconception and prenatal patients in the clinical setting. Am J Obstet Gynecol 2012;207:463–70.

66

Precocious puberty

A 5-year-old girl is brought to your office by her mother because of pubertal changes. The mother denies that the girl has had any vaginal bleeding, but she is worried about breast development and hair growth. Physical examination shows Tanner stage III breasts, pubic hair, and axillary hair. Her basal luteinizing hormone (LH) level is 1.7 international units/L and increases to 21 international units/L on a gonadotrophin-releasing hormone (GnRH) stimulation test. Her bone age development is 8 years. The best next step is

(A) reassurance
(B) 17α-hydroxyprogesterone level measurement
(C) karyotyping
(D) pelvic ultrasonography
* (E) brain magnetic resonance imaging

Precocious puberty is defined as development of pubertal changes at an age younger than population norms. The normal progression of puberty starts with breast budding (thelarche) followed by growth of pubic and axillary hair (adrenarche) and onset of menses (menarche) 2–3 years after initiation of breast development. The average age at thelarche is 10 years and the average age at menarche is 12.5 years. Development generally occurs at an earlier age among African American girls compared with white girls. Pubic hair and axillary hair typically are not observed until girls reach Tanner stage III breast development. Normal puberty can begin as young as age 6 years among African American girls and as young as age 7 years among white girls. Onset of puberty before this age range, abnormal rate or sequence of progression of puberty, accelerated linear growth (height), or advanced bone age are all factors that suggest a need for evaluation of precocious puberty.

Precocious puberty can be classified as either central precocious puberty or peripheral precocious puberty. Central precocious puberty is GnRH-dependent and is caused by early reactivation of the hypothalamic–pituitary–gonadal axis. Pattern and timing of pubertal events typically occurs in a normal sequence, with accelerated linear growth for age, advanced bone age, and pubertal levels of follicle-stimulating hormone (FSH), LH, and estradiol. Diagnosis of central precocious puberty is made by measuring LH levels before and after GnRH stimulation. Stimulated LH levels above 5–8 international units/L suggest central precocious puberty. In contrast, with peripheral precocious puberty, LH and FSH levels are in the prepubertal range (less than 0.1 international units/L) at baseline and do not increase with GnRH stimulation.

The described patient has central precocious puberty. Most cases of this condition are idiopathic. However, cranial and pituitary magnetic resonance imaging is necessary to evaluate for an organic cause. Hamartomas of the tuber cinereum are the type of central nervous system tumor that most frequently causes precocious puberty in very young children. Other central nervous system tumors that have been associated with central precocious puberty are listed in Box 66-1.

Peripheral precocious puberty is GnRH-independent and is caused by excess estrogen or androgen exposure from gonadal, adrenal, or external sources. The peripheral source of hormones is more likely to cause deviations from the normal sequence and pace of puberty. Levels of LH are in the normal preadolescent range and do not respond to stimulation with GnRH.

Ultrasonography is indicated for girls with peripheral precocious puberty to look for large functioning follicular cysts or ovarian tumors. Granulosa cell tumors may

BOX 66-1

Central Nervous System Aberrations Associated With Central Precocious Puberty

- Hamartomas of the tuber cinereum
- Astrocytoma
- Ependymoma
- Pinealoma
- Optic glioma
- Hypothalamic glioma
- Hydrocephalus
- Cysts
- Trauma
- Inflammatory disease
- Congenital midline defects

cause isosexual precocious puberty, whereas Sertoli–Leydig cell tumors and gonadoblastomas may produce androgens and cause contrasexual precocious puberty (virilization) in girls. Recurrent ovarian cysts may be associated with McCune–Albright syndrome, a cause of peripheral precocious puberty that is manifested by a triad of peripheral precocious puberty, café au lait skin pigmentation, and fibrous dysplasia of the bone. Although ultrasonography may show maturation of internal genitalia in central precocious puberty, it would not be the best next step for the described patient.

Nonprogressive premature thelarche generally is benign and self-limited, likely as a result of FSH-driven ovarian cyst formation and increasing estradiol levels. Expectant management may be appropriate, but progression to pubic hair is inconsistent with isolated premature thelarche and requires further evaluation, as seen in the described patient. Accelerated growth velocity and rapid bone maturation, as observed in this patient, can result in reduced adult height. Evaluation is necessary, primarily to identify and treat underlying factors that may be life threatening. Treatment can allow such patients to be normalized to peers and can enable attainment of appropriate adult height. Use of a GnRH analog is an effective therapy in increasing adult height for girls with early-onset central precocious puberty (age younger than 6 years). Reassurance alone would not be appropriate for the described patient because a significant underlying condition may not be detected, and the opportunity for treatment would be missed.

Late-onset congenital adrenal hyperplasia (CAH) is part of the differential diagnosis of peripheral precocious puberty, and the condition may present as isolated premature adrenarche, with early onset of pubic hair, axillary hair, mild acne, and body odor. The most common form results from a deficiency of 21-hydroxylase and can be diagnosed by measurement of 17α-hydroxyprogesterone levels. The premature adrenarche of CAH results from a peripheral (adrenal) source of increased androgens. Therefore, LH levels would be in the prepubescent range and would not respond to GnRH stimulation. In addition, CAH typically is not associated with early thelarche. Although specific genetic mutations have been associated with central precocious puberty, karyotyping is not part of the standard evaluation of precocious puberty.

Carel JC, Eugster EA, Rogol A, Ghizzoni L, Palmert MR, Antoniazzi F, et al. Consensus statement on the use of gonadotropin-releasing hormone analogs in children. ESPE-LWPES GnRH Analogs Consensus Conference Group. Pediatrics 2009;123:e752–62.

Fuqua JS. Treatment and outcomes of precocious puberty: an update. J Clin Endocrinol Metab 2013;98:2198–207.

Harrington J, Palmert MR. Definition, etiology, and evaluation of precocious puberty. In: Post TW, editors. UpToDate. Waltham (MA): UpToDate; 2016.

Neely EK, Crossen SS. Precocious puberty. Curr Opin Obstet Gynecol 2014;26:332–8.

67

Markers for ovarian cancer screening

A 64-year-old woman has had vague left lower quadrant pain for 2 weeks. Her medical history is unremarkable. On examination, you palpate a 4-cm mass in the left adnexa. You order pelvic ultrasonography that reveals a complex cystic ovarian mass with increased vascularity. As a result of these findings, you order additional testing to assess the risk of malignancy. The ovarian mass risk algorithm that incorporates measurement of serum CA 125 and human epididymis secretory protein 4 is

* (A) Risk of Ovarian Malignancy Algorithm
(B) International Ovarian Tumor Analysis
(C) Risk of Malignancy Index
(D) Risk of Ovarian Cancer Algorithm

Several algorithms have been proposed to help predict which ovarian masses are malignant. Most of these approaches are not designed for primary ovarian screening. Instead, most of these protocols have been developed to further evaluate a mass that is identified by ultrasonography. The benefit of a correct preoperative assignment as benign or malignant is that women with a malignancy will be referred for surgical management by a gynecologic oncologist or other specifically trained surgeon. Women who have been diagnosed with ovarian malignancy and have surgery performed by nongynecologic oncology surgeons may undergo inadequate surgical staging or suboptimal removal of tumor, which in turn affects prognosis.

Assessment of CA 125 levels has traditionally been used as a serum marker for ovarian cancer. CA 125 is elevated in less than one half of cases of early ovarian cancer, though, and it is not expressed at all in approximately 20% of epithelial ovarian malignancies. Human epididymis secretory protein 4 is overexpressed in ovarian cancer cells. It has been shown to be more specific for malignancies than CA 125. Therefore, many clinicians measure human epididymis secretory protein 4 when serum CA 125 levels are elevated to reduce the false-positive rate. This may be especially helpful in premenopausal women who are likely to have elevated CA 125 as a result of a benign condition.

The Risk of Ovarian Malignancy Algorithm uses a logistic regression model that incorporates serum levels of CA 125 and human epididymis secretory protein 4 in a woman with a pelvic mass. This approach was studied prospectively in a multicenter trial. The algorithm categorizes women as high risk or low risk based on levels of these serum markers and menopausal status. Overall, the approach was associated with a sensitivity of 88.7% and a specificity of 74.7%. In postmenopausal women only, the sensitivity was 92.3%, and the negative predictive value was 92.6%. If the Risk of Ovarian Malignancy Algorithm is combined with an initial clinical assessment incorporating imaging, the screening performance is improved.

The International Ovarian Tumor Analysis group is a collaborative endeavor from several international ultrasonography centers that have compiled a set of simple rules by which to classify an adnexal mass as malignant or benign. No serum markers are used in this protocol. A variety of defining features, such as presence of papillary projections and septal thickness, are assessed. This group uses five features to categorize a mass as malignant or benign (Table 67-1). A tumor is defined as benign if one or more of the benign features is present and no malignant features are present. Conversely, a tumor is defined as malignant if one or more malignant features are identified, with no benign features. If none of these features are present, or if features from both lists are present, the tumor is unclassified. A systematic review of published reports of prospective studies using this algorithm to identify malignant tumors concluded that sensitivity and specificity in premenopausal women were 89% and 97%, respectively. In postmenopausal women, sensitivity and specificity were both 94%. Approximately 20% of tumors were not classifiable preoperatively as either benign or malignant.

A commonly used clinical approach to the preoperative evaluation of an ovarian mass forms the foundation for the Risk of Malignancy Index. This protocol uses ultrasonography and CA 125 levels in addition to the patient's menopausal status. These three factors are multiplied together, and if the threshold score is met, the index is considered positive. Several studies have shown this approach outperforms clinical judgment in terms of correct preoperative prediction of malignancy and that more patients would be referred appropriately to a gynecologic oncologist if this approach was used.

The Risk of Ovarian Cancer Algorithm uses a two-stage approach and is a screening protocol, as opposed to an evaluation of an examination-detected mass. This

TABLE 67-1. Five Ultrasonographic Features Used to Classify Ovarian Tumors by Malignant or Benign

Malignant	Benign
Irregular solid tumor	Unilocular cyst
Ascites	Largest solid component is less than 7 mm
At least four papillary structures	Acoustic shadows
Irregular multilocular–solid tumor with largest diameter at least 100 mm	Smooth multilocular tumor less than 100 mm in largest diameter
Very high color content on color Doppler ultrasonography	No detectable blood flow on Doppler ultrasonography

Modified from Nunes N, Ambler G, Foo X, Naftalin J, Widschwendter M, Jurkovic D. Use of IOTA simple rules for diagnosis of ovarian cancer: meta-analysis. Ultrasound Obstet Gynecol 2014;44:503–14.

protocol makes use of the fact that, in many early ovarian malignancies, the longitudinal increase in serum CA 125 can identify early-stage malignancy, even if the absolute value is within normal limits. Initial studies using this approach demonstrate promise in terms of sensitivity and specificity in the identification of early-stage ovarian cancer.

No perfect method exists to distinguish consistently between benign and malignant ovarian masses. The various aforementioned models work with similar effectiveness, but none has been shown to be clearly superior to experience and clinical judgment.

Bristow RE, Smith A, Zhang Z, Chan DW, Crutcher G, Fung ET, et al. Ovarian malignancy risk stratification of the adnexal mass using a multivariate index assay. Gynecol Oncol 2013;128:252–9.

Lu KH, Skates S, Hernandez MA, Bedi D, Bevers T, Leeds L, et al. A 2-stage ovarian cancer screening strategy using the Risk of Ovarian Cancer Algorithm (ROCA) identifies early-stage incident cancers and demonstrates high positive predictive value. Cancer 2013;119:3454–61.

Moore RG, Hawkins DM, Miller MC, Landrum LM, Gajewski W, Ball JJ, et al. Combining clinical assessment and the Risk of Ovarian Malignancy Algorithm for the prediction of ovarian cancer. Gynecol Oncol 2014;135:547–51.

Nunes N, Ambler G, Foo X, Naftalin J, Widschwendter M, Jurkovic D. Use of IOTA simple rules for diagnosis of ovarian cancer: meta-analysis. Ultrasound Obstet Gynecol 2014;44:503–14.

van den Akker PA, Aalders AL, Snijders MP, Kluivers KB, Samlal RA, Vollebergh JH, et al. Evaluation of the Risk of Malignancy Index in daily clinical management of adnexal masses. Gynecol Oncol 2010;116:384–8.

68

Office simulation emergency drill

You work in an obstetrics and gynecology practice with three other physicians and two advanced nurse practitioners. Three patients in the past month experienced vasovagal episodes during loop electrosurgical excision procedures, and there were no formal protocols in place to dictate how to manage such an emergency situation. Because of the desire to improve patient safety, your office is planning to create a policy manual, perform mock drills, and incorporate safety checklists. The first step in creating an office safety program is to

(A) certify health care providers in advanced cardiac life support
* (B) designate a medical director for safety
(C) have a debriefing session
(D) find someone to act as a patient for mock drills
(E) create an office policy and procedure manual

Most health care in the United States is provided in the ambulatory setting. In 2010, there were 900 million visits to physicians' offices compared with one million hospital discharges. Despite this great difference between care settings, most patient safety research has been performed in hospital environments. The Agency for Healthcare Research and Quality found that only 10% of patient safety studies have been performed in the outpatient setting. In an active primary care office, emergency situations are to be expected, and physicians and their staff must be prepared to handle acute situations effectively to optimize outcomes. Understanding the importance of patient safety, the American College of Obstetricians and Gynecologists published its *Report of the Presidential Task Force on Patient Safety in the Office Setting* in 2010. This publication is intended to help implement patient safety initiatives in the office setting.

Because of patient, physician, and insurance payer preferences, an increasing number of procedures that previously were performed in regulated surgical centers are now being done in the office. This trend toward more outpatient procedures is anticipated to continue. Although a patient is undergoing a procedure in the office as opposed to a hospital, she should expect the same level of safety.

Hospitals have many protocols in place to evaluate patient safety. Some of these initiatives include patient safety teams, safety reporting systems, root cause analyses, and culture surveys. Crew resource management programs have become popular initiatives for hospital units to improve teamwork, communication, and patient safety. Ambulatory practices should consider these programs in order to improve safety in the office setting.

Designating a medical director with specific patient-safety responsibilities is the first step that office practices must take in creating a formal safety program. The medical director ensures that everyone who works in the office understands his or her role in regard to patient safety. The medical director should lead regular meetings to evaluate the current status of protocols and the overall safety environment of the office.

The depth of anesthesia level provided at the office should dictate resuscitative training in accordance with American Society of Anesthesiologists guidelines. In a level I facility (local anesthesia with minimal preoperative oral anxiolytic medication), someone who is trained in basic life support should be immediately available until the last patient is discharged. Ideally, all office employees should be trained in basic life support regardless of their responsibilities. In a level II office (moderate sedation), at least one obstetrician–gynecologist or other health care provider with training in advanced cardiac life support should be readily available at all times. However, this would not be the first step when initiating an office safety program.

A debriefing session should occur after each procedure is completed. The discussion should include whether all equipment was functioning, what went well, and what could be improved for future procedures. A debriefing session does not need to involve the entire office staff. Only those directly involved with the procedure should participate.

High-reliability organizations such as airlines and nuclear power plants have used mock drills and simulations to better prepare for infrequent emergencies. Because medicine has the potential for such emergencies, mock drills have become a mainstay in patient safety programs. Drills should be conducted at least quarterly with all office staff present, and each individual's role must be defined clearly. Drills give the office staff an opportunity to review all steps of the emergency protocol and may help identify corrections to be made to the protocol. Some examples of mock drills in the office setting include vasovagal episode, allergic reaction, and uterine hemorrhage. The American College of Obstetricians and Gynecologists' *Report of the Presidential Task Force on Patient Safety in the Office Setting* includes a complete list of suggested drills to be conducted. Having a team member portray a patient is effective.

An office policy and procedure manual is essential in any office where surgery is performed. Surgical safety checklists should be used for each procedure, which will minimize the chance of error. However, before writing a policy and procedure office manual, a medical director must be chosen to direct this activity.

American College of Obstetricians and Gynecologists. Quality and safety in women's health care. 2nd ed. Washington, DC: American College of Obstetricians and Gynecologists; 2010.

Erickson TB, Kirkpatrick DH, DeFrancesco MS, Lawrence HC 3rd. Executive summary of the American College of Obstetricians and Gynecologists Presidential Task Force on Patient Safety in the Office Setting: reinvigorating safety in office-based gynecologic surgery. Obstet Gynecol 2010;115:147–51.

Gandhi TK, Lee TH. Patient safety beyond the hospital. N Engl J Med 2010;363:1001–3.

Toback SL. Medical emergency preparedness in office practice. Am Fam Physician 2007;75:1679–84.

69

Extended-cycle contraception

A 27-year-old healthy nulligravid woman with a history of regular menses and primary dysmenorrhea reports that her symptoms have improved since she began taking continuous extended-cycle combination oral contraceptives (OCs) 12 months ago. She generally is happy with the regimen; however, she is bothered by light but irregular bleeding that started a few months ago. Her physical examination is normal, and a urine pregnancy test result is negative. The best initial approach for her irregular bleeding is to

* (A) stop taking the OC for 3–4 days
(B) continue the current regimen
(C) add conjugated estrogen
(D) switch to progestin-only OCs
(E) double the dosage for 10 days

As many as 90% of women experience dysmenorrhea at some point in their lives. Hormonal contraceptives have been associated with a reduction in menstruation-related pain in up to 75% of women with dysmenorrhea. The use of continuous combination OCs is a safe and effective option for the treatment of dysmenorrhea. Studies have noted decreased menstrual pain scores in women who take extended-cycle regimens (84 days) compared with traditional 21-day or 24-day regimens. Although all women who use extended-cycle or continuous combination OCs may experience breakthrough or unscheduled bleeding more frequently than patients taking cyclic combined OCs, this adverse effect usually diminishes after 6 months of use. However, some women experience breakthrough bleeding that develops after or extends past the initial 6 months of use. It is important to evaluate the patient for common causes of abnormal bleeding, such as infection, cervical lesions, and pregnancy.

The described patient has a history of regular menses and of recent-onset irregular bleeding, which in an otherwise healthy 27-year-old would not be expected to indicate serious uterine pathology. Studies of women who used continuous combination OCs with a 3–4-day drug-free interval during a 5-month period reported less irregular bleeding and fewer bleeding days overall than women without a drug-free interval. The Centers for Disease Control and Prevention recommends a 3–4-day hiatus for women with breakthrough bleeding related to the continuous use of combination OCs. This would be the appropriate strategy for the described patient because it allows the endometrium to proliferate from endogenous estradiol production. If the patient's symptoms persist after a 3–4-day pill-free interval, further evaluation or management could be considered. Note that to maintain contraceptive efficacy, the patient should have at least 21 days of continuous exposure to combination OCs and a pill-free interval no greater than 7 days. With 3 months of irregular bleeding, continued observation is likely to lead to patient frustration and possible nonadherence or cessation of the regimen. The mechanism of breakthrough bleeding is related to endometrial atrophy; however, supplementation with conjugated estrogen has not been recommended for women who experience breakthrough bleeding while taking combination OCs (Fig. 69-1).

Primary dysmenorrhea is related to a cascade of biochemical events beginning with ovulation, production, and withdrawal of progesterone and followed by the formation of endometrial prostaglandins that increase uterine contractility and pain. Even with near-perfect use, women ovulate during up to 50% of cycles while taking a progestin-only OC, which theoretically would make this choice less appealing for the treatment of primary dysmenorrhea. Doubling the dose of the contraceptive for 10 days would not be expected to improve endometrial atrophy and has not been shown to decrease breakthrough bleeding. All women taking OCs should be instructed about the proper timing and administration of combination OCs because missed pills are the most common cause of OC-related irregular bleeding.

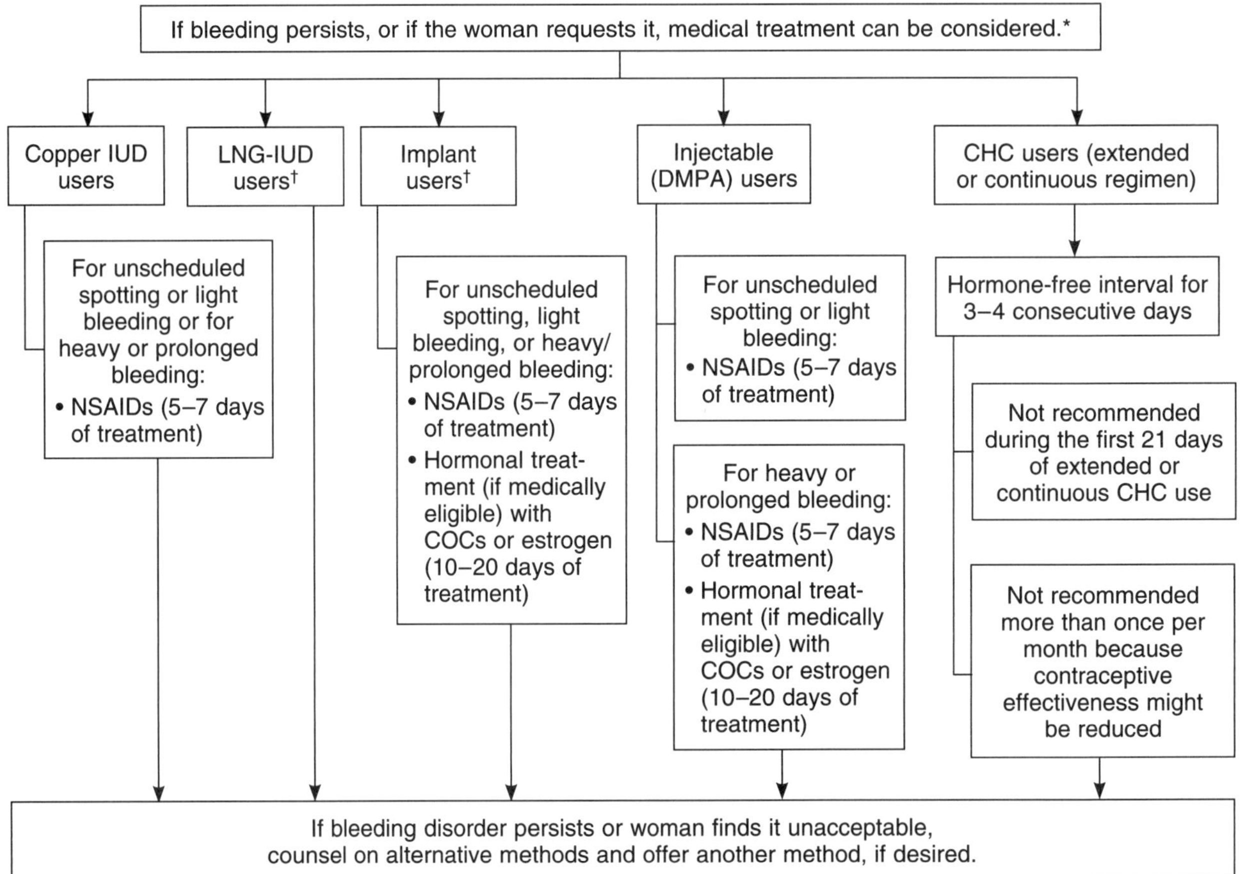

FIGURE 69-1. Management of women with bleeding irregularities while using contraception. Abbreviations: CHC, combined hormonal contraceptive; COC, combined oral contraceptive; DMPA, depot medroxyprogesterone acetate; IUD, intrauterine device; LNG, levonorgestrel; NSAIDs, nonsteroidal antiinflammatory drugs. *If clinically warranted, evaluate for underlying condition. Treat the condition or refer for care. †Heavy or prolonged bleeding, either unscheduled or menstrual, is common. (Appendix E in Division of Reproductive Health, National Center for Chronic Disease Prevention and Health Promotion, Centers for Disease Control and Prevention (CDC). U.S. selected practice recommendations for contraceptive use, 2013: adapted from the World Health Organization selected practice recommendations for contraceptive use, 2nd edition. MMWR Recomm Rep 2013;62(RR-05):1–60.)

Edelman A, Micks E, Gallo MF, Jensen J, Grimes DA. Continuous or extended cycle vs. cyclic use of combined hormonal contraceptives for contraception. Cochrane Database of Systematic Reviews 2014, Issue 7. Art. No.: CD004695. DOI: 10.1002/14651858.CD004695.pub3.

Godfrey EM, Whiteman MK, Curtis KM. Treatment of unscheduled bleeding in women using extended- or continuous-use combined hormonal contraception: a systematic review. Contraception 2013;87: 567–75.

U.S. Selected Practice Recommendations for Contraceptive Use, 2013: adapted from the World Health Organization selected practice recommendations for contraceptive use, 2nd edition. Division of Reproductive Health, National Center for Chronic Disease Prevention and Health Promotion, Centers for Disease Control and Prevention. MMWR Recomm Rep 2013;62(RR-05):1–60.

70

Hematuria in a nonpregnant reproductive-aged woman

A 46-year-old woman, gravida 4, para 4, underwent a hysterectomy 8 years ago. She experiences urinary stress incontinence with coughing; her symptoms worsened recently after she had a cold. She states that she has not experienced dysuria, gross hematuria, or flank pain. She has no other medical issues. She has a 12-pack-per-year smoking history. A pelvic examination demonstrates pelvic relaxation but is otherwise normal. A urine specimen is collected and office point-of-care testing detects microhematuria. The best next step is

(A) urine cytology
* (B) microscopic urinalysis
(C) computed tomography urography
(D) cystoscopy
(E) renal ultrasonography

Approximately 5% of individuals with microscopic hematuria will have an underlying malignancy. A woman has an approximately 1 in 90 lifetime risk of developing bladder cancer. Although the diagnosis is more common in men, more than 17,000 U.S. women are diagnosed with bladder cancer each year. Age is an important risk factor, and approximately 7% of women with bladder cancer are diagnosed between ages 45 years and 54 years. White race is associated with a twofold increased risk of bladder cancer. Genetic factors can increase a woman's risk; defects in the retinoblastoma gene, the phosphatase and tensin (*PTEN*) gene mutation (Cowden disease), and hereditary nonpolyposis colon cancer (Lynch syndrome) all have been associated with a higher risk of bladder cancer. Smoking is the most important risk factor for the development of bladder cancer because the carcinogens are concentrated in the urine. Smokers are three times more likely to develop bladder cancer than nonsmokers. Figure 70-1 shows the incidence of bladder cancer by age and sex per 100,000 people in the United States.

Hematuria is a fairly common finding and can range from visible (gross) hematuria to microscopic hematuria. In young women, hematuria typically is transient and of no consequence; however, in women older than 35 years,

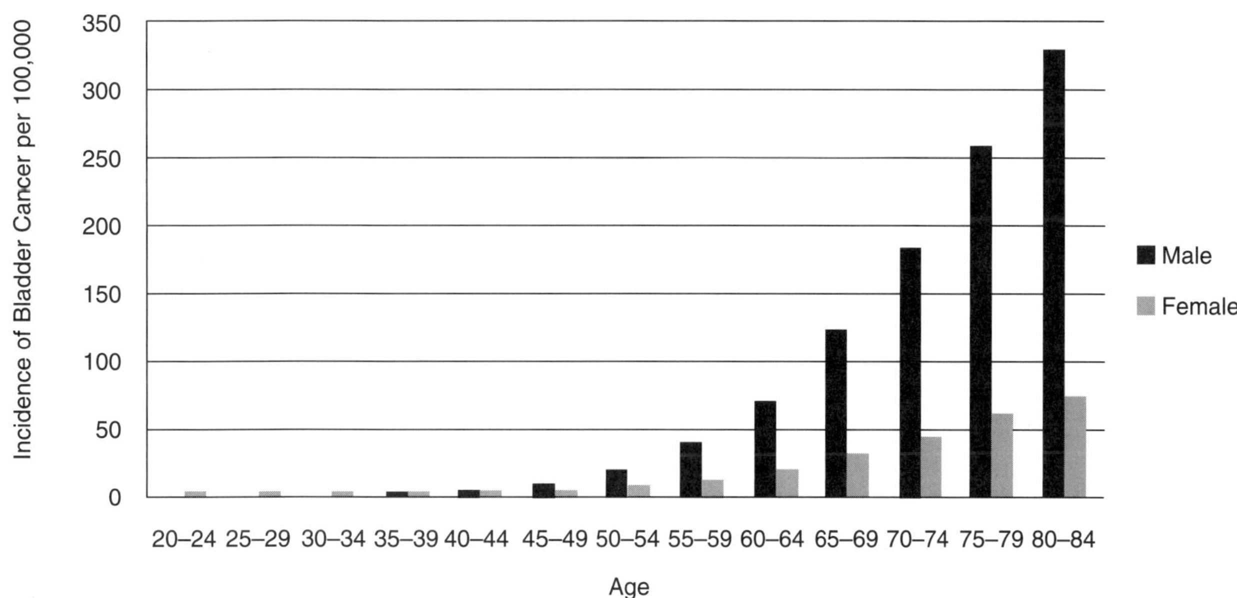

FIGURE 70-1. Incidence of bladder cancer by age and sex per 100,000 in the United States. (Adapted from Cancer of the urinary bladder. In: Howlader N, Noone AM, Krapcho M, Miller D, Bishop K, Altekruse SF, et al, editors. SEER cancer statistics review, 1975-2013. Bethesda (MD): National Cancer Institute; 2016. Available at: http://seer.cancer.gov/csr/1975_2013/results_merged/sect_27_urinary_bladder.pdf. Retrieved June 17, 2016.)

it can be a symptom of underlying malignancy. Gross hematuria usually represents a urologic condition, although urine can be discolored by other substances, such as myoglobin (crush injuries or rhabdomyolysis), beeturia (from eating beets), porphyria, or some medications (eg, rifampin, cyclophosphamide, or chlorpromazine hydrochloride). Microscopic hematuria may have a source from anywhere in the urologic system. A urine dipstick is very sensitive and can detect as few as one or two erythrocytes per high-power field. Microscopic hematuria is defined by three or more erythrocytes per high-power field on a fresh clean-catch urine sample.

Transient hematuria may occur in 6–39% of the general population; in women, it can be caused by menstruation, recent exercise, sexual activity, viral infections, nephrolithiasis, or trauma. Urinary tract infection or urethritis from a sexually transmitted infection can cause hematuria. A history of dysuria or urinary frequency is suggestive of a urinary tract infection. Urinary stones usually are accompanied by pain, and pyelonephritis is accompanied by fever. If these conditions are present or a thorough history suggests a cause for hematuria that does not need to be treated, then the urinalysis should be repeated in 48 hours. If microscopic hematuria persists over two out of three successive urinalyses, then other causes should be sought.

Blood is filtered in the kidney by the glomerulus. The presence of urinary erythrocytes indicates that there is some source for the erythrocytes within the kidney or distal renal collection system. The presence of protein, which also is filtered by the glomerulus, indicates likely intrinsic renal disease. In these cases, examination of the urinary sediment will reveal casts (tube-shaped particles that develop in the distal tubule or renal collecting system that may consist of erythrocytes, leukocytes, renal cells, proteins, or fat). Immunoglobulin A nephropathy is the most common glomerular disease that can cause hematuria. Less frequent causes include thin basement membrane disease, hereditary nephritis (Alport syndrome), and mild focal glomerulonephritis. In such cases, the next step in management would be microscopic examination of the urine. Urine dipstick testing can detect blood below the threshold of microscopic hematuria; the presence of crystals or bacteria will suggest benign causes of hematuria. For cases in which microscopic hematuria is confirmed, examination of the urinary sediment for casts may suggest renal disease, which would prompt evaluation by a nephrologist. Figure 70-2 shows an algorithmic approach to microscopic hematuria in adults.

The described patient is at increased risk of bladder cancer because she is older than 35 years and has a history of smoking. If microscopic hematuria is confirmed on urinalysis, then she should be referred for cystoscopy and radiologic evaluation of the urinary tract. A woman who has been diagnosed with persistent microscopic hematuria and has risk factors should be evaluated for bladder cancer. Microscopic urinalysis is the single most important test in the evaluation of microscopic hematuria; it will confirm hematuria and identify women with glomerular or nonglomerular disease. Urine cytology is not indicated at this point in the workup (Fig. 70-2).

Cohen RA, Brown RS. Microscopic hematuria. N Engl J Med 2003:348:2330–8.

Davis R, Jones JS, Barocas DA, Jones JS, Barocas DA, Castle EP, et al. Diagnosis, evaluation and follow-up of asymptomatic microhematuria (AMH) in adults: AUA guideline. American Urological Association. J Urol 2012;188:2473–81.

McDonald MM, Swagerty D, Wetzel L. Assessment of microscopic hematuria in adults. Am Fam Physician 2006;73:1748–54.

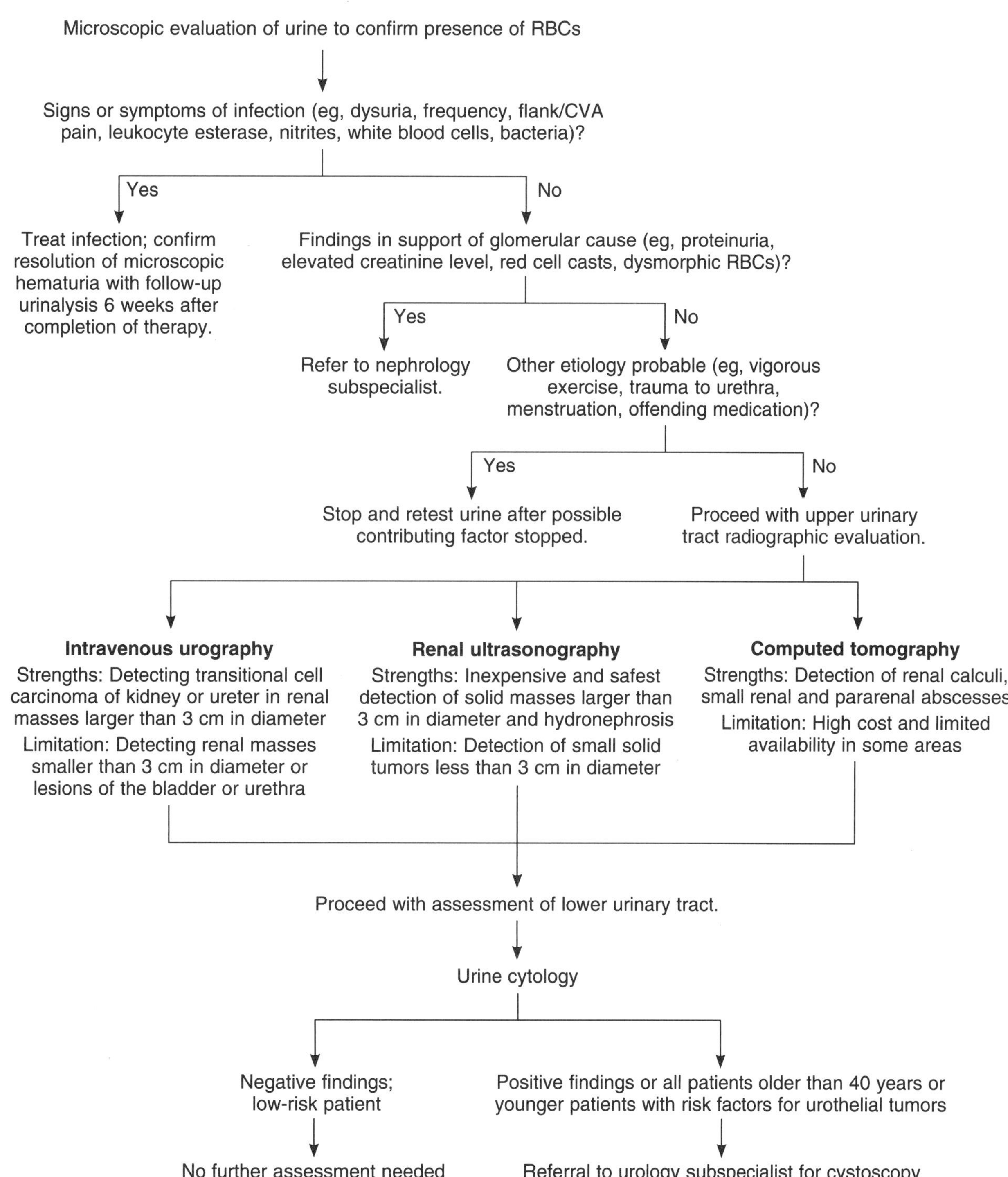

FIGURE 70-2. Algorithmic approach to microscopic hematuria in adults. Abbreviations: CVA, costovertebral angle; RBCs, red blood cells. (McDonald MM, Swagerty D, Wetzel L. Assessment of microscopic hematuria in adults. Am Fam Physician 2006;73:1748–54.)

71

Noncontraceptive benefits of intrauterine devices

A 30-year-old woman, gravida 2, para 2, visits your office for her annual well-woman examination. She and her partner have been using male condoms since the birth of her last child, and she is interested in a longer-acting method of contraception. She asks if using a levonorgestrel intrauterine device (IUD) would offer any health benefits besides birth control. You counsel her that in addition to decreasing menstrual flow and associated anemia, an IUD will most significantly reduce her risk of developing

(A) endometrial polyp
* (B) endometrial cancer
(C) leiomyoma growth
(D) ovarian cancer
(E) ovarian cysts

The noncontraceptive benefits of various forms of birth control can be a strong inducement to start or continue a particular contraceptive method. A patient's desire for improvement of heavy menstrual bleeding, the potential for reduction in dysmenorrhea, or a family history of cancer may have a significant effect on her choice of contraception. Although most published research focuses on the noncontraceptive benefits of combination hormonal oral contraceptive pills (OCPs), there also is evidence suggesting benefits with IUDs, particularly IUDs that contain levonorgestrel. The levonorgestrel IUD has a U.S. Food and Drug Administration indication to treat heavy menstrual bleeding.

One of the most common noncontraceptive reasons to use certain contraceptive methods is improvement in bleeding. A systematic review and meta-analysis found that the levonorgestrel IUD was associated with significant reductions in menstrual blood loss and improvement in quality of life. A Cochrane Review found that the levonorgestrel IUD is a more effective treatment for heavy bleeding than norethindrone, with higher satisfaction and continuation rates. The levonorgestrel IUD is effective in reducing abnormal uterine bleeding from ovulatory and endometrial sources. However, it has no effect on development or treatment of structural causes of heavy bleeding, such as polyps.

Similarly, data are limited about the efficacy of hormonal treatment for uterine leiomyomas. The outcomes of control of bleeding symptoms and control of leiomyoma growth are not synonymous and may be different with use of the levonorgestrel IUD. In one study, the levonorgestrel IUD reduced overall uterine volume without affecting the size of the leiomyomas themselves. At this point, there is no clear association between levonorgestrel IUD use and reduced leiomyoma growth.

Risk reduction of ovarian cancer is one of the most powerful noncontraceptive benefits of combination OCPs. Use of combination OCPs decreases the risk of ovarian cancer by 30% or more; the longer the duration of combination OCP use, the greater the risk reduction. The mechanism for ovarian cancer risk reduction is presumed to be the marked reduction in ovulation. The levonorgestrel IUD, however, only occasionally leads to anovulatory cycles and derives its contraceptive efficacy from other mechanisms. Consequently, no relationship has been noted between levonorgestrel IUD use and ovarian cancer risk. In the same way, because the levonorgestrel IUD does not consistently suppress ovulation, it does not lead to a reduction in ovarian cyst formation; in fact, persistence of ovarian cysts is a known adverse effect.

The levonorgestrel IUD achieves its strongest noncontraceptive effects locally. Concentrations of progestin in the endometrium are several hundredfold higher than those seen with oral progestin therapy. The degree of endometrial protection is so high that the levonorgestrel IUD can be used as the progestin component in hormone replacement therapy, and a systematic review found its use effective for treatment of hyperplasia without atypia. The copper IUD and the levonorgestrel IUD are effective in reducing incidence of endometrial cancer. Thus, use of any IUD leads to a reduction in risk of endometrial cancer. Therefore, the patient should be counseled that, in addition to decreasing menstrual flow and associated anemia, use of a levonorgestrel IUD offers the strongest risk reduction of endometrial cancer.

Beining RM, Dennis LK, Smith EM, Dokras A. Meta-analysis of intrauterine device use and risk of endometrial cancer. Ann Epidemiol 2008;18:492–9.

Castellsague X, Diaz M, Vaccarella S, de Sanjose S, Munoz N, Herrero R, et al. Intrauterine device use, cervical infection with human papillomavirus, and risk of cervical cancer: a pooled analysis of 26 epidemiological studies. Lancet Oncol 2011;12:1023–31.

Lindh I, Milsom I. The influence of intrauterine contraception on the prevalence and severity of dysmenorrhea: a longitudinal population study. Hum Reprod 2013;28:1953–60.

Noncontraceptive uses of hormonal contraceptives. ACOG Practice Bulletin No. 110. American College of Obstetricians and Gynecologists. Obstet Gynecol 2010;115:206–18.

72

Expedited partner therapy

A 19-year-old nonpregnant nulligravid woman comes to your office for her first well-woman examination. She reports that she has been in a monogamous relationship for the past 2 months. You screen her for sexually transmitted infections (STIs), and her test results are positive for chlamydial infection. You provide her with immediate antibiotic therapy, and she requests testing for her boyfriend who does not have a health care provider. In accordance with the Centers for Disease Control and Prevention (CDC) guidelines, the step that you should take is to

(A) give her a laboratory slip for him to be tested
(B) refer the partner to a local health care provider who cares for men
* (C) provide prompt treatment for her partner
(D) have her return in 4 weeks for test of cure

Sexually transmitted infections pose a significant health risk for women, particularly young females aged 15–24 years, who are disproportionately affected compared with females in other age groups. *Chlamydia trachomatis* is the most frequently reported STI in the United States, with the highest prevalence rates noted in individuals younger than 24 years. Chlamydial infection can present with mucopurulent cervicitis, abnormal vaginal discharge, or irregular intermenstrual vaginal bleeding. However, asymptomatic infection is quite common and contributes to profound morbidity, including preventable infertility, pelvic inflammatory disease, and ectopic pregnancy in affected women. Because of the high prevalence rates, the potential for active infection in the absence of symptoms, and widespread availability of highly effective treatment strategies, routine annual screening is recommended for all sexually active women younger than 25 years. Additionally, routine screening is recommended in high-risk older women, including those who have a new sex partner, a sex partner with concurrent partners, or a sex partner who has an STI.

Urogenital infection in women can be diagnosed by urine testing or swab specimens collected from the vagina or endocervix. Culture, direct immunofluorescence, enzyme-linked immunoassay, nucleic acid hybridization tests, and nucleic acid amplification tests (NAATs) all are available for the detection of *C trachomatis* by endocervical swab specimens. The NAATs are the most sensitive tests and are considered first-line testing; NAATs are endorsed by the U.S. Food and Drug Administration for use with endocervical swabs, vaginal swabs, and urine specimens. Although clinician-collected vaginal swabs are used most commonly, self-collected vaginal swab specimens are equivalent in sensitivity and specificity to those collected using NAATs and often are preferred by younger women. First-void urine specimens can be considered in adolescents who are reluctant to have a pelvic examination; however, this modality may miss up to 10% of infections.

One of the contributing factors to the current prevalence rate is the high rate of reinfection from an untreated partner. Rates of reinfection within 12 months of an initial chlamydial infection range from 14% to 26%. All sex partners should be referred for evaluation, testing, and presumptive treatment if there has been sexual contact with the patient during the 60 days preceding the patient's onset of symptoms or confirmed diagnosis. If the patient has had no partners in that time frame, the most recent partner should be notified. If the most recent sexual contact was more than 60 days ago, that individual is considered at risk and should be treated accordingly.

Although providing the patient's partner with a laboratory slip to be tested is an important initial step, it is not the most appropriate course of treatment because it does not address the critical need to provide treatment for a presumptive infection. Additionally, the patient's partner has no established care with an obstetrician–gynecologist or health care provider and would have no one with whom to follow up if he received a positive test result. Similarly, referring the partner to a local health care provider does not ensure that he will be seen or that he will receive timely therapy.

In accordance with current CDC guidelines, if the obstetrician–gynecologist or health care provider is concerned that a sex partner is unable to access prompt evaluation and appropriate treatment services, timely treatment by expedited partner therapy should be considered as permitted by state and local laws. Expedited partner therapy refers to the clinical practice of treating the sex partners of patients in whom an STI has been diagnosed without requiring an examination beforehand. This is particularly critical for partners who are unlikely or unable to receive in-person evaluation and appropriate therapy. Additionally, current evidence demonstrates that expedited partner therapy decreases reinfection rates compared with routine partner referrals for evaluation and treatment. Expedited partner therapy is endorsed by national organizations, including the American College of Obstetricians and Gynecologists, the American Medical Association, the Society for Adolescent Health and Medicine, the American Academy of Pediatrics, the CDC, and the American Bar Association.

A number of barriers to expedited partner therapy exist, including the concern obstetrician–gynecologists and other health care providers have regarding missed opportunities to screen for human immunodeficiency virus (HIV) infection, fear of legal ramifications on the part of the obstetrician–gynecologist, issues related to billing and reimbursement, and reluctance to prescribe medications that can result in adverse drug reactions and antibiotic resistance. However, such barriers are outweighed by the significant benefits of expedited partner therapy and can be reduced through the implementation of practice protocols, hospital guidelines, and accompanying algorithms. Guidelines are subject to change and clinicians should refer to CDC recommendations for guidance regarding state and local regulations for provision of expedited partner therapy. Additionally, having partners accompany patients when they return for treatment is an alternative strategy that can be used to ensure partner therapy.

Once the clinician has assessed the risk of intimate partner violence associated with partner notification, this patient's partner should be offered expedited partner therapy if it is permissible according to his or her state's rules or regulations regarding this practice. Of note, expedited partner therapy is not intended for use in cases of suspected child abuse, sexual assault, or other circumstances in which the patient's safety could be at risk.

Individuals who are treated for chlamydial infection should abstain from intercourse for 7 days after single-dose therapy or until completion of a 7-day regimen. Test-of-cure (repeated testing 3–4 weeks after completing therapy) is not recommended for individuals appropriately treated with the recommended or alternative regimens unless symptoms persist, therapeutic adherence is in question, or reinfection is suspected. Because the described patient is receiving appropriate therapy and is requesting partner therapy, a test of cure in 4 weeks is not indicated. However, given the high rates of reinfection, all women should be offered repeat testing 3 months after treatment and whenever they seek medical care within the following 3–12 months.

The use of NAATs for the detection of *C trachomatis* at less than 3 weeks after completion of therapy is not recommended because nonviable organisms may persist and lead to a false-positive test result. The one exception to nonroutine test-of-cure testing is pregnancy. Because of the potential for adverse maternal and fetal sequelae related to active maternal chlamydial infection, women diagnosed during pregnancy require a test of cure 1 month after treatment, a repeat test 3 months after treatment and, in the case of high-risk patients, rescreening during the third trimester.

American College of Obstetricians and Gynecologists. Guidelines for women's health care: a resource manual. 4th edition. Washington, DC: American College of Obstetricians and Gynecologists; 2014.

Expedited partner therapy in the management of gonorrhea and chlamydia by obstetrician–gynecologists. Committee Opinion No. 632. American College of Obstetricians and Gynecologists. Obstet Gynecol 2015;125:1526–8.

Workowski KA, Bolan GA. Sexually transmitted diseases treatment guidelines, 2015. Centers for Disease Control and Prevention [published erratum appears in MMWR Recomm Rep 2015;64:924]. MMWR Recomm Rep 2015;64:1–137.

73

Prophylaxis for deep vein thrombosis

A 29-year-old woman, gravida 3, para 3, had a normal spontaneous vaginal delivery 6 weeks ago and has come to your office for a postpartum visit. She has completed childbearing and desires laparoscopic tubal ligation. Her past medical history is significant for obesity and smoking five cigarettes daily. She has been using low-dose combination oral contraceptive pills (OCPs) for contraception. You schedule her for laparoscopic bilateral tubal ligation and inform her that the surgery should take less than 30 minutes. She prefers to avoid injectable medications. The appropriate prophylaxis for venous thromboembolism prevention in this case is

* (A) mechanical prophylaxis
(B) discontinue OCPs
(C) early mobilization
(D) aspirin

Multiple studies have shown that appropriate thromboprophylaxis reduces all forms of venous thromboembolism, including deep vein thrombosis (DVT) and pulmonary embolism (PE). The most common preventable cause of hospital death is PE. In the United States, PE accounts for approximately 100,000 deaths annually. In 2001, the Agency for Healthcare Research and Quality reported that the appropriate use of thromboprophylaxis is a priority safety practice. Patients undergoing gynecologic surgeries should be assessed preoperatively for their risk of venous thromboembolism and given thromboprophylaxis based on risk stratification.

The prevalence of DVT is 15–40% in patients who undergo major gynecologic surgery without thromboprophylaxis. Formation of a venous thromboembolism is multifactorial and includes hypercoagulability, endothelial injury, and venous stasis (referred to as the Virchow triad). Risk factors for venous thromboembolism are shown in Box 73-1. The described patient has multiple risk factors, including obesity, tobacco use, postpartum status, and use of combination OCPs. Given that she is younger than 40 years and is undergoing minor surgery, she would be considered to be at moderate risk (Appendix G) and without prophylactic measures would have a 10–20% risk of developing a DVT and 1–2% risk of clinical PE. Although some obstetrician–gynecologists and other health care providers would stop the OCPs, the risk of unintended pregnancy has to be weighed against the risk of hypercoagulability.

As the complexity of the surgery and the age of the patient increase in the setting of additional risk factors, the recommendations for prevention of venous thromboembolism escalate to include mechanical prophylaxis and increasing doses of anticoagulation (Appendix G). Because the described patient is considered to be at moderate risk, unfractionated heparin, low-molecular-weight heparin, or mechanical prophylaxis are all options for venous thromboembolism prophylaxis. Mechanical

BOX 73-1

Risk Factors for Venous Thromboembolism

- Surgery
- Trauma (major or lower extremity)
- Immobility, paresis
- Malignancy
- Cancer therapy (hormonal, chemotherapy, or radiotherapy)
- Previous venous thromboembolism
- Increasing age
- Pregnancy and the postpartum period
- Estrogen-containing OCP or hormone therapy
- Selective estrogen receptor modulators
- Acute medical illness
- Heart or respiratory failure
- Inflammatory bowel disease
- Myeloproliferative disorders
- Paroxysmal nocturnal hemoglobinuria
- Nephrotic syndrome
- Obesity
- Smoking
- Varicose veins
- Central venous catheterization
- Inherited or acquired thrombophilia

Abbreviation: OCP, oral contraceptive pill.

Geerts WH, Pineo GF, Heit JA, Bergqvist D, Lassen MR, Colwell CW, et al. Prevention of venous thromboembolism: the Seventh ACCP Conference on Antithrombotic and Thrombolytic Therapy. Chest 2004;126(suppl): 338S–400S. Copyright 2004, with permission from Elsevier.

prophylaxis with graduated compression stockings or intermittent pneumatic compression devices increases venous flow and, therefore, reduces stasis. Mechanical prophylaxis is preferred in women with a high risk of bleeding or as an adjunct to anticoagulant-based prophylaxis. It also is the best option in this patient who prefers to avoid injectable medications. Pneumatic compression should be started preoperatively, maintained intraoperatively, and continued until hospital discharge.

Early and aggressive mobilization would be sufficient for this patient if she did not have additional risk factors. The American College of Chest Physicians does not recommend aspirin as the sole prophylaxis for venous thromboembolism for any patient group.

Kearon C, Akl EA, Ornelas J, Blaivas A, Jimenez D, Bounameaux H, et al. Antithrombotic Therapy for VTE Disease: CHEST Guideline and Expert Panel Report. Chest 2016;149:315–52.

Prevention of deep vein thrombosis and pulmonary embolism. ACOG Practice Bulletin No. 84. American College of Obstetricians and Gynecologists. Obstet Gynecol 2007;110:429–40.

74

Labial adhesions in the pediatric patient

An active and playful 3-year-old girl received a recent diagnosis from her pediatrician of labial agglutination (Fig. 74-1; see color plate). Her mother is concerned because the pediatrician recommends no treatment, yet she feels that her daughter's vulva does not look "normal." The girl has not been scratching the area, is fully potty trained, and is able to urinate without difficulty. After confirming the diagnosis, you explain that you recommend

(A) application of estrogen cream
(B) surgical separation of the labial adhesions
(C) application of betamethasone cream
* (D) continued observation
(E) gentle labial traction to be performed daily

Labial agglutination is a common finding in girls younger than 2 years, with a reported incidence of 1% to as high as 10%. Adhesions may be minimal and filmy or may result in near-complete obliteration of the vulvar vestibule. The etiology of labial agglutination is unknown but thought to be related to low estrogen levels. Girls with labial agglutination typically are asymptomatic; however, severe adhesions can result in diminished or diverted urinary stream and, rarely, may be associated with urinary tract infection (UTI). Girls with recurrent UTIs and labial agglutination should undergo the recommended evaluation for children with recurrent UTIs who do not have labial agglutination. Lichen sclerosus and genital trauma should be considered in the differential diagnosis. Labial agglutination typically resolves spontaneously with the initial endogenous estrogen production at around age 5–6 years; therefore, treatment is reserved for symptomatic patients. Examples of symptoms caused by labial agglutination include inability to potty train, which may involve trapping urine, resulting in postvoid accidents and difficulty directing the urine stream when voiding.

Application of estrogen cream is the initial treatment of choice for patients with symptoms associated with labial agglutination. Topical estrogen is applied twice daily to the white or gray median raphe of the adhesion until resolution of symptoms. Avoiding irritants and soaking in clean, warm bathwater also are beneficial. Patients should be monitored frequently during this time for improvement. Successful labial separation has been reported in 80–100% of girls treated with estrogen with an average length of treatment of 2–4 months. Potential adverse effects associated with the use of topical estrogen cream include thelarche and vaginal bleeding. Failure of treatment is thought to be associated with improper estrogen application. Once separated, a film of bland ointment should be applied to the labia each day. One study of 100 children between the ages of 3 months and 10 years noted a 41% recurrence rate after topical estrogen therapy.

Routine manual labial traction is not recommended because tearing of the adhesion can lead to reformation. At this point, there is very limited data supporting the role of betamethasone in the treatment of symptomatic labial agglutination. Girls with complete labial agglutination and failed medical management with estrogen may be considered for surgical separation. Recurrence of labial agglutination has been noted in up to 10% of girls who undergo surgical separation. Continued observation is the appropriate management decision for this asymptomatic patient with labial agglutination.

Berenson AB, Heger AH, Hayes JM, Bailey RK, Emans SJ. Appearance of the hymen in prepubertal girls. Pediatrics 1992;89:387–94.

Kumetz LM, Quint EH, Fisseha S, Smith YR. Estrogen treatment success in recurrent and persistent labial agglutination. J Pediatr Adolesc Gynecol 2006;19:381–4.

Mayoglou L, Dulabon L, Martin-Alguacil N, Pfaff D, Schober J. Success of treatment modalities for labial fusion: a retrospective evaluation of topical and surgical treatments. J Pediatr Adolesc Gynecol 2009;22:247–50.

Schober J, Dulabon L, Martin-Alguacil N, Kow LM, Pfaff D. Significance of topical estrogens to labial fusion and vaginal introital integrity. J Pediatr Adolesc Gynecol 2006;19:337–9.

Tebruegge M, Misra I, Nerminathan V. Is the topical application of oestrogen cream an effective intervention in girls suffering from labial adhesions? Arch Dis Child 2007;92:268–71.

75

Infertility workup

A 25-year-old nulligravid woman comes to your office with her husband. The couple has been unable to become pregnant despite 1 year of unprotected, properly timed intercourse. As part of their infertility evaluation, you order a semen analysis. The sample shows 3 mL of ejaculate containing 50 million spermatozoa, of which 5% have normal morphology with 32% total motility and 60% vitality. The result that is abnormal is

* (A) 32% total motility
(B) 5% normal morphology
(C) 60% vitality
(D) 50 million spermatozoa per ejaculate
(E) 3 mL volume ejaculate

For healthy couples, the probability of a pregnancy in a given reproductive cycle—referred to as fecundability—is approximately 20–25%. Fecundity is the probability that a live birth will result from a single cycle. With unprotected intercourse, properly timed around ovulation, 60% of couples will get pregnant within 6 months, 84% within 12 months, and 92% within 2 years. *Infertility* in women younger than 35 years is defined as the inability to become pregnant despite unprotected, properly timed intercourse for 12 months. In women aged 35 years and older, *infertility* is defined as the inability to become pregnant after 6 months of unprotected, properly timed intercourse. Up to 15% of couples in the United States experience infertility. Among infertile couples, infertility is secondary to female factor in approximately 40% of cases, to male factor in approximately 30%, and is unexplained in approximately 30%.

The goal of an infertility evaluation is to determine the cause of the infertility and assess reproductive potential. Components of an infertility evaluation include history and physical examination, semen analysis, assessment of ovulatory function (basal body temperature curves, ovulation predictor kits, day-21 serum progesterone), ovulatory reserve (day-3 follicle-stimulating hormone levels, estradiol, or antimüllerian hormone), and evaluation of tubal patency and the endometrial cavity (hysterosalpingography). Additional testing may include ultrasonography and laparoscopy for select patients.

Semen analysis is the principal screening tool for male factor infertility and should be obtained after 72 hours of sexual abstinence. Normal values are determined based on population norms in fertile men whose partners became pregnant in 12 months or less. According to the World Health Organization, the lower reference limits (5th percentile) for fertile men are as follows: sperm concentration of 15 million spermatozoa/mL, 39 million spermatozoa per ejaculate, 32% progressive motility, 40% total motility, 4% normal morphology, 58% vitality, and 1.5 mL of ejaculate. Values falling below the 5th percentile are considered abnormal. In the semen analysis results for the described patient's husband, the only value that is abnormal is the total motility of 32%. All other values reported are normal. An abnormal semen analysis should be repeated.

Evaluation of male factor infertility includes assessment of vital signs, body mass index (calculated as weight in kilograms divided by height in meters squared [kg/m^2]), arm span, gynecomastia, thyroid gland, secondary sexual characteristics, abdominal masses, inguinal hernias, undescended testes, presence of vas deferens, intact perineal sensation, and sphincter tone. Laboratory assessment should include a complete blood count and infectious studies such as hepatitis B, hepatitis C, human immunodeficiency virus (HIV), and *Chlamydia trachomatis*.

Cooper TG, Noonan E, von Eckardstein S, Auger J, Baker HW, Behre HM, et al. World Health Organization reference values for human semen characteristics. Hum Reprod Update 2010;16:231–45.

Hull MG, Glazener CM, Kelly NJ, Conway DI, Foster PA, Hinton RA, et al. Population study of causes, treatment, and outcome of infertility. Br Med J (Clin Res Ed) 1985;291:1693–7.

Kamel RM. Management of the infertile couple: an evidence-based protocol. Reprod Biol Endocrinol 2010;8:21.

76

Lynch syndrome

A premenopausal 51-year-old woman undergoes endometrial biopsy secondary to irregular spotting. The biopsy report reveals grade 2 endometrial adenocarcinoma. Because of the patient's age, the pathologist reflexively ordered immunohistochemical testing on the biopsy specimen, which revealed absence of *MLH1* protein expression. The patient reports a family history of colorectal cancer in her father and a paternal uncle, both diagnosed in their 60s. Your patient underwent colonoscopy 2 years ago, with no abnormalities identified. Because of her biopsy report, she is scheduled for exploratory laparotomy, total abdominal hysterectomy, bilateral salpingo-oophorectomy (BSO), and surgical staging. The best next step in her evaluation is

(A) colonoscopy
(B) germline mutation testing of mismatch repair genes
(C) obtain immunohistochemical testing result of her father's colon cancer
* (D) perform *MLH1* methylation studies on her endometrial biopsy
(E) refer for genetic counseling

Lynch syndrome is an inherited cancer predisposition syndrome of relevance to gynecologists because endometrial cancer is a common feature. This syndrome, formerly known as hereditary nonpolyposis colorectal cancer, is inherited in an autosomal dominant pattern and is highly penetrant. It is reported to account for 2–3% of all cases of endometrial cancer and 2–4% of all cases of colorectal cancer. The most common malignancies manifested in patients with Lynch syndrome (Appendix F) and the lifetime risks of developing those malignancies are shown in Table 76-1. Traditional risk factors for endometrial cancer, such as obesity and anovulation, do not play a major role in the development of this malignancy in women with Lynch syndrome. In addition, women with Lynch syndrome develop endometrial cancer at a younger age than the general population.

Lynch syndrome results from a mutation in one of several mismatch repair genes. These genes, and the relative proportion of Lynch syndrome patients carrying mutations for each, are *MLH1* (42%), *MSH2* (33%), *MSH6* (18%), and *PMS2* (7.5%). In addition to these four major genes, a small fraction of Lynch syndrome patients may have deletions in *EpCAM*, which in turn inactivates *MSH2*. The risk of developing endometrial cancer varies among the four mismatch repair genes that are associated with Lynch syndrome. The mismatch repair system is an important safeguard at the cellular level to correct single-base errors arising during DNA replication.

In many women who have a Lynch syndrome mutation, endometrial cancer is the sentinel malignancy, and it is important to recognize relevant clinical features so that appropriate genetic testing is performed. A list of clinical and family history features that should trigger consideration of a Lynch syndrome diagnosis is shown in Box 76-1. The diagnosis of Lynch syndrome may be made based on clinical features, and various criteria have been created to assist the clinician in making this diagnosis. However, strict application of any of these sets of criteria will result in missing a substantial number of patients who actually do carry a mismatch repair gene mutation. For this reason, many authorities advocate a broader approach to identification of Lynch syndrome patients and use tumor testing as a triage method to identify at-risk individuals. This tumor testing involves immunohistochemical testing for the four mismatch repair proteins. If all four proteins are present in the tumor, Lynch syndrome

TABLE 76-1. Cancer Risks in Individuals Aged 70 Years or Younger With Lynch Syndrome Compared With the General Population

Cancer Site	Cumulative Risk (%) to Age 70 Years in Patients With Lynch Syndrome
Colon	52–82
Endometrial	25–60
Stomach	6–13
Small bowel	3–6
Hepatobiliary	1.4–4
Urologic (transitional cell)	1–4
Ovarian	4–12
Other: pancreas, breast, prostate, glioblastoma	Unknown

Kohlmann W, Gruber SB. Lynch syndrome. In: Pagon RA, Adam MP, Ardinger HH, Wallace SE, Amemiya A, Bean LJH, et al, editors. GeneReviews [internet]. Seattle (WA): University of Washington; 1993–2015. Available at: http://www.ncbi.nlm.nih.gov/books/NBK1211. Retrieved June 12, 2016.

BOX 76-1

Clinical Features That Suggest Further Testing for Lynch Syndrome Is Warranted

1. Colorectal cancer diagnosed before age 50 years
2. Presence of synchronous or metachronous CRC or other LS-associated tumor
3. Colorectal cancer with any of the following histologic features: tumor-infiltrating lymphocytes, peritumoral lymphocytes, Crohn-like lymphocytic reaction, mucinous/signet ring differentiation, or medullary growth pattern diagnosed before age 60 years
4. Patients with endometrial or CRC **and** a first-degree relative with a LS-associated tumor diagnosed before age 50 years **or** with two or more first-degree or second-degree relatives with LS-associated tumor, regardless of age

Abbreviations: CRC, colorectal cancer; LS, Lynch syndrome.

Adapted from Lynch syndrome. Practice Bulletin No. 147. American College of Obstetricians and Gynecologists. Obstet Gynecol 2014;124:1042–54.

is ruled out. If one or more proteins are missing, then further analysis is warranted. There is no benefit to repeat immunohistochemical testing.

Many authorities recommend immunohistochemical testing only for women who are younger than 60 years and in whom endometrial cancer has been diagnosed. Absence of one or more mismatch repair proteins on tumor slides helps identify which genes should be evaluated. Figure 76-1 demonstrates this algorithm. However, as multigene panels are becoming more commonplace, most patients believed to have Lynch syndrome will have genetic assessment of all relevant genes.

Approximately 20–30% of cases of endometrial cancer with absence of *MLH1* on immunohistochemical testing are due to *MLH1* methylation. In general, these patients need no further evaluation for Lynch syndrome mutations. Performing this step will prevent many women from being tested inappropriately for Lynch syndrome mutations, which would add unnecessary costs to the health care system. Another risk of overtesting is the likelihood of identifying a variant of undetermined significance in one of the mismatch repair genes. This can create clinical uncertainty and increased anxiety for the patient and her family. Therefore, correct identification of the appropriate candidates for germline testing is important. Box 76-1 shows clinical features that suggest when further testing for Lynch syndrome is warranted.

Identification of Lynch syndrome is critical to determine the need for additional screening and surveillance of other organs at risk of malignancy, specifically the large bowel. Individuals diagnosed with Lynch syndrome should undergo colonoscopy with resection of polyps every 1–2 years. Evidence-based screening protocols for endometrial cancer have not yet been established. Ultrasonography and histologic sampling have been promoted as potential methods. Ultrasonography may be less reliable than endometrial biopsy, especially in premenopausal women.

Medical risk-reducing strategies directed at lowering endometrial cancer risk are less well studied. Whether progestins provide the same degree of protection in women who have Lynch syndrome as they do in women with no mismatch repair gene mutations is uncertain. More research is needed on this topic, but in the meantime, use of oral contraceptive pills, a progestin-containing intrauterine device, or injectable progestins are reasonable measures.

Most authorities recommend risk-reducing surgery, specifically total abdominal hysterectomy and BSO, for women with Lynch syndrome because screening for early endometrial cancer or ovarian cancer still is unproved. Guidelines typically suggest that this surgery should be done at age 35–45 years or when childbearing is completed. Ovarian cancer and endometrial cancer appear at younger ages in women with Lynch syndrome than in the general population, so a delay in total abdominal hysterectomy and BSO is not recommended.

The best way to further assess the described patient's risk of having Lynch syndrome is to analyze her endometrial tumor for *MLH1* methylation. If present, she does not need to undergo additional germline mutation testing. Her family history of colorectal cancer does not fit criteria for the diagnosis of Lynch syndrome based on this information alone. She may benefit from genetic counseling for reassurance purposes, but further germline

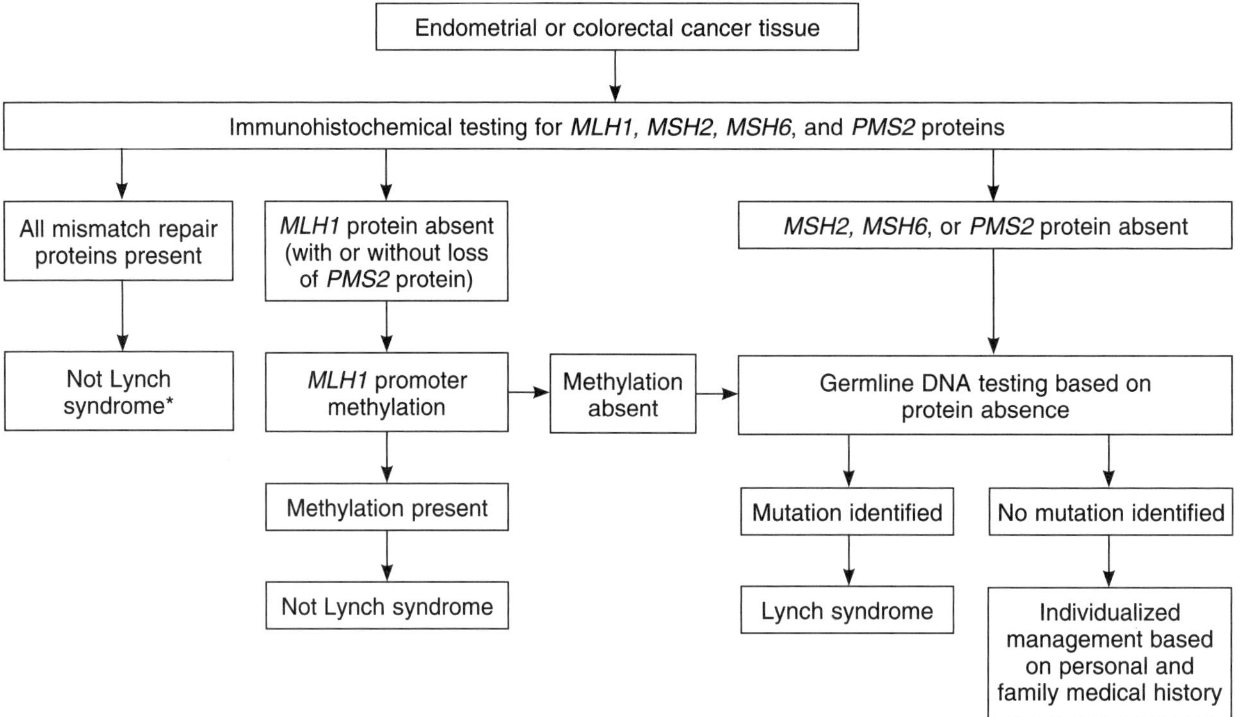

FIGURE 76-1. Immunohistochemistry-based endometrial or colorectal tumor testing for mismatch repair gene expression to assess for the possibility of Lynch syndrome. *The scenario in which the presence of all four mismatch repair proteins does not rule out Lynch syndrome is the relatively uncommon situation in which a deleterious mutation allows the production of a full-length but nonfunctional mismatch repair protein. Given this possibility, in the setting of a very high clinical suspicion of Lynch syndrome and normal immunohistochemical testing results, the tumor can be evaluated further by microsatellite instability testing. (Lynch syndrome. Practice Bulletin No. 147. American College of Obstetricians and Gynecologists. Obstet Gynecol 2014;124:1042–54.)

mutation testing would not be warranted unless *MLH1* hypermethylation studies were negative. Based on her family history alone, regular colonoscopy screening at 5–10-year intervals is indicated.

Buchanan DD, Tan YY, Walsh MD, Clendenning M, Metcalf AM, Ferguson K, et al. Tumor mismatch repair immunohistochemistry and DNA *MLH1* methylation testing of patients with endometrial cancer diagnosed at age younger than 60 years optimizes triage for population-level germline mismatch repair gene mutation testing. J Clin Oncol 2014;32:90–100.

Dempsey KM, Broaddus R, You YN, Noblin SJ, Mork M, Fellman B, et al. Is it all Lynch syndrome?: An assessment of family history in individuals with mismatch repair-deficient tumors. Genet Med 2015;17:476–84.

Lynch HT, Snyder CL, Shaw TG, Heinen CD, Hitchins MP. Milestones of Lynch syndrome: 1895-2015. Nat Rev Cancer 2015;15:181–94.

Lynch syndrome. Practice Bulletin No. 147. American College of Obstetricians and Gynecologists. Obstet Gynecol 2014;124:1042–54.

77

Shingles and postherpetic neuralgia

A 60-year-old woman with no prior significant medical problems presents with a 48-hour history of an erythematous rash with clusters of clear vesicles isolated to the right midabdomen area in the T10 dermatome. She reports that the rash was preceded by intense itching and tingling in the same area for several days, but now the pain is severe: 8 out of 10 on a pain scale. To treat her pain and accelerate her healing, you prescribe hydrocodone and

(A) varicella zoster virus (VZV) vaccine
(B) oral corticosteroids
* (C) valacyclovir
(D) amitriptyline hydrochloride
(E) lidocaine gel

The lifetime risk of reactivation of a VZV infection is 10–20%. The primary infection is varicella, or chickenpox, which typically is seen only in unvaccinated children because of the childhood vaccine that became available in 1995. Approximately 90% of the adult U.S. population, however, has serologic evidence of VZV infection from natural immunity. After the acute infection, the virus remains dormant in the sensory dorsal nerve root ganglia adjacent to the spinal cord. Reactivation can cause a secondary infection called herpes zoster, or shingles, which is more common in older adults and immunocompromised individuals. The risk of reactivation is related to decreasing cell-mediated immune responses, a result of processes associated with aging, immunosuppression, or medical treatments. Clinical manifestations follow a dermatomal distribution of the involved sensory nerve root, with the most common dermatomes being thoracic, cervical, and ophthalmic. A prodromal presentation of pain, pruritus, and abnormal skin sensations typically precedes the rash by days or weeks. The rash is painful and pruritic with erythema and clustered vesicular eruptions. Complete healing of the rash occurs within 2–4 weeks, although some patients have permanent scarring and pigmentation changes.

After resolution of the rash, nerve injury can precipitate a chronic debilitating pain called postherpetic neuralgia (PHN). Although there are multiple definitions, pain that persists past 30 days of onset of the rash can be considered PHN. The chances of developing PHN vary from 8% to 70%, with older age being one of the most significant risk factors. Postherpetic neuralgia can significantly affect quality of life and last for months or years. Other complications of zoster include secondary infections, eye involvement (herpes zoster ophthalmicus), encephalitis, and palsies. These complications tend to be more severe in immunocompromised individuals.

Early treatment (within 72 hours) of an acute zoster infection is effective in decreasing new lesion formation and resolving acute pain, as well as limiting viral shedding, which can reduce the amount of damage to neurons. Treatment with a combination of analgesics and antiviral agents, such as valacyclovir, typically are used for acute outbreaks. Several studies have shown that treatment with valacyclovir or famciclovir is superior to treatment with acyclovir. There is no evidence that longer courses of antiviral therapy reduce disease sequelae. Even though only approximately 50% of patients present within 72 hours of rash appearance, all symptomatic patients should be offered treatment.

The described patient should receive antiviral and pain management therapy. Although supplemental systemic corticosteroids in some studies have been shown to accelerate the rate of cutaneous healing and to reduce acute pain and development of PHN, a meta-analysis (including five randomized controlled trials of antiviral therapy alone versus antiviral therapy with corticosteroids) failed to demonstrate any benefit to the addition of steroids in the prevention of PHN or other secondary outcomes. However, it also was concluded that there was no evidence of any greater risks with the coadministration of steroids. Further randomized controlled trials are needed to establish any significant benefit to the addition of corticosteroids for acute symptom control.

Treatment of PHN involves a chronic pain therapy approach, including analgesics (opioids), tricyclic antidepressants (most commonly amitriptyline), and gabapentin. Topical analgesics in the form of lidocaine patches or capsaicin creams have demonstrated efficacy, and gabapentin and lidocaine patches are approved by the U.S. Food and Drug Administration for use for PHN. Lysine is a popular complementary and alternative medical remedy, but scientific evidence to support a beneficial effect is lacking.

Other therapies without data on effectiveness include nerve blocks, neuromodulation techniques, intrathecal anesthetics, and botulinum toxin.

A licensed VZV vaccine has demonstrated effectiveness in preventing zoster and reducing the severity and duration of pain in those whose infections are reactivated. Additionally, the vaccine has been shown to significantly decrease the chances of developing PHN. Current recommendations from the Advisory Committee on Immunization Practices include vaccination for all adults aged 60 years and older because of the increased risk of reactivation with age and higher risk of progression to PHN. The vaccine can be administered to those individuals who have had a previous episode of herpes zoster virus infection, but it is not indicated for the treatment of acute zoster or to prevent PHN after an acute reactivation has occurred. The zoster vaccine is a live, attenuated vaccine with an approximately 14-fold higher concentration than the regular varicella vaccine.

Gnann JW Jr, Whitley RJ. Clinical practice. Herpes zoster. N Engl J Med 2002;347:340–6.

Hales CM, Harpaz R, Ortega-Sanchez I, Bialek SR. Update on recommendations for use of herpes zoster vaccine. Centers for Disease Control and Prevention. MMWR Morb Mortal Wkly Rep 2014;63:729–31.

Harpaz R, Ortega-Sanchez IR, Seward JF. Prevention of herpes zoster: recommendations of the Advisory Committee on Immunization Practices (ACIP). Advisory Committee on Immunization Practices, Centers for Disease Control and Prevention. MMWR Recomm Rep 2008;57:1–30; quiz CE2–4.

Oxman MN, Levin MJ, Johnson GR, Schmader KE, Straus SE, Gelb LD, et al. A vaccine to prevent herpes zoster and postherpetic neuralgia in older adults. Shingles Prevention Study Group. N Engl J Med 2005;352:2271–84.

Whitley RJ, Volpi A, McKendrick M, Wijck A, Oaklander AL. Management of herpes zoster and post-herpetic neuralgia now and in the future. J Clin Virol 2010;48(suppl):S20–8.

78
Office safety

A 30-year-old nulligravid white woman comes to your office for her annual well-woman examination, and she tells you that she would like to become pregnant within a year. You order a rubella titer and carrier screening tests for cystic fibrosis and spinal muscular atrophy. She returns to your office 3 months later suspecting she is pregnant. You confirm that she is now at 6 weeks of gestation. While reviewing the medical record, your medical assistant notices that when the test results came in, you forwarded the chart to your nurse, who left a message for the patient regarding the results. However, the patient did not return the call to the nurse and was not notified of the results. The carrier screening test results were notable for positive carrier status for cystic fibrosis. Follow-up of medical test results is the responsibility of the

(A) patient
(B) laboratory
(C) office nurse
(D) referring physician
* (E) ordering physician

The failure to evaluate and communicate critical test results may be expected to adversely affect patient care and outcomes. All medical test results must be communicated to patients in a timely fashion, even those that are not designed to manage or diagnose acute or serious illnesses. Missed diagnoses and delayed therapy are real issues directly related to the failure of laboratory and imaging testing follow-up.

The importance of reliable and timely reporting of medical test results was recognized as one of the Joint Commission's National Patient Safety Goals. The exact incidence and effects of missed test results are unknown; however, the rate of failed follow-up in a large study of 4,500 patients from academic and community practices was 7.1%. Although patients should be encouraged to follow up all test results and office clinical personnel may assist with the workflow, it is the physician who bears the legal responsibility of communicating test results to the patient.

Results may be shared electronically, by mail, or verbally, and communications should be designed so that patients understand the results and instructions. Written records shared with patients may be preferable; studies have shown that patients who receive important results verbally may be unable to process the information in the moment that it is delivered. Confirmation that the patient has received critical lab reports and associated recommendations is imperative and should be documented in the patient's medical record.

Individual practices should involve clinic stakeholders in creating policies that delineate standard tracking and reminder systems workflow, individual responsibilities, and process monitoring. Policies should outline the method of communication, the timeline for reporting critical and noncritical results, and expectations for documentation.

Callen JL, Westbrook JI, Georgiou A, Li J. Failure to follow-up test results for ambulatory patients: a systematic review. J Gen Intern Med 2012;27:1334–48.

Casalino LP, Dunham D, Chin MH, Bielang R, Kistner EO, Karrison TG, et al. Frequency of failure to inform patients of clinically significant outpatient test results [published erratum appears in Arch Intern Med 2009;169:1626]. Arch Intern Med 2009;169:1123–9.

Singh H, Vij MS. Eight recommendations for policies for communicating abnormal test results. Jt Comm J Qual Patient Saf 2010;36:226–32.

Tracking and reminder systems. Committee Opinion No. 546. American College of Obstetricians and Gynecologists. Obstet Gynecol 2012;120:1535–7.

79

Methods to increase lactation

A 28-year-old woman, gravida 1, para 1, was recently diagnosed with severe preeclampsia at 28 weeks of gestation. She underwent cesarean delivery because of malpresentation. Her newborn is now 3 weeks old. She is aware of the benefits of human breast milk and is concerned that she is not producing enough milk. In an effort to promote better breastfeeding, she has been pumping eight times a day with a hospital-grade pump combined with hand expression of milk. She has met with the lactation support specialist. She is trying to get 7–8 hours of sleep per night and is getting skin-to-skin contact with her newborn. She requests information about additional interventions to increase her breast milk supply. You tell her that in the United States, no medications have been approved by the U.S. Food and Drug Administration (FDA) to increase breast milk supply but that the off-label treatment that would best increase her milk supply is

(A) bromocriptine
* (B) metoclopramide
(C) fenugreek
(D) intranasal oxytocin

The American College of Obstetricians and Gynecologists and the American Academy of Pediatrics recommend breastfeeding or the provision of human breast milk for newborns to promote neonatal and maternal health. Box 79-1 shows newborn breastfeeding goals for the United States by the year 2020. Breastfeeding supports optimal growth and development of the infant while decreasing the risk of a variety of other diseases. Benefits to the infant include reduction in gastrointestinal and respiratory infections as well as decreased otitis media. A particular advantage for the premature infant is that breastfeeding helps to prevent necrotizing enterocolitis. Breastfeeding also provides the woman with health advantages, including decreased postpartum hemorrhage and postpartum depression as well as improved weight control and lower rates of breast cancer, hypertension, diabetes mellitus, and hyperlipidemia. The obstetrician–gynecologist or other obstetric care provider should begin to promote breastfeeding during the antenatal period. Other measures shown to increase the success rate of breastfeeding include initiation of breastfeeding within the first hour of birth, free access to the breast with frequent feedings, and skin-to-skin contact with the baby.

Providing human breast milk to the premature infant presents some special challenges. The fetus typically gains a significant amount of weight during the third trimester and does not have the additional caloric requirements related to temperature regulation and respiration while in utero. For these reasons, it is typical to fortify breast milk to meet these caloric needs. Women with a newborn in the neonatal intensive care unit should be encouraged to initiate pumping within 6–12 hours of delivery and pump frequently (8–12 times per day) to completely empty the breasts and stimulate breast milk production. There are

BOX 79-1

Healthy People 2020 Targets for Breastfeeding*

Increase the proportion of infants who are
- ever breastfed (81.9%)
- breastfed at 6 months (60.6%)
- breastfed at 1 year (34.1%)
- exclusively breastfed through 3 months (46.2%)
- exclusively breastfed through 6 months (25.5%)

Increase the number of employers with on-site lactation support (38%)

Reduce the proportion of breastfed newborns who receive formula supplementation within the first 2 days of life (14.2%)

Increase the proportion of live births that occur in facilities that provide recommended care for lactating women and their infants (8.1%)

*Healthy People 2020 targets are shown parenthetically.

Centers for Disease Control and Prevention. Breastfeeding report card: United States 2014. Atlanta (GA): CDC; 2014. Available at: https://www.cdc.gov/breastfeeding/pdf/2014breastfeedingreportcard.pdf. Retrieved June 18, 2016.

qualitative differences in the foremilk and the hindmilk, the latter being higher in protein, fatty acids, energy, and fat-soluble multivitamins. The hindmilk has a higher viscosity and is more difficult to express with an electric pump. Hand expression of breast milk is more effective in releasing the hindmilk, and the combination of hand expression with electric pumping has shown a benefit in neonatal weight gain.

Other measures associated with successfully breastfeeding a premature infant include increased skin-to-skin contact; reduction of stress; and careful attention to diet, sleep, and pumping schedules. Despite these interventions, some women have difficulty maintaining their own breast milk supply. Galactagogues are medications that can increase the breast milk supply. Metoclopramide, which is a galactagogue, is a dopamine antagonist used to promote stomach emptying and gastrointestinal motility. In standard dosage, metoclopramide has been shown to increase breast milk supply by 52–93%. The FDA lists a "black-box" warning for tardive dyskinesia with use of metoclopramide, which can be irreversible and is related to the duration of therapy. Therefore, the FDA recommends use of this agent for no more than 12 weeks. The use of metoclopramide to increase breast milk supply, like the use of all galactagogues, typically has been limited to 7–14 days, after which it is unlikely to become beneficial. The medication is able to cross the woman's blood–brain barrier, which can promote an acute dystonic reaction, usually in the first 24–48 hours of treatment. Metoclopramide would be the best option for the described patient.

Bromocriptine is a dopamine agonist. Its use would suppress the production of prolactin and diminish breast milk supply.

Fenugreek (*Trigonella foenum-graecum*) is an herbal supplement most commonly used as an antidiabetic and antilipidemic compound. Fenugreek contains phytoestrogens and diosgenin, which are reported to increase milk supply within 24–72 hours. Well-controlled studies on these herbal galactagogues are lacking. Adverse effects include nausea, diarrhea, and exacerbation of asthma.

Oxytocin promotes release of prolactin in the anterior pituitary and is an important hormone for promotion of the breast milk let-down reflex. Historically, intranasal administration of oxytocin has been used for labor induction. There has been a resurgence of interest in its use for the treatment of migraines, autism, and alcohol dependence. Randomized controlled studies have demonstrated no difference in milk production or quality with intranasal oxytocin use.

Abdulwadud OA, Snow ME. Interventions in the workplace to support breastfeeding for women in employment. Cochrane Database of Systematic Reviews 2012, Issue 10. Art. No.: CD006177. DOI: 10.1002/14651858.CD006177.pub3.

Breastfeeding and the use of human milk. Section on Breastfeeding. Pediatrics 2012;129:e827–41.

Breastfeeding in underserved women: increasing initiation and continuation of breastfeeding. Committee Opinion No. 570. American College of Obstetricians and Gynecologists. Obstet Gynecol 2013;122:423–8.

Forinash AB, Yancey AM, Barnes KN, Myles TD. The use of galactogogues in the breastfeeding mother. Ann Pharmacother 2012;46: 1392–404.

Ingram J, Taylor H, Churchill C, Pike A, Greenwood R. Metoclopramide or domperidone for increasing maternal breast milk output: a randomised controlled trial. Arch Dis Child Fetal Neonatal Ed 2012;97:F241–5.

Lessen R, Kavanagh K. Position of the academy of nutrition and dietetics: promoting and supporting breastfeeding. J Acad Nutr Diet 2015;115:444–9.

Osadchy A, Moretti ME, Koren G. Effect of domperidone on insufficient lactation in puerperal women: a systematic review and meta-analysis of randomized controlled trials. Obstet Gynecol Int 2012;2012:642893.

Underwood MA. Human milk for the premature infant. Pediatr Clin North Am 2013;60:189–207.

80

Failed pregnancy of unknown location

A 37-year-old woman, gravida 4, para 3, comes to your office with left lower quadrant pain, vaginal spotting, and a positive pregnancy test. Her last menstrual period was 6 weeks ago, and she tells you that the current pregnancy is unplanned but highly desired. Examination reveals a temperature of 37.0°C (98.6°F), heart rate of 65 beats per minute, and blood pressure of 132/80 mm Hg. Her abdomen is soft with no associated tenderness. Pelvic examination reveals a 6-week-sized uterus and is otherwise unremarkable. Transvaginal ultrasonography demonstrates an empty uterus. A 2.5-cm anechoic mass is observed in the left adnexa separate from the ovary. There is no evidence of free fluid. Laboratory results include a quantitative serum β-hCG level of 2,560 mIU/mL; on repeat testing 48 hours later, the β-hCG level is 2,500 mIU/mL, and repeat transvaginal ultrasonography is unchanged. Her blood type is AB positive. The most appropriate next step in her management is

(A) repeat serum β-hCG level in 48 hours
* (B) uterine evacuation
(C) methotrexate
(D) diagnostic laparoscopy
(E) progesterone level

Ectopic pregnancy accounts for approximately 2% of pregnancies in the United States and is the leading cause of maternal mortality in the first trimester, accounting for 10% of all pregnancy-related deaths. Although the incidence of ectopic pregnancy has remained stable over the past two decades, the associated mortality rate has decreased to 0.5 deaths per 1,000 pregnancies, largely because of early diagnosis and appropriate treatment. Complications associated with ectopic pregnancy can be reduced effectively and often eliminated by early diagnosis and intervention. Early detection is possible with improved capabilities of current diagnostic tools, and it enables successful medical management before the onset of rupture. However, with the advances of modern technology and management, obstetrician–gynecologists and other health care providers are now faced with the perils of misinterpretation of serial β-hCG values, overinterpretation of a single ultrasonographic examination, and inappropriate use of methotrexate.

The described patient has a *pregnancy of unknown location*, defined as a clinical scenario of a positive β-hCG level test result and nondiagnostic transvaginal ultrasonography. A total of 50–70% of these pregnancies will resolve spontaneously. An additional 30% go on to be diagnosed as intrauterine pregnancies and 7–20% as ectopic pregnancies. However, "pregnancy of unknown location" is a descriptive term or a classification rather than a final diagnosis; once a pregnancy of unknown location has been deemed nonviable, a definitive location for the pregnancy must be determined. The discriminatory zone for β-hCG is linked closely to the accuracy of ultrasonography as well as the available laboratory assays. This number ranges between 1,500 mIU/mL and 2,500 mIU/mL in the literature and ultimately will vary between institutions.

The diagnosis of ectopic pregnancy relies on serial β-hCG levels in conjunction with transvaginal ultrasonography findings. At serum β-hCG levels above the discriminatory zone, an intrauterine gestational sac should be visualized. A true gestational sac possesses a double decidual sign and often is located eccentrically within the endometrial cavity. This is in contrast with a pseudogestational sac observed with an ectopic pregnancy. The presence of a true intrauterine gestational sac essentially excludes the presence of an ectopic pregnancy; however, careful consideration should be given to the possibility of a heterotopic pregnancy in high-risk patients. In patients with a pregnancy of unknown location, β-hCG levels should be trended, and an appropriate rise is an increase of at least 53% in 48 hours. In a patient with a pregnancy of unknown location who has an inappropriate trend and a persistently empty uterus with β-hCG levels greater than 2,500 mIU/mL, the pregnancy can be confidently determined to be nonviable.

The described patient's β-hCG levels are clearly abnormal and, thus, given her symptoms and the presence of an adnexal mass, repeating a serum β-hCG level in another 48 hours would not be the most appropriate next step in her management. Although the differential diagnosis still includes failed intrauterine pregnancy and ectopic pregnancy, a delay in making a definitive diagnosis could result in avoidable rupture of an ectopic pregnancy. This patient can be classified as having a nonviable pregnancy of unknown location. A presumed diagnosis of an ectopic pregnancy will be incorrect in approximately 27–50% of cases. Such a diagnosis would result in inappropriate administration of methotrexate in 40% of failed intrauterine pregnancies. Inappropriate administration of methotrexate can have catastrophic outcomes for patients, including inadvertent exposure of a fetus to methotrexate and iatrogenic complications related to the chemotherapeutic medication's effect on rapidly proliferating tissues such as the bone marrow, respiratory epithelium, and the buccal and intestinal mucosa. Ultrasonographic findings that are nondiagnostic in conjunction with absolute and serial β-hCG levels may be associated with but cannot definitively predict an accurate final diagnosis.

Although this patient's ultrasonographic findings demonstrate an adnexal mass, which could indicate an ectopic pregnancy, preliminary ultrasonographic reports suggestive of ectopic pregnancy can be incorrect in 11% of cases. This mass could represent other etiologies, including a hemorrhagic cyst or paratubal cyst. Given the patient's hemodynamic stability and an unconfirmed diagnosis of an ectopic pregnancy, performing a diagnostic laparoscopy would be premature and could expose her to potential complications of unnecessary surgery.

The described patient has already demonstrated a β-hCG trend consistent with a nonviable pregnancy; therefore, a progesterone level test is not indicated because it will not provide any additional information regarding pregnancy viability. Furthermore, serum progesterone has limited use with respect to distinguishing a nonviable intrauterine pregnancy from an ectopic pregnancy. The most appropriate course of action for this patient is to perform uterine evacuation to exclude a failed intrauterine pregnancy.

Surgical evacuation of the uterus is a useful diagnostic tool for a woman with a nonviable pregnancy of unknown location and can be therapeutic as well. Evacuation of the uterus with misoprostol is inappropriate in the absence of confirmation of the location of the failed pregnancy.

Barnhart KT. Clinical practice. Ectopic pregnancy. N Engl J Med 2009;361:379–87.

Medical management of ectopic pregnancy. ACOG Practice Bulletin No. 94. American College of Obstetricians and Gynecologists. Obstet Gynecol 2008;111:1479–85.

Medical treatment of ectopic pregnancy: a committee opinion. Practice Committee of the American Society for Reproductive Medicine. Fertil Steril 2013;100:638–44.

Rubal L, Chung K. Do you need to definitively diagnose the location of a pregnancy of unknown location? The case for "yes." Fertil Steril 2012;98:1078–84.

Seeber, BE. What serial hCG can tell you, and cannot tell you, about an early pregnancy. Fertil Steril 2012;98:1074–7.

Shaunik A, Kulp J, Appleby DH, Sammel MD, Barnhart KT. Utility of dilation and curettage in the diagnosis of pregnancy of unknown location. Am J Obstet Gynecol 2011;204:130.e1–6.

81

Chronic cough in women treated with antihypertensive medication

A 54-year-old postmenopausal woman presents for her annual well-woman examination. She reports a 3-month history of a nonproductive cough with no associated triggers. She has not experienced fever, shortness of breath, chest pain, or heartburn. She has a history of hypertension and has been taking captopril for the past year. She has a 20-pack-per-year history of smoking. You obtain a chest X-ray, which is negative. The next best step in management is

(A) computed tomography (CT) scan of chest
(B) pulmonary function test
(C) histamine-2 receptor antagonist
* (D) change in antihypertensive medication
(E) allergy testing

Coughing is one of the most common symptoms for which patients seek medical care in the United States. Most cases of *chronic cough*, defined as a cough lasting longer than 8 weeks, are due to upper airway cough syndrome (from postnasal drip), asthma, or gastroesophageal reflux disease (GERD). One study found that these disorders were responsible for chronic chough in 99.4% of patients who were nonsmokers, did not use an angiotensin-converting enzyme (ACE) inhibitor, and had a normal chest X-ray. The character of the cough (eg, productive versus dry, "barking," "honking") is not helpful in differentiating the possible causes. The initial approach is based on identifying and treating illnesses that could trigger the cough reflex.

The most common symptoms of GERD are heartburn, regurgitation, and dysphagia; less common manifestations include bronchospasm, laryngitis, and chronic cough. A diagnosis of GERD can be made based on symptoms and response to a histamine-2 receptor antagonist or proton pump inhibitor. Upper endoscopy with biopsies can be reserved for patients who do not respond to empiric treatment or when the diagnosis is uncertain. Initiation of a histamine-2 receptor antagonist may be second-line treatment for the described patient, but because she lacks the classic symptoms of GERD, it is not the best next step in management.

New-onset cough in a postmenopausal woman who smokes may signify lung cancer or other chest masses. The most common symptoms of lung cancer are cough, weight loss, dyspnea, and chest pain. Most patients with lung cancer have advanced disease at the time of diagnosis. Therefore, patients with symptoms suggestive of primary or metastatic lung cancer should undergo expedient imaging with chest X-ray. Mediastinal masses can present in a variety of ways. Patients may be symptomatic and exhibit such symptoms as cough, hemoptysis, shortness of breath, pain, dysphagia, hoarseness, and facial or upper extremity swelling resulting from superior vena cava syndrome. The masses also may be asymptomatic and suspected based upon abnormalities in a chest X-ray performed for symptoms or for other reasons (such as preoperative evaluation). A chest CT scan with intravenous contrast typically is used to evaluate chest X-ray abnormalities. Given that the described patient had a negative chest X-ray, a chest CT scan is not indicated at this time.

Asthma may develop at any age, although new-onset asthma is less frequent in older adults than in other age groups. Patients may report a pattern of respiratory symptoms that occur with exposure to triggers (eg, allergens, exercise, or upper respiratory infection) and resolve with trigger avoidance or asthma medication. The classic symptoms of asthma are wheeze, cough (often worse at night), and shortness of breath or difficulty breathing. Asthma may be the cause of the described patient's cough, but it is a less likely cause in the absence of other symptoms, so pulmonary function testing is not helpful at this stage of her evaluation.

Allergic rhinitis presents with episodes of sneezing, rhinorrhea, nasal obstruction, and nasal itching; other common symptoms include postnasal drip, cough, irritability, and fatigue. Episodes may be intermittent or persistent and range in severity from mild to moderate–severe (with sleep disturbances and impairment in daily activities including work and school). Allergic rhinitis rarely presents for the first time in older adults unless there is a significant change in exposures (eg, a new pet or a move to a different climate). Therefore, in the described patient, empiric treatment for allergies or referral for allergy testing is not indicated.

A chronic dry cough is a common adverse effect of taking an ACE inhibitor and will occur in 5–35% of patients. This cough may present up to 6–12 months after medication initiation. Switching treatment from one

ACE inhibitor to another is not effective because cough is a class adverse effect. When ACE inhibitor use is discontinued, improvement of the cough generally occurs within 1–4 weeks. In some patients, however, resolution of the cough may take a few months. The best next step in management for the described patient, who developed a cough while using the ACE inhibitor captopril, is to replace the captopril with another antihypertensive medication, such as an angiotensin receptor blocker, and be reevaluated in 3 months. The patient also should be counseled on smoking cessation. Appendix E shows an algorithm for the diagnostic approach to chronic cough.

Bezalel S, Mahlab-Guri K, Asher I, Werner B, Sthoeger ZM. Angiotensin-converting enzyme inhibitor-induced angioedema. Am J Med 2015;128:120–5.

Iyer VN, Lim KG. Chronic cough: an update. Mayo Clin Proc 2013;88:1115–26.

Morice AH, Fontana GA, Sovijarvi ARA, Pistolesi M, Chung KF, Widdicombe J, et al. The diagnosis and management of chronic cough. Eur Respir J 2004;24:481–92.

Terasaki G, Paauw DS. Evaluation and treatment of chronic cough. Med Clin North Am 2014;98:391–403.

82

Risks of untreated asymptomatic bacteriuria in pregnancy

A 23-year-old woman, gravida 1, para 0, at 10 weeks of gestation has a routine urinary culture at the time of her initial visit. Although she has reported no urinary symptoms, the results show 100,000 organisms/mL of *Escherichia coli*. You recommend a 7-day course of nitrofurantoin because this treatment has been shown to decrease the risk of subsequent acute pyelonephritis. This treatment also will decrease the risk of

(A) chronic renal insufficiency
* (B) preterm delivery
(C) neonatal meningitis
(D) preeclampsia

Urinary tract infections (UTIs) are among the most common bacterial infections. Such infections can be divided into upper or lower UTIs. Women are at particularly high risk because of the shortened urethra and the close proximity of the urethra to the genitalia. Cystitis is an infection of the lower urinary tract with associated symptoms of dysuria, frequency, urgency and, occasionally, suprapubic tenderness.

Urinary tract infections are further subdivided into complicated and uncomplicated cases. Most reproductive-aged women will have an uncomplicated UTI, which will respond to a short (3-day) course of antibiotics. Complicated UTI cases, including those involving pregnant patients, typically require a longer course of treatment. A patient may have asymptomatic bacteriuria with a significant bacterial load in the urine but lack symptoms. Studies using quantitative bacterial culture have defined significant bacteriuria as greater than 100,000 organisms per milliliter in a single voided midstream collection.

Population studies indicate that approximately 5% of the general population and 2–10% of pregnant women will have asymptomatic bacteriuria. The belief that asymptomatic bacteriuria leads to chronic renal disease or hypertensive disease has been disproved and, thus, screening of the general population is not recommended. Significant health risks remain in certain high-risk populations (ie, elderly, pregnant, immunosuppressed, recently catheterized), and quantitative culture is encouraged. During pregnancy, up to 30% of women with asymptomatic bacteriuria may develop acute pyelonephritis which, if left untreated, can go on to cause maternal septicemia, renal failure, respiratory insufficiency, and preterm labor. Preterm delivery and low birth weight have been associated with asymptomatic bacteriuria; treatment can decrease these risks. The association of infection of the maternal urinary tract with preterm labor is thought to be mediated by prostaglandins and other cytokines. Chorioamnionitis and resultant fetal infections can be a complication of pyelonephritis, but this is infrequent. There are no direct fetal risks, such as neonatal sepsis or meningitis, from infection of the maternal urinary tract.

The most common causative agent of UTI in women is *E coli* (75–90%). The remaining cases are caused by other *Enterobacteriaceae*, such as *Klebsiella pneumoniae*, and gram-positive bacteria, such as *Staphylococcus saprophyticus, Enterococcus faecalis*, and *Streptococcus agalactiae* (group B streptococci). Urine dipstick testing for nitrites and leukocyte esterase is a rapid and inexpensive method to diagnose a UTI, and it often is used in nonpregnant women. Because of the significant risks to pregnant women, culture remains the criterion standard. Local sensitivity profiles will largely guide antibiotic treatment choices. Standard treatment with 7–10 days of antibiotics has been shown to be effective in preventing upper UTIs; suppressive antibiotics through the duration of the pregnancy are not indicated. Screening for and treatment of asymptomatic bacteriuria during pregnancy will prevent maternal complications of upper UTIs and decrease the risk of preterm labor. Unlike UTIs, pyelonephritis requires suppressive therapy throughout the remainder of pregnancy. Asymptomatic bacteria without progression to more systemic illness has not been associated with renal insufficiency or preeclampsia.

Hooton TM. Clinical practice. Uncomplicated urinary tract infection. N Engl J Med 2012;366:1028–37.

Nicolle LE. Asymptomatic bacteriuria--important or not? N Engl J Med 2000;343:1037–9.

Treatment of urinary tract infections in nonpregnant women. ACOG Practice Bulletin No. 91. American College of Obstetricians and Gynecologists. Obstet Gynecol 2008;111:785–94.

Vazquez JC, Abalos E. Treatments for symptomatic urinary tract infections during pregnancy. Cochrane Database of Systematic Reviews 2011, Issue 1. Art. No.: CD002256. DOI: 10.1002/14651858.CD002256.pub2.

Widmer M, Lopez I, Gülmezoglu AM, Mignini L, Roganti A. Duration of treatment for asymptomatic bacteriuria during pregnancy. Cochrane Database of Systematic Reviews 2015, Issue 11. Art. No.: CD000491. DOI: 10.1002/14651858.CD000491.pub3.

83

Methotrexate use in ectopic pregnancy

A 22-year-old woman, gravida 1, comes to your office with mild pelvic pain and vaginal spotting. Her last menstrual period was 6 weeks ago. Her serum β-hCG level is 3,000 mIU/mL, and her serum progesterone level is 4 ng/mL. No intrauterine pregnancy is seen on transvaginal ultrasonography. After counseling, you initiate single-dose methotrexate therapy. Four days later, her β-hCG level is 4,500 mIU/mL. She continues to have mild pelvic pain. The best next step in management is

(A) pelvic ultrasonography
(B) suction curettage
(C) repeat methotrexate
* (D) serum β-hCG level measurement in 3 days
(E) laparoscopy

Methotrexate therapy for suspected ectopic pregnancy has an overall success rate of 70–95% and is dependent on the treatment regimen used, gestational age, and initial β-hCG level. Absolute contraindications to methotrexate use include breastfeeding; immunodeficiency; hepatic, renal, or hematologic dysfunction; pulmonary disease, peptic ulcer disease, and known sensitivity to methotrexate. Relative contraindications include an adnexal mass larger than 3.5 cm in diameter, the presence of fetal cardiac activity, and a β-hCG level of 6,000–15,000 mIU/mL.

The diagnosis of an ectopic pregnancy can be made by the absence of an intrauterine gestational sac on ultrasonography when the β-hCG level is within or greater than the "discriminatory zone" of 1,500–2,500 mIU/mL, depending on the institution. If the β-hCG level is higher than the discriminatory zone and the transvaginal ultrasonography examination is nondiagnostic (ie, no pregnancy can be identified), an ectopic pregnancy is likely. There is little use to repeating the pelvic ultrasonography for this patient without significant change in her symptoms suggesting a ruptured ectopic pregnancy.

Serum progesterone measurement may aid in the diagnosis of an ectopic pregnancy. A low serum progesterone level (below 5 ng/mL) is diagnostic of an abnormal pregnancy but does not distinguish between a failed intrauterine pregnancy and an ectopic pregnancy. Endometrial sampling can help with this distinction by confirming the presence or absence of intrauterine chorionic villi. In the described patient, with an ultrasonographic result highly suspicious for ectopic pregnancy and undergoing methotrexate therapy, there is no need for confirmatory sampling with a suction curettage.

There are three described protocols for methotrexate dosage: 1) single dose, 2) two dose, and 3) fixed multidose. The single-dose regimen is the simplest and most commonly used protocol, but up to 40% of patients will require additional doses. The fixed multidose regimen may be more appropriate for women with more advanced gestations and those with embryonic cardiac activity but requires folinic acid rescue to minimize adverse effects. The two-dose regimen maximizes the methotrexate dose without the need for folinic acid rescue or more obstetrician–gynecologist or other health care provider visits because the second dose is given on day 4. After administration of the single methotrexate dose, the β-hCG level may rise between days 0 and 4; this increase alone is not an indication for repeat methotrexate dosage.

Patients who undergo methotrexate therapy for a presumed ectopic pregnancy should be counseled about expected adverse effects. Abdominal pain may continue to be present or even increase after methotrexate administration, likely from the cytotoxic effects of the drug on the trophoblast tissue causing tubal abortion. In the absence of signs and symptoms of tubal rupture and significant hemoperitoneum, this pain can be managed expectantly with hemoglobin and ultrasonographic monitoring. The described patient is not experiencing pain consistent with tubal rupture, so there is no need for surgical exploration at this time.

The serum β-hCG level should be expected to decrease by at least 15% from day 4 to day 7 after methotrexate administration. The β-hCG levels then can be measured weekly until reaching nonpregnant levels. If the decrease is less than 15%, or if β-hCG levels plateau or increase during surveillance, the methotrexate dose can be repeated. In the current scenario, the obstetrician–gynecologist or other health care provider can stay the course and draw the next β-hCG level in 3 days—on day 7—unless the patient's clinical presentation worsens.

Bachman EA, Barnhart K. Medical management of ectopic pregnancy: a comparison of regimens. Clin Obstet Gynecol 2012;55:440–7.

Capmas P, Bouyer J, Fernandez H. Treatment of ectopic pregnancies in 2014: new answers to some old questions. Fertil Steril 2014;101: 615–20.

Cecchino GN, Araujo Junior E, Elito Junior J. Methotrexate for ectopic pregnancy: when and how. Arch Gynecol Obstet 2014;290:417–23.

Medical management of ectopic pregnancy. ACOG Practice Bulletin No. 94. American College of Obstetricians and Gynecologists. Obstet Gynecol 2008;111:1479–85.

84

Clostridium difficile infection

A 19-year-old nulligravid woman was discharged from the hospital 3 days ago for treatment of a tubo-ovarian abscess. She received 7 days of intravenous gentamicin and clindamycin and was converted to oral amoxicillin–clavulanate before discharge. She returns to the emergency department with a temperature of 38.3°C (101°F), nausea, and abdominal pain with watery diarrhea. A *Clostridium difficile* test result is positive. Her white blood cell count is 16.2 g/dL. Abdominal films show multiple air–fluid levels but no suggestion of dilated bowel loops. In addition to continuing her current antibiotic regimen for the tubo-ovarian abscess, the treatment that will offer the lowest risk of recurrence of *C difficile* is

(A) oral neomycin
(B) oral metronidazole
(C) oral vancomycin
(D) fecal transplant
* (E) oral fidaxomicin

C difficile, a gram-positive, spore-forming bacteria, has become a leading cause of hospital-associated gastrointestinal illness. *C difficile* infections cost the U.S. health care system an estimated $3.2 billion annually. The bacteria are noninvasive; however, toxins produced by the bacterium can cause a spectrum of disease, from asymptomatic carriage through mild diarrhea to colitis and pseudomembranous colitis. At the extreme end of the spectrum, patients can develop toxic megacolon, which is a surgical emergency.

C difficile infections may manifest with watery diarrhea but are rarely associated with the passage of blood. Symptoms of fever, cramping, and abdominal discomfort, as well as an elevated white blood cell count, are present in less than one half of cases. Approximately 1–2% of healthy adults will be colonized with *C difficile*. Colonization rates increase in proportion to the length of hospitalization, with rates of 7–26% in acute care facilities and 57% among the elderly in long-term care facilities. The normal gut flora prevents colonization with

C difficile. Antibiotic use can alter the colonic microbiome and increase susceptibility to colonization with *C difficile*. Rates of *C difficile* infections have increased dramatically since 1990 for reasons that are not well understood. Possible factors may include changing antibiotic prescribing practices, a trend toward hospitalization of older and sicker patients, and widespread use of alcohol-based hand sanitizers, which do not adequately treat the infectious spores.

Practically all antibiotics have been implicated as a risk factor for *C difficile* infection. The diagnosis of *C difficile* infection should be considered in patients with three or more unformed stools within 24 hours and recent antibiotic exposure. Infection can be confirmed by testing for the toxin through the polymerase chain reaction test, cytotoxic neutralization assay, or toxigenic culture. Screening tests for glutamate dehydrogenase, an enzyme produced by *C difficile*, have been introduced; glutamate dehydrogenase testing has a high negative predictive value, but positive results still require confirmation of toxin production.

For patients in whom *C difficile* infection has been diagnosed, the inciting antibiotics should be discontinued with a few exceptions. Protocols for isolation and strict hand washing with soap and water should be initiated.

Disease severity is graded mild if there is only the presence of diarrhea. A *C difficile* infection severity index score also has been used (Table 84-1). Severe and complicated disease criteria would include patients with intensive care unit admission, mental status change, hypotension, ileus, white blood cell count greater than 35 g/dL or less than 2.0 g/dL, elevated lactate level, and fever with a temperature of 38.5°C (101.3°F) or higher. Among patients with a severe *C difficile* infection, hypoalbuminemia (less than 3 g/dL), white blood cell count greater than 15.0 g/dL, and abdominal distention predict patients that are likely to need intensive care unit admission or colectomy.

Several antibiotics have been useful in the treatment of *C difficile* infection. The most commonly used are metronidazole, vancomycin, and fidaxomicin. Fidaxomicin, a poorly absorbed oral macrocyclic antibiotic, has efficacy similar to oral vancomycin. Ideally, patients who have a *C difficile* infection should discontinue all other antibiotics; in some cases, however, the clinical condition of the patient will mandate that the antibiotics be continued. The described patient will need to continue antibiotics for the treatment of the tubo-ovarian abscess, and she has a severe form of disease that puts her at a higher risk of recurrence. Treatment of *C difficile* infections while continuing antibiotic use delays resolution of diarrhea and is associated with a lower cure rate and higher recurrence rate. Treatment with fidaxomicin has been shown to have a higher cure rate and lower recurrence rate in patients with a severe *C difficile* infection and who are receiving concomitant antibiotics. Because of cost considerations, fidaxomicin use often is limited to patients at high risk of recurrence (eg, patients of advanced age, who have a severe *C difficile* infection, or who are on concomitant antibiotic therapy). Fidaxomicin would be the best choice for this patient because of the improved cure rate and lower recurrence rate of *C difficile* infection.

Oral metronidazole is less expensive than commercially available oral vancomycin preparations. Patients with a mild *C difficile* infection are treated with oral metronidazole. Lack of response to therapy within 5–7 days should prompt replacement of oral metronidazole with oral vancomycin. For severe *C difficile* infections, oral vancomycin is clinically superior to oral metronidazole, with a cure rate of 97% versus 76%, respectively. Patients with severe disease should have initial therapy with oral vancomycin; however, this would not be the preferred treatment for the described patient because of her high risk of recurrence due to her use of concomitant antibiotics. Neomycin (an aminoglycoside) has been used to prevent infections during gastrointestinal surgeries but is not recommended for treatment of gram-positive *C difficile*. A cost-effective alternative is to compound vancomycin for oral use from the intravenous form of the medication. Restoration of the normal gut flora with fecal microbiota transplantation has been effective for refractory cases of *C difficile* infection and is recommended

TABLE 84-1. Severity Scoring Index for *Clostridium difficile* Infection*

Variable	Points
Fever (38°C)	1
Ileus (diagnosed by clinical or radiographic findings)	1
Systolic blood pressure less than 100 mm Hg†	1
Leukocytosis†	
WBC less than 15,000/mm^3	0
WBC equal to or greater than 15,000/mm^3, less than 30,000/mm^3	1
WBC greater than 30,000/mm^3	2
CT scan findings (thickened colonic wall, colonic dilatation, ascites)‡	0
No findings	1
One finding	1
Two or more findings	2

Abbreviations: CT, computed tomography; WBC, white blood cell.

*A score equal to or greater than 2 is indicative of severe *Clostridium difficile* infection.

†Any single reading within 3 days of *Clostridium difficile* infection diagnosis.

‡Obtaining a CT scan is not mandatory.

Modified from Fujitani S, George WL, Murthy AR. Comparison of clinical severity score indices for *Clostridium difficile* infection. Infect Control Hosp Epidemiol 2011;32:220–8.

after the third recurrence. Despite these treatments and control measures, a recurrence rate of 15–25% of *C difficile* has been reported.

Cohen SH, Gerding DN, Johnson S, Kelly CP, Loo VG, McDonald LC, et al. Clinical practice guidelines for *Clostridium difficile* infection in adults: 2010 update by the Society for Healthcare Epidemiology of America (SHEA) and the Infectious Diseases Society of America (IDSA). Society for Healthcare Epidemiology of America, Infectious Diseases Society of America. Infect Control Hosp Epidemiol 2010;31:431–55.

Fujitani S, George WL, Murthy AR. Comparison of clinical severity score indices for *Clostridium difficile* infection. Infect Control Hosp Epidemiol 2011;32:220–8.

Le F, Arora V, Shah DN, Salazar M, Palmer HR, Garey KW. A real-world evaluation of oral vancomycin for severe *Clostridium difficile* infection: implications for antibiotic stewardship programs. Pharmacotherapy 2012;32:129–34.

Louie TJ, Miller MA, Mullane KM, Weiss K, Lentnek A, Golan Y, et al. Fidaxomicin versus vancomycin for *Clostridium difficile* infection. OPT-80-003 Clinical Study Group. N Engl J Med 2011;364:422–31.

Mullane KM, Miller MA, Weiss K, Lentnek A, Golan Y, Sears PS, et al. Efficacy of fidaxomicin versus vancomycin as therapy for *Clostridium difficile* infection in individuals taking concomitant antibiotics for other concurrent infections [published erratum appears in Clin Infect Dis 2011;53:1312]. Clin Infect Dis 2011;53:440–7.

Nelson RL, Kelsey P, Leeman H, Meardon N, Patel H, Paul K, et al. Antibiotic treatment for *Clostridium difficile*-associated diarrhea in adults. Cochrane Database of Systematic Review 2011, Issue 9. Art. No.: CD004610. DOI: 10.1002/14651858.CD004610.pub4.

Surawicz CM, Brandt LJ, Binion DG, Ananthakrishnan AN, Curry SR, Gilligan PH, et al. Guidelines for diagnosis, treatment, and prevention of *Clostridium difficile* infections. Am J Gastroenterol 2013;108:478,98; quiz 499.

85

Colon cancer screening in postmenopausal women

A 58-year-old woman visits you for a well-woman examination. Her internist ordered fecal occult blood testing approximately 2 years ago, but she has had no other colon cancer screening. Her family history is negative for colon cancer. She exercises regularly and does not smoke. You counsel her about the various approaches to colon cancer screening and the benefits and limitations of each approach. The most appropriate management of this patient is

(A) office-based rectal examination with guaiac testing every year
(B) computed tomography (CT) colonography every 5 years
(C) fecal DNA testing every 5 years
* (D) colonoscopy every 10 years
(E) flexible sigmoidoscopy every 10 years

Colorectal cancer is the third leading cause of cancer death in women. Effective screening for colorectal cancer is available in many forms, each with its own benefits and limitations. Colonoscopy has been associated with an 83% reduction in mortality from colon cancer, the highest reported rate of the various screening modalities. Colonoscopy offers the single best approach in terms of allowing for complete visualization of the entire length of the colon and for the ability to resect polyps. Adenomatous polyps are the most common precancerous lesions, and resecting them decreases the risk of colorectal cancer.

The American College of Obstetricians and Gynecologists (the College) and the U.S. Preventive Services Task Force (USPSTF) recommend colonoscopy (or other colorectal cancer screening modalities) beginning at age 50 years. The College recommends that screening begin at age 45 years in African Americans because of this group's higher colorectal cancer incidence rate. In general, patients are advised to undergo this procedure every 10 years unless findings such as identification of polyps at the time of the procedure mandate otherwise. Family history and other factors also can affect the interval between colonoscopy procedures. Of importance, colonoscopy not only detects colorectal cancer, it also detects polyps that may be precursors to neoplasia, particularly adenomatous polyps. The prevalence of large polyps (1 cm or larger) in women aged 50–54 years has been found to be approximately 4%, and the incidence of polyps of any size is up to 25%. Because polyps can be resected at the time of the colonoscopy, this intervention also is important in risk-reduction strategies. Other noninvasive means of screening do not have this feature and, thus, abnormalities found by those techniques ultimately will result in a colonoscopy to allow for biopsy, resection, or both. Colonoscopy does, however, have its limitations: malignancies and polyps greater than 10 mm sometimes are missed. Adequacy of bowel preparation and endoscopist experience have been cited as important in the sensitivity of colonoscopy.

Flexible sigmoidoscopy every 5 years also has been demonstrated to be an effective screening modality and offers the ability to resect precancerous lesions, but it is limited because the instrument typically does not reach beyond 40 cm. The advantage of flexible sigmoidoscopy over colonoscopy is that it can be performed without sedation and has a lower rate of perforation. The USPSTF recommends that if flexible sigmoidoscopy is chosen as the screening modality, high-sensitivity fecal occult blood testing should be performed every 3 years as well. However, with the increasing availability of colonoscopy, fewer sigmoidoscopies are being performed in the United States.

The other aforementioned screening modalities do not permit direct visualization of the lesions and, if results are abnormal, would lead to a need for colonoscopy. However, for individuals who might otherwise forego screening because of aversion to the invasiveness of colonoscopy, one of the other screening modalities may be more acceptable to the patient.

Computed tomography colonography, sometimes called "virtual colonoscopy," involves CT imaging of the large bowel after bowel prep, similar to colonoscopy. Ingested contrast material aids in the visualization of colonic lesions. A sensitivity of 90% has been reported for CT colonography for detection of polyps of at least 1 cm in size. One unique feature of CT colonography is the potential for identifying extracolonic lesions. Many of these are benign findings, yet they result in patient anxiety and increased evaluation costs. Additionally, there is radiation exposure from this modality, with the median exposure at 10 mSv, a level that has been deemed to increase malignancy risk by a factor of 1 in 2,000 (compared with background malignancy risk of approximately 1 in 20). This form of colonography is less readily available and is not covered by many insurance plans.

Fecal DNA tests (and fecal immunochemical testing) are noninvasive modalities that detect somatic DNA mutations or blood from the lower gastrointestinal tract in a stool specimen. These tests generally are shown to be more acceptable to patients given the lower intrusiveness. However, they must be repeated more frequently. Fecal DNA testing is too new to have been shown to reduce mortality and has not yet received a recommendation from most authorities. Additionally, the cost of this test is substantially higher than other stool-based assays.

In-office rectal examination with guaiac testing has been demonstrated to have poor sensitivity and specificity. It is no longer recommended by any professional organization for detection of colorectal neoplasia.

The College and the USPSTF advise cessation of routine colorectal cancer screening at age 75 years. Because the interval between polyp appearance and transformation to malignant neoplasm is thought to be several years, this is a reasonable stance. However, with increasing life expectancy among women, study of colorectal cancer screening efficacy in geriatric populations is warranted.

Anderson JC, Shaw RD. Update on colon cancer screening: recent advances and observations in colorectal cancer screening. Curr Gastroenterol Rep 2014;16:403.

Colorectal cancer screening strategies. Committee Opinion No. 609. American College of Obstetricians and Gynecologists. Obstet Gynecol 2014;124:849–55.

Screening for colorectal cancer: U.S. Preventive Services Task Force recommendation statement. U.S. Preventive Services Task Force. Ann Intern Med 2008;149:627–37.

86

Informed consent

A 43-year-old woman, gravida 2, para 2, has chronic pelvic pain due to endometriosis. She has completed childbearing and desires definitive therapy. You discuss with her the risks and benefits of hysterectomy as well as the alternative treatment options available to her. During the informed consent process, she is adamant that she desires a laparoscopic hysterectomy. She asks you how many of these procedures you have performed in your career. Additionally, she wants to know how many complications you have experienced. As part of informed consent, answering her questions truthfully is an example of

(A) autonomy
(B) comprehension
(C) free consent
* (D) disclosure
(E) confidentiality

Ethics has been an important aspect in medicine for thousands of years, as is evidenced by the Hippocratic Oath, which sets expectations for the ethical behavior of physicians. As the modern health care model has progressed from a paternalistic view to a shared decision-making model, principle-based ethics has become the mainstay of medical ethics. The main components of principle-based ethics include respect for patient autonomy, beneficence, nonmaleficence, and justice. Autonomy allows the patient to make choices based on her personal values and beliefs. Beneficence means "the doing of good"; this concept means that the physician should act in the patient's best interests to provide the optimal medical outcome. Nonmaleficence, commonly known as *primum non nocere* (first do no harm), is an accepted expectation in the patient–physician relationship. Justice is the obligation to treat all patients who share the same medical problem equally. This is a difficult ethical principle because resources and access to health care vary widely across the United States.

Disclosure goes beyond reviewing risks and benefits of a procedure with a patient. During the informed consent process, physicians also must disclose any personal or economic interests that may influence their judgment and all diagnostic tests that may rule out a possible condition. Physicians also are required to disclose risks associated with refusal of treatment. During the informed consent conversation, the described patient introduces the concept of disclosure when she inquires about the obstetrician–gynecologist's level of experience with laparoscopic hysterectomy. The requirement for a physician to answer questions regarding experience and success rates as part of informed consent was brought forth in the case *Johnson v. Kokemoor*, 545 N.W.2d 495 (1996).

Although informed consent often is regarded as just a legal document that a patient signs before a procedure, it is actually a process of information exchange that allows patients and physicians to form a collaborative relationship. Through this communication, the patient is given autonomy. During the informed consent process, autonomy allows the patient to consider all risks and benefits in order to make the best decision for her care.

Informed consent also involves comprehension and free consent. Comprehension includes the patient's awareness and ability to understand the risks and benefits of the proposed procedure, as well as the alternatives to the procedure. Many patients have a limited understanding of medicine, so it is imperative for the physician to afford time for the patient and her family to ask questions and to have the questions answered in a way that they can understand. Free consent is the ability of the patient to make the medical decisions herself and not be coerced by others.

Confidentiality is not part of the informed consent process; however, it is a common ethical issue in obstetrics and gynecology. Part of patient autonomy is the right to privacy. Discussion between the physician and the patient must be confidential, and any information disclosed to the physician must remain protected. Without assurance of confidentiality, the patient may not share critical medical information that would optimize her care. Although confidentiality must be upheld most of the time, legal exceptions are made in cases of sexually transmitted infection reporting and child abuse.

Avery DM. Summary of informed consent and refusal. Am J Clin Med 2009;6(3):28–9.

Ethical decision making in obstetrics and gynecology. ACOG Committee Opinion No. 390. American College of Obstetricians and Gynecologists. Obstet Gynecol 2007;110:1479–87.

Informed consent. ACOG Committee Opinion No. 439. American College of Obstetricians and Gynecologists. Obstet Gynecol 2009; 114:401–8.

Murray B. Informed consent: what must a physician disclose to a patient? Virtual Mentor 2012;14:563–6.

O'Connor E, Rossom RC, Henninger M, Groom HC, Burda BU. Primary care screening for and treatment of depression in pregnant and postpartum women: evidence report and systematic review for the US Preventive Services Task Force. JAMA 2016;315:388–406.

87

Urge incontinence

A 69-year-old woman, gravida 5, para 4, is referred to you by her primary care physician for evaluation of prolapse noted on examination. The patient has not noticed a vaginal bulge. She does not have any urine leakage when she coughs or sneezes. However, she states that she has to urinate frequently and often cannot get to the bathroom on time, leaking a small amount soon after the urge strikes. She plans her daily activities around where she knows she can find a clean bathroom and often leaks as soon as she puts the key in her front door on arriving home. She wakes approximately three times a night to void. She has no dysuria. She is not sexually active. She is otherwise healthy and is not taking any medications. She is 1.68 m (66 in.) tall and weighs 79 kg (175 lb), so her body mass index (calculated as weight in kilograms divided by height in meters squared [kg/m^2]) is 28.2. Pelvic examination shows normal external female genitalia, atrophic vaginal mucosa, first-degree cystocele, normal-sized uterus, and no adnexal masses. A urinalysis is negative. The best next step for the management of her bladder symptoms is

* (A) behavior modification
(B) a continence pessary
(C) antimuscarinic therapy
(D) onabotulinumtoxinA
(E) vaginal estrogen therapy

Urinary urge incontinence is the involuntary leakage of urine associated with a sudden compelling desire to void. *Overactive bladder* is defined by the International Continence Society as urinary urgency, typically accompanied by frequency and nocturia, with or without urge incontinence, in the absence of urinary tract infection or other pathology. Overactive bladder can be diagnosed when these symptoms are self-reported as bothersome. The described patient has overactive bladder. The minimum evaluation includes history, physical examination, and urinalysis to rule out evidence of infection or hematuria.

Behavioral therapy, including bladder training, pelvic floor muscle training, and fluid management, should be offered as first-line therapy to all patients with overactive bladder. Such interventions are risk free and do not interfere with subsequent treatment options. Although behavioral therapy interventions may not result in complete resolution of symptoms, they can result in significant improvement in symptoms and quality of life. Weight loss is an important component and an effective strategy for incontinence treatment in overweight and obese women. The Program to Reduce Incontinence by Diet and Exercise study enrolled overweight and obese women with 10 or more urinary incontinence episodes per week and showed that weight reduction of 5–10% was sufficient for significant improvement in urinary incontinence. Furthermore, a secondary cohort analysis showed a $327 savings per woman per year in incontinence management.

Continence pessaries are a therapy for stress incontinence and are thought to work by augmenting urethral closure during increases in abdominal pressure. In a randomized trial comparing behavioral therapy with continence pessary or with a combination of both in patients with stress incontinence, behavioral therapy was found to be associated with fewer incontinence episodes and better patient satisfaction at 3 months. Combined therapy was not superior to behavioral therapy. Treatment group differences did not persist at 12 months.

Although a number of antimuscarinic or anticholinergic medications are used to treat urge incontinence or overactive bladder, they are not the best first-line therapy. A meta-analysis of 50 randomized trials involving more than 27,000 women showed only modest improvement in symptoms, with 1.73 fewer episodes of incontinence per day and 2.06 fewer voids per day from a baseline of 2.79 and 11.28, respectively. No one antimuscarinic medication was found to be superior to others. Most of the studies were of fair or poor quality, industry sponsored, and relatively short term. When taking into account the effect of placebo, the net effect of antimuscarinic therapy was reduction by less than one episode of incontinence per day and by just over one void per day. Dry mouth, constipation, and vision changes were the most common adverse effects, although study withdrawal was infrequent. Such symptoms may be less with extended-release or transdermal formulations. Antimuscarinic medications should be avoided in patients with narrow-angle glaucoma, impaired gastric emptying, or a history of urinary retention, and in patients taking oral potassium chloride supplements.

OnabotulinumtoxinA has been found to have comparable efficacy to antimuscarinic therapy in a head-to-head trial. In 2013, onabotulinumtoxinA was approved by the U.S. Food and Drug Administration for the treatment of overactive bladder. It is a second-line treatment option for patients who have not had success with behavior modification techniques. Women considering this treatment for overactive bladder must be counseled about risks of urinary retention, urinary tract infection, hematuria, pain, and transient body weakness. The trial comparing anticholinergic medication with onabotulinumtoxinA found similar improvements in overactive bladder in patients treated with a daily anticholinergic medication and patients treated with a single intradetrusor injection of onabotulinumtoxinA. Patients treated with onabotulinumtoxinA had higher cure rates. Complications of urinary retention and urinary tract infection occurred in 5% and 33%, respectively, of patients who received onabotulinumtoxinA. Figure 87-1 shows the pattern for intradetrusor onabotulinumtoxinA injections for the treatment of overactive bladder or detrusor overactivity associated with a neurologic condition.

Although the bladder and urethra have a rich supply of estrogen receptors, making it biologically feasible that estrogen therapy would affect urinary symptoms, trials have found an increase in incontinence with oral estrogen replacement therapy. Vaginal estrogen therapy has not been well studied for this purpose.

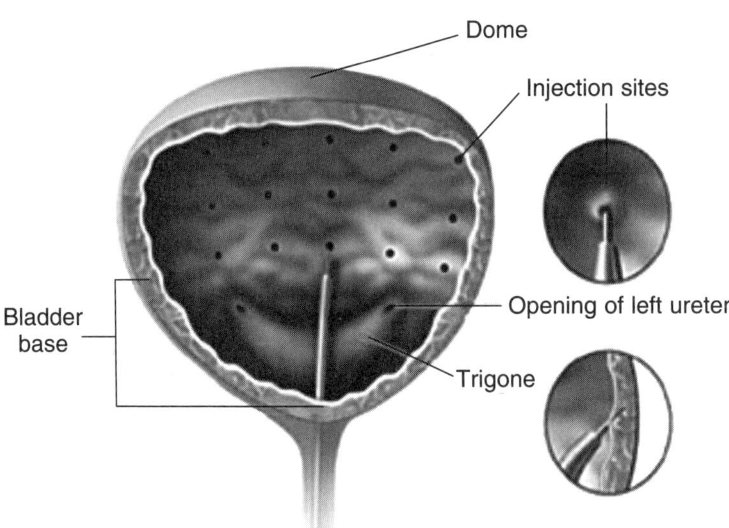

FIGURE 87-1. Pattern for intradetrusor onabotulinumtoxinA injections for the treatment of overactive bladder or detrusor overactivity associated with a neurologic condition. OnabotulinumtoxinA and the bladder. (Reprinted with permission from the Botox Full Prescribing Information. Irvine, CA. Allergan. Available at: http://www.allergan.com/assets/pdf/botox_pi.pdf. Retrieved June 1, 2016.)

Abrams P, Cardozo L, Fall M, Griffiths D, Rosier P, Ulmsten U, et al. The standardisation of terminology in lower urinary tract function: report from the standardisation sub-committee of the International Continence Society. Standardisation Sub-Committee of the International Continence Society. Urology 2003;61:37–49.

Gormley EA, Lightner DJ, Burgio KL, Chai TC, Clemens JQ, Culkin DJ, et al. Diagnosis and treatment of overactive bladder (non-neurogenic) in adults: AUA/SUFU guideline. American Urological Association and Society of Urodynamics, Female Pelvic Medicine & Urogenital Reconstruction. J Urol 2012;188:2455–63.

OnabotulinumtoxinA and the bladder. Committee Opinion No. 604. American College of Obstetricians and Gynecologists. Obstet Gynecol 2014;123:1408–11.

Reynolds WS, McPheeters M, Blume J, Surawicz T, Worley K, Wang L, et al. Comparative effectiveness of anticholinergic therapy for overactive bladder in women: a systematic review and meta-analysis. Obstet Gynecol 2015;125:1423–32.

Richter HE, Burgio KL, Brubaker L, Nygaard IE, Ye W, Weidner A, et al. Continence pessary compared with behavioral therapy or combined therapy for stress incontinence: a randomized controlled trial. Pelvic Floor Disorders Network. Obstet Gynecol 2010;115:609–17.

Subak LL, Marinilli Pinto A, Wing RR, Nakagawa S, Kusek JW, Herman WH, et al. Decrease in urinary incontinence management costs in women enrolled in a clinical trial of weight loss to treat urinary incontinence. Program to Reduce Incontinence by Diet and Exercise. Obstet Gynecol 2012;120:277–83.

Visco AG, Brubaker L, Richter HE, Nygaard I, Paraiso MF, Menefee SA, et al. Anticholinergic therapy vs. onabotulinumtoxinA for urgency urinary incontinence. Pelvic Floor Disorders Network. N Engl J Med 2012;367:1803–13.

Wing RR, Creasman JM, West DS, Richter HE, Myers D, Burgio KL, et al. Improving urinary incontinence in overweight and obese women through modest weight loss. Program to Reduce Incontinence by Diet and Exercise. Obstet Gynecol 2010;116:284–92.

88

Treatment of psychiatric disorder during pregnancy

A 28-year-old woman, gravida 3, para 2, comes to your office for a prenatal visit at 37 weeks of gestation. She wishes to discuss the safety of medications used to treat bipolar disorder during pregnancy and lactation. She has used carbamazepine in the past but did not like the adverse effects. She has been adamant about refusing all medications during pregnancy in order to minimize fetal exposure. She tells you that her psychiatrist recommends medication initiation immediately after delivery. She plans to breastfeed and would like your advice about which mood stabilizer would be the most appropriate to take while breastfeeding. Based on available data, you suggest that she take

(A) lithium carbonate
* (B) valproic acid
(C) lamotrigine
(D) quetiapine

Bipolar disorder is characterized by depressive episodes in addition to manic (bipolar disorder, type I) or hypomanic (bipolar disorder, type II) episodes. Most women who will be affected have onset of the disorder in their teens or early 20s. The estimated lifetime prevalence of bipolar spectrum disorder in the United States is 4.4%. This disorder tends to affect men and women equally, although women are more likely to experience depressive episodes, rapid cycling (four or more mood episodes over a year), or mixed episodes (depressive and manic symptoms simultaneously).

Symptoms of bipolar disorder during pregnancy tend to be depressive. Misclassification of bipolar disorder as major depressive disorder is common and can result in inappropriate treatment and worsening of the condition. Bipolar disorder and depression should be treated during pregnancy when the benefits of treatment outweigh potential risks.

The biggest risks of leaving maternal depression untreated or treated subtherapeutically are suicide and homicide. Inadequately treated maternal psychiatric illness may result in nonadherence to prenatal care; increased alcohol, tobacco, and drug abuse; and postnatal complications. Prepregnancy counseling for the patient preferably should be performed in a multidisciplinary fashion that includes her primary care provider, psychiatrist or psychologist, and an obstetrician. Women who choose to discontinue their mood stabilizer treatment before or during early pregnancy have twice the risk of recurrence compared with women who continue their treatment. A woman whose mood is considered stable and who desires pregnancy should discuss options with her psychiatrist and an obstetrician before discontinuing any medications.

Patients with bipolar disorder are at a high risk of postpartum depression as well as postpartum psychosis. Awareness of the risks is crucial, and treatment should be used as necessary. Sleep deprivation can be destabilizing for patients with bipolar disorder, so the postpartum period makes these patients especially vulnerable to relapse. Those who experience episodes of mental illness during pregnancy are more likely to have a recurrence in subsequent pregnancies.

Typically, the drug treatment regimen for patients with bipolar disorder includes mood stabilizers. In general, single-medication regimens are preferred over multiple-dose regimens, and medication selection should take into consideration the severity of maternal illness, history of efficacy, frequency of mood episodes, and reproductive safety information (such as the resources at the following websites: http://www.reprotox.org and http://depts.washington.edu/terisweb). All psychotropic medications that have been studied to date cross the placenta and have been isolated in amniotic fluid as well as in breast milk.

Although most medications are transferred through breast milk, most are found at low levels, and the benefits of breastfeeding should be weighed against the potential risk to the neonates of medication exposure. Valproic acid generally is considered to be safe for breastfeeding women; therefore, it is the best option to safely treat the described patient's bipolar disorder and to try to avoid an exacerbation of postpartum depression. Of the 41 woman–infant nursing pairs studied, only one adverse event of fetal thrombocytopenia and anemia has been reported with maternal use of valproic acid. It is considered lactation risk category L2 (safer).

Lithium should only be given to women with caution because it has been shown to transfer to infants, resulting in blood concentrations of up to one half of therapeutic levels. Therefore, it is considered lactation risk category L4 (possibly hazardous). Ten mother–infant nursing pairs were studied for lithium exposure, and adverse events (including cyanosis and electrocardiographic changes) were noted in two children. Lamotrigine has been found to transfer to infants through breast milk, resulting in serum concentrations in infants that have the potential to reach therapeutic levels; lamotrigine is considered lactation risk category L3 (moderately safe). Quetiapine, an atypical antipsychotic, is considered lactation risk category L4. If a nursing infant develops symptoms suggestive of medication exposure, then breastfeeding should be discontinued.

Becker MA, Weinberger TE, Denysenko L, Kunkel EJS. Mood disorders. In: Berghella V, editor. Maternal–fetal evidence based guidelines. 2nd ed. New York (NY): Informa Healthcare; 2012. p. 138–52.

Doering PL, Stewart RB. The extent and character of drug consumption during pregnancy. JAMA 1978;239:843–6.

Hostetter A, Ritchie JC, Stowe ZN. Amniotic fluid and umbilical cord blood concentrations of antidepressants in three women. Biol Psychiatry 2000;48:1032–4.

Merikangas KR, Jin R, He JP, Kessler RC, Lee S, Sampson NA, et al. Prevalence and correlates of bipolar spectrum disorder in the world mental health survey initiative. Arch Gen Psychiatry 2011;68:241–51.

Newport DJ, Hostetter A, Arnold A, Stowe ZN. The treatment of postpartum depression: minimizing infant exposures. J Clin Psychiatry 2002;63 Suppl 7:31–44.

REPROTOX: an information system on environmental hazards to human reproduction and development. Available at: http://www.reprotox.org/. Retrieved June 15, 2016.

Sachs HC. The transfer of drugs and therapeutics into human breast milk: an update on selected topics. Committee On Drugs. Pediatrics 2013;132:e796–809.

Sharma V, Burt VK, Ritchie HL. Bipolar II postpartum depression: Detection, diagnosis, and treatment. Am J Psychiatry 2009;166: 1217–21.

TERIS: teratogen information system and the on-line version of Shepard's catalog of teratogenic agents. Available at: http://depts.washington.edu/terisweb/teris/. Retrieved June 15, 2016.

Use of psychiatric medications during pregnancy and lactation. ACOG Practice Bulletin No. 92. American College of Obstetricians and Gynecologists. Obstet Gynecol 2008;111:1001–20.

Viguera AC, Whitfield T, Baldessarini RJ, Newport DJ, Stowe Z, Reminick A, et al. Risk of recurrence in women with bipolar disorder during pregnancy: prospective study of mood stabilizer discontinuation. Am J Psychiatry 2007;164:1817–24; quiz 1923.

89

Dyspareunia in menopause

A 68-year-old woman, gravida 3, para 3, comes to your office very upset about the discomfort she experiences with sexual activity. After being widowed at age 48 years, she has recently met a new partner with whom she is sexually active. Sexual activity is very uncomfortable for her and occasionally results in postcoital spotting. She has tried vaginal lubricants but reports that her entire vagina still feels sore and irritated. On physical examination, the labia appear pale and thin with minimal hair. The introitus does not appear narrowed, and the vaginal epithelium is thin and smooth with small fissures at the perineum. On speculum examination, there is scant but normal-appearing mucus at the cervical os and no bleeding. The option most likely to result in improvement of her symptoms is

* (A) vaginal estrogen
(B) dilator therapy
(C) acyclovir
(D) vaginal moisturizer
(E) vaginal clindamycin

Dyspareunia affects women across the age spectrum but is as high as 40% among postmenopausal women. Clinical presentations can vary, with either superficial or deep pain being described. Although both types of pain are common, superficial pain is more prevalent, especially in postmenopausal patients. The most likely reason for this pain is vaginal atrophy (also called atrophic vaginitis) from the hypoestrogenic state associated with menopause (as well as breastfeeding). This hypoestrogenic state causes numerous physiologic changes that can result in vaginal irritation and dyspareunia (Fig. 89-1). The external genitalia lose superficial epithelial cells, which causes tissue thinning, dryness, and decreased elasticity, resulting in increased fissures and tearing. The labia majora also lose subcutaneous fat, which can lead to narrowing and shortening of the vagina. Vaginal secretions decrease and the environment becomes more alkaline, increasing susceptibility to urogenital infections. The most effective treatment to reverse these effects is vaginal estrogen, which works to restore the vaginal tissue to a premenopausal state. Although systemic estrogen also is effective, vaginal application appears to be slightly more effective and to

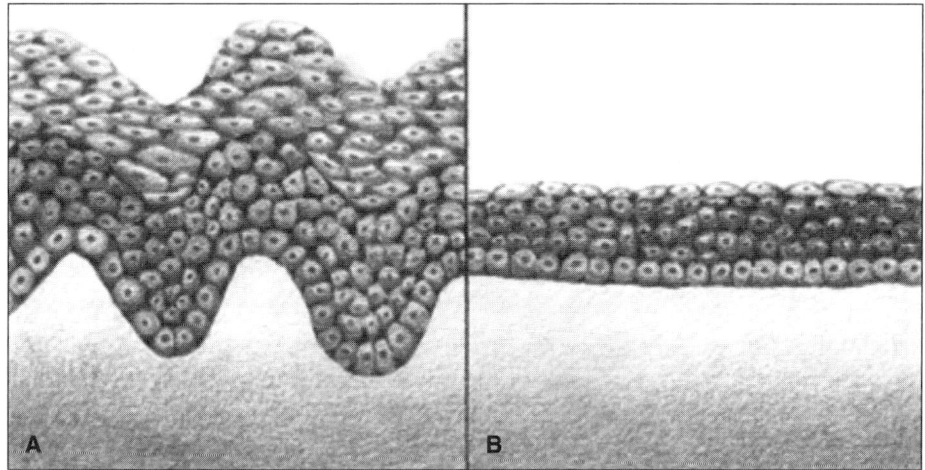

FIGURE 89-1. Effects of estrogen on the vaginal mucosa. **A.** Vaginal lining with estrogen. **B.** Vaginal lining in hypoestrogenic state. (North American Menopause Society. Changes in the vagina and vulva. Mayfield Heights (OH): NAMS; 2016. Available at: http://www.menopause.org/for-women/sexual-health-menopause-online/changes-at-midlife/changes-in-the-vagina-and-vulva. Retrieved June 16, 2016. Reprinted with permission of the North American Menopause Society and Juliet Sweany, illustrator.)

have decreased risks (mainly cardiovascular); therefore, it should be recommended to the described patient.

Although atrophy also can result in vaginal narrowing, dilator therapy usually is not needed in multiparous women with a normal vaginal size on examination who have not undergone vaginal or vulvar surgery. In the absence of such surgeries, the ability to do a bimanual examination and easily pass two fingers generally suggests a vaginal width that should be adequate for sexual activity. However, if vaginal estrogen improves tissue health and the patient still reports dyspareunia with penetration, vaginal dilator therapy may be beneficial.

Although acyclovir is the first-line treatment for genital herpes lesions, the described patient does not have any findings consistent with herpes. Genital herpes, associated more commonly with herpes simplex type 2, often causes tingling or burning pain before the appearance of lesions. Lesions are typically vesicular or in clusters of inflamed papules and can be extremely painful.

Nonhormonal water-based or silicone-based vaginal lubricants or moisturizers can be beneficial in improving dyspareunia associated with vaginal dryness and atrophy but are unlikely to be as effective as vaginal estrogen. Lubricants are used with sexual activity to minimize friction and associated discomfort from decreased natural secretions. Vaginal moisturizers work to trap moisture and provide more long-term relief from vaginal dryness. Limited data suggest that both of these over-the-counter products may be helpful in managing vaginal dryness, itching, and dyspareunia. However, in the described patient who already has fissures and thinned tissue and has not responded to vaginal lubricants, it is likely that hormonal treatment will be needed to provide symptom relief.

Vaginal clindamycin is second-line treatment for bacterial vaginosis and probably would not prove beneficial for this patient. Although patients with bacterial vaginosis may report dyspareunia, it is uncommon with bacterial vaginosis alone. Typically, patients report vaginal discharge, odor, or both. On examination, the discharge usually is off-white, thin, and homogeneous with a classic "fishy smell" that often is noticed after sexual activity. Although oral metronidazole is the first-line treatment, many patients do not tolerate it well and prefer a vaginal treatment. Vaginal clindamycin is well tolerated but also has been associated with increased resistance after treatment. This treatment is not an appropriate option for this patient, who has no abnormal discharge or odor concerning for bacterial vaginosis.

Grant MD, Marbella A, Wang AT, Pines E, Hoag J, Bonnell C, et al. Menopausal symptoms: Comparative effectiveness of therapies. comparative effectiveness review no. 147. Rockville (MD): Agency for Healthcare Research and Quality; 2015. Available at: https://effectivehealthcare.ahrq.gov/ehc/products/353/2051/menopause-report-150305.pdf. Retrieved June 15, 2016.

Kao A, Binik YM, Kapuscinski A, Khalife S. Dyspareunia in postmenopausal women: a critical review. Pain Res Manag 2008;13:243–54.

Management of menopausal symptoms. Practice Bulletin No. 141. American College of Obstetricians and Gynecologists. Obstet Gynecol 2014;123:202–16.

Rahn DD, Carberry C, Sanses TV, Mamik MM, Ward RM, Meriwether KV, et al. Vaginal estrogen for genitourinary syndrome of menopause: a systematic review. Society of Gynecologic Surgeons Systematic Review Group. Obstet Gynecol 2014;124:1147–56.

90

Low back pain

An otherwise healthy 47-year-old woman comes to your office with severe low back pain. She reports onset 2 days ago after a yoga class. She did not experience loss of consciousness or other symptoms. She is ambulatory but walks slowly. She states that the pain is exacerbated by leaning forward. She has no incontinence or urinary retention. The most appropriate next step in her management is

(A) narcotic analgesics
(B) computed tomography scan
(C) magnetic resonance imaging scan
* (D) neurologic examination
(E) massage therapy

Low back pain is a common reason for physician visits and results in tremendous economic burden in the United States, estimated at $50 million annually. At least 80% of the population reports low back pain at some point in their lifetime, and approximately 25% report low back pain lasting more than 1 day in the past 3 months. Approximately 2% of the U.S. workforce is compensated for back injuries each year. Most individuals with acute back pain will spontaneously recover with no further interventions. However, up to one third will report some level of persistent pain 1 year after an acute episode.

A focused physical examination, including neurologic examination, can identify the subset of patients in whom further evaluation in the form of imaging is appropriate. Identifying motor deficits at more than one spinal level, fecal incontinence, saddle anesthesia, or bladder dysfunction indicates severe neurologic deficits. Side-to-side comparison of sensation to light touch and sharp prick should be performed. The neurologic examination should include evaluation of knee strength and reflexes (assessing L4). Foot dorsiflexion strength assesses L5. Foot plantar flexion and ankle reflexes assess the S1 nerve root. More than 90% of symptomatic lumbar disk herniation occurs at L4/L5 and L5/S1.

Most patients recover from back pain within 1 month and will do better with recommendations to remain active rather than resting in bed. Patients should be encouraged to return to normal activities as soon as possible. Nonnarcotic analgesics, exercise, and application of heat generally are viewed as first-line interventions.

Prescribing opioids may be a component of short-term management of back pain but generally should be avoided. There is only weak evidence supporting the use of opioids for back pain, and most are from chronic pain studies. It is not proven that opioid use leads to more rapid recovery or return to work. Opioid sales in the United States have quadrupled between 1999 and 2010, as have admissions to substance treatment programs. The risk of opioid dependence is substantial and can occur with only 1–3 months of daily use. Alternatives to opioids should be considered first-line therapies. Acetaminophen or nonsteroidal antiinflammatory drugs generally are the preferred therapies.

Alternatives to use of opioid analgesics include tricyclic antidepressants, exercise, cognitive behavior therapy, spinal manipulation, acupuncture, and massage therapy in the event that the initial course of treatment does not provide sufficient relief. In addition, assessment by a pain specialist is advisable if it appears that long-term use of opioids may ensue.

Guidelines exist for appropriate use of medical imaging in evaluation of low back pain. In most instances, imaging should be avoided. No studies demonstrate improved patient outcomes with computed tomography or magnetic resonance imaging scans, and many radiographic abnormalities may be identified that have poor or no correlation with the patient's symptoms. Findings such as disk bulge or facet joint arthritis are identified frequently in asymptomatic patients. Despite these facts, imaging is ordered in 25% of low back pain consultations, and this figure is increasing.

Guidelines for further assessment have been recommended by the American College of Physicians and the American Pain Society. Diagnostic imaging is recommended only for those patients who have severe or progressive neurologic deficits or who demonstrate features consistent with a serious underlying condition. Diagnoses to consider under these circumstances include vertebral infection, cauda equina syndrome, or malignancy with impending spinal cord compression. Magnetic resonance imaging is the preferred imaging modality for evaluation of the spinal soft tissues and spinal canal. If there is suspicion of vertebral fracture, such as trauma or osteoporotic fracture, then plain radiography is the imaging modality of choice.

Other indications for a more serious underlying disorder include age older than 50 years, systemic symptoms (such as fever or chills), history of malignancy, night pain, immunosuppression, prolonged corticosteroid use, or trauma. With these features, further diagnostic workup may be warranted.

Chou R, Qaseem A, Owens DK, Shekelle P. Diagnostic imaging for low back pain: advice for high-value health care from the American College of Physicians. Clinical Guidelines Committee of the American College of Physicians [published erratum appears in Ann Intern Med 2012;156:71]. Ann Intern Med 2011;154:181–9.

Deyo RA, Von Korff M, Duhrkoop D. Opioids for low back pain. BMJ 2015;350:g6380.

Patrick N, Emanski E, Knaub MA. Acute and chronic low back pain. Med Clin North Am 2014;98:777,89, xii.

Traeger AC, Hubscher M, Henschke N, Moseley GL, Lee H, McAuley JH. Effect of primary care-based education on reassurance in patients with acute low back pain: systematic review and meta-analysis. JAMA Intern Med 2015;175:733–43.

91

Thrombophilia in a nonpregnant woman

A 21-year-old white woman comes to your office for contraceptive counseling. She elects to start combination oral contraceptives (OCs). She has no significant medical history and is taking no medications. On questioning about her family history, she tells you that her sister was recently diagnosed with a pulmonary embolism 3 days after a cesarean delivery and is now taking warfarin. Her mother has no history of thromboembolic disorders, but her father died suddenly from a stroke at age 50 years. The most likely thrombophilia to be found in this patient is

(A) prothrombin gene mutation (*G20210A*)
(B) antithrombin III deficiency
* (C) factor V Leiden
(D) protein C deficiency
(E) protein S deficiency

The most common inherited thrombophilia in women of European ancestry is factor V Leiden mutation. The heterozygous state is present in approximately 5% of this population and in approximately 3% of African Americans whose ancestors are not recent immigrants. Patients with this mutation are resistant to the normal proteolysis of factor V by activated protein C. Although the heterozygous state accounts for 40% of all venous thromboembolic disease during pregnancy, the absolute increased risk of venous thromboembolism in these patients is 5–12 in 1,000 deliveries compared with a risk of 0.5–2 in 1,000 deliveries in normal pregnancies. This risk, however, increases to 15 in 1,000 deliveries if the patient also has a first-degree relative with a history of venous thromboembolism and increases to a 10% risk if a heterozygous patient has a personal history of a venous thromboembolic event. Similarly, the risks of venous thromboembolism in patients who are heterozygous for factor V Leiden and who also are taking estrogen-containing combination OCs are further increased by family and personal history. The other common inherited thrombophilias and their prevalence in the general population are shown in Table 91-1.

The prothrombin *G20210A* gene mutation is a point mutation that results in elevated circulating levels of prothrombin. Protein C and protein S deficiencies are diagnosed by functional assays because multiple different mutations have been identified, all of which can result in altered activity. Antithrombin III deficiency can occur because of either reduced antigen production or reduced activity of abnormal antigen. The American College of Obstetricians and Gynecologists does not support testing for methylenetetrahydrofolate reductase polymorphisms or measurement of fasting homocysteine levels in a thrombophilia work up because there is insufficient evidence for either an increased risk of venous thromboembolism or treatment that affects outcome.

Use of combination OCs is a known risk factor for venous thromboembolism. Estrogen increases the production of clotting factors VII and X and fibrinogen. Although the magnitude of venous thromboembolism is increased about fourfold in users compared with nonusers, the absolute risk is still considerably lower than in women who have a normal pregnancy. Before starting a patient on an estrogen-containing OC, it is important to consider risk-to-benefit ratios of taking the combination OC relative to the risks if the patient were to become pregnant and the risks associated with other contraceptive alternatives. Risk factors for venous thromboembolism are listed in Box 91-1. A personal history of a documented venous thromboembolism is a contraindication to an estrogen-containing OC, although debate exists about the use of a combination OC in a patient with a personal history of venous thromboembolism who also is receiving effective anticoagulation treatment.

Likewise, an increased risk of venous thromboembolism is seen in women with any of the common hereditary thrombophilias (Appendix D). Estimates of the magnitude of this increased risk in women who are heterozygous for factor V Leiden range from eightfold to 30-fold. In spite of this increased risk and the prevalence of factor V Leiden carrier status of approximately 5% in the United States, routine screening of a general population for a thrombophilia before the initiation of combination OCs has not been shown to be effective. This is because most carriers will not develop venous thromboembolism, and venous thromboembolism leading to a fatal event is uncommon in reproductive-aged women. The described patient had a family history of a sister with a pregnancy-related pulmonary embolism and a father who had a sudden fatal stroke at age 50 years, both of which would constitute reasons to perform thrombophilia testing before starting her on an estrogen-containing OC.

TABLE 91-1. Prevalence (%) of Inherited Thrombophilias in the General Population

Thombophilia Type	Prevalence
Factor V Leiden heterozygote	1–15
Factor V Leiden homozygote	<1
Prothrombin gene mutation heterozygote	2–5
Prothrombin gene mutation homozygote	<1
Factor V Leiden/prothrombin double heterozygote	0.01
Antithrombin III deficiency	0.02
Protein C deficiency	0.2–0.4
Protein S deficiency	0.03–0.13

Modified from Inherited thrombophilias in pregnancy. Practice Bulletin No. 138 American College of Obstetricians and Gynecologists. Obstet Gynecol 2013;122:706–17.

BOX 91-1

Risk Factors for Thromboembolic Disease

- Strong risk factors (odds ratio greater than 10)
  - Fracture (hip or leg)
  - Hip or knee replacement
  - Major general surgery
  - Major trauma
  - Spinal cord injury
- Moderate risk factors (odds ratio 2–9)
  - Arthroscopic knee surgery
  - Central venous lines
  - Chemotherapy
  - Oral contraceptive therapy
  - Paralytic stroke
  - Pregnancy (postpartum)
  - Previous venous thromboembolism
  - Thrombophilia
- Weak risk factors (odds ratio less than 2)
  - Bed rest more than 3 days
  - Immobility due to sitting (eg, prolonged car or air travel)
  - Increasing age
  - Laparoscopic surgery (eg, cholecystectomy)
  - Obesity
  - Pregnancy (antepartum)
  - Varicose veins

Anderson FA Jr, Spencer FA. Risk factors for venous thromboembolism. Circulation 2003;107:I9–16.

Inherited thrombophilias in pregnancy. Practice Bulletin No. 138. American College of Obstetricians and Gynecologists. Obstet Gynecol 2013;122:706–17.

Silver R, Lockwood C. Thrombosis, thrombophilia, and thromboembolism. Clin Update Womens Health Care 2016;XV (3):1–70.

92

Contraceptive choice for an adolescent with migraines

A 16-year-old nulligravid adolescent girl visits your office for contraceptive counseling. She thinks she may want to use oral contraceptives (OCs) like her sister and knows that she does not want a device that "goes inside my body." She has a history of migraine headaches without aura, which she controls with over-the-counter analgesics. She sees a dermatologist for moderate acne, for which she uses a topical treatment. She smokes half a pack of cigarettes per day. Her body mass index (calculated as weight in kilograms divided by height in meters squared [kg/m^2]) is 38. The most appropriate contraceptive method for her is

(A) male condoms
* (B) combination hormonal OCs
(C) contraceptive patch
(D) depot medroxyprogesterone acetate (DMPA)
(E) progesterone-only pill

Multiple methods of birth control are available to adolescents, and studies have confirmed the importance of patient choice regarding contraceptive selection. An adolescent (or an adult woman) is more likely to continue a method of birth control that she chooses for herself. Best practices in contraceptive counseling call for nonbiased counseling about the various options that a patient is eligible to receive. An obstetrician–gynecologist or other health care provider should not restrict contraceptive options based on beliefs that are not evidence based, such as restricting certain methods because of age, parity, or medical history. The Centers for Disease Control and Prevention Medical Eligibility Criteria guidelines for contraceptive use are publically available.

Many adolescents engage in high-risk sexual behaviors that place them at high risk of contracting a sexually transmitted infection. Consequently, all adolescents should be counseled about safer sexual behaviors and condom usage for prevention of sexually transmitted infections. Male condoms are a male partner-controlled method of contraception, and many teenagers have difficulty negotiating condom use. In addition, condoms are a less effective method of contraception (18% failure rate with typical use) than other choices, making it a less-than-optimal primary contraceptive method for the described patient.

The contraceptive patch contains norelgestromin and ethinyl estradiol. Each patch is used for 1 week, with three patches used consecutively, followed by a patch-free week that causes a withdrawal bleed in most cycles. It is unclear if the patch has higher failure rates in obese women. Because the described patient has an elevated body mass index, the patch is a possible but not optimal choice of contraception for her.

Depot medroxyprogesterone acetate comes in two formulations: an intramuscular dose and a subcutaneous dose. Although DMPA has a low failure rate when injections are given on time and the subcutaneous form can be self-administered, there are concerns about bone loss with prolonged use of DMPA, particularly in adolescents, but no evidence of increased fracture risk. For women younger than 18 years, the benefits of using DMPA generally outweigh the known or theoretical risks (World Health Organization and Centers for Disease Control and Prevention category 2). Although DMPA is also category 1 for obesity, obese adolescents who used DMPA have been shown to be more likely to gain weight than obese nonusers, obese combination hormonal OC users, and nonobese DMPA users, making DMPA category 2 for obese teenagers. For this reason, DMPA is a possible choice but not the best choice for the described patient.

The progesterone-only pill is available in one formulation in the United States (ie, norethindrone). Although the progesterone-only pill is considered to have equal effectiveness to combination OCs, it must be taken at the same time every day to be effective. Additionally, it is less likely to help control acne than a pill that contains estrogen. For these reasons, the progesterone-only pill is not the optimal choice for this adolescent patient with moderate acne.

More than one half of sexually active female adolescents have used combination hormonal OCs. In addition to contraception, use of a combination OC can provide multiple noncontraceptive benefits that can encourage continuation of the method, such as a reduction in dysmenorrhea and acne. The described patient has no contraindications to combination OC use (category 2 for migraines without aura in women younger than 35 years; category 2 for obesity; and category 2 for smoking in women younger than 35 years), making it the best contraceptive method for her at this time. However, because the typical-use pregnancy rate is 7%, it also is important that the patient be counseled carefully about establishing a successful strategy to take her pills daily and make a plan for what to do when she misses pills.

Chang CL, Donaghy M, Poulter N. World Health Organisation Collaborative Study of Cardiovascular Disease and Steroid Hormone Contraception. Migraine and stroke in young women: case control study. BMJ 1999;318:13–8.

Depot medroxyprogesterone acetate and bone effects. Committee Opinion No. 602. American College of Obstetricians and Gynecologists. Obstet Gynecol 2014;123:1398–402.

Understanding and using the U.S. Medical Eligibility Criteria for Contraceptive Use, 2010. Committee Opinion No. 505. American College of Obstetricians and Gynecologists. Obstet Gynecol 2011; 118:754–60.

U.S. Medical Eligibility Criteria for Contraceptive Use, 2010. Centers for Disease Control and Prevention. MMWR Recomm Rep 2010; 59(RR-4):1–86.

93

Ultrasonography in adnexal torsion

A 25-year-old nulligravid woman reports acute onset of severe right lower quadrant pain 24 hours ago after a strenuous workout. The pain has been constant and is associated with nausea and intermittent emesis. She has tried nonsteroidal antiinflammatory drugs with no improvement in her symptoms. She has not had a fever or chills but does report loss of appetite. Upon examination, she appears very uncomfortable. She has a temperature of 37.0°C (98.6°F), a heart rate of 102 beats per minute, and blood pressure of 115/72 mm Hg. Abdominal examination shows tenderness to palpation in the right lower quadrant with voluntary guarding but no rebound tenderness. Pelvic examination reveals an enlarged right ovary with focal tenderness. Laboratory studies reveal a negative pregnancy test, negative urinalysis, and white blood cell count of 14 g/dL. Ultrasonography of the pelvis reveals a 4-cm heterogeneous mass with normal Doppler flow (Fig. 93-1). The best next step in management is

(A) follow-up in 48 hours
(B) computed tomography (CT) scan
* (C) laparoscopy
(D) inpatient observation
(E) combination oral contraceptives (OCs)

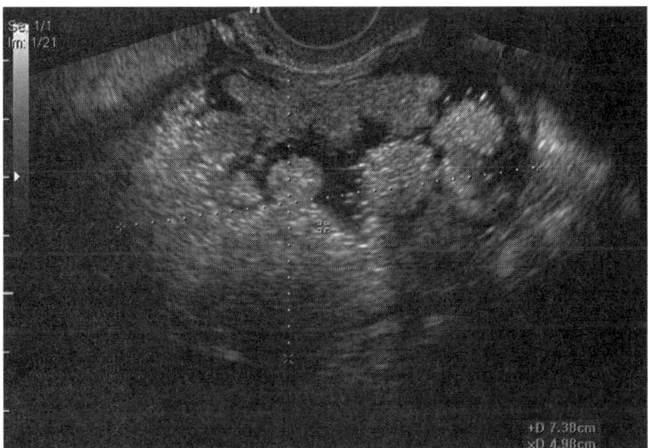

FIGURE 93-1. Image was kindly provided by James Shwayder, MD.

Pelvic pain occurs frequently in women of all ages and is a common reason for them to seek medical care. Whether the pain is acute or chronic, there is a wide spectrum of causes for pelvic pain, and a thorough history and physical examination are critical components of the diagnostic evaluation. Torsion is defined as complete or partial rotation of the adnexa around its vascular pedicle, resulting in diminished blood flow to the affected ovary. Adnexal torsion is the fifth most common gynecologic emergency, and diagnosis can be difficult because there are varying clinical presentations and radiological findings. The prevalence is highest in prepubertal girls and during pregnancy and the puerperium because of tissue laxity. Clinical symptoms often include abrupt onset of pelvic pain, nausea, vomiting, tachycardia, and even a low-grade fever. However, patients may present with atypical symptoms that can lead to missed or delayed diagnosis.

Ultrasonography has many advantages in the acute evaluation of pelvic pain, given its high sensitivity, relatively low cost, lack of ionizing radiation, and widespread availability. For these reasons, ultrasonography remains the imaging modality of choice for women with pelvic pain. However, the appearance of adnexal torsion on ultrasonography is highly variable. Varying appearances on ultrasonography include an enlarged, edematous ovary or a twisted pedicle demonstrated as "whirlpool" in grey scale and color Doppler studies. Furthermore, ultrasonography is not always reliable in the absence of an enlarged ovary. Given the described patient's symptoms of abrupt onset of pain, nausea and vomiting, and an enlarged and tender ovary, adnexal torsion is the most likely diagnosis despite the presence of Doppler flow to the affected ovary. Although abnormal or absent Doppler signals are noted in most cases of adnexal torsion, loss of Doppler flow may be a late sign in the clinical presentation. Therefore, the diagnosis of torsion is largely a clinical one, and presence of Doppler signals within the ovary does not exclude ovarian torsion. Although pain management is an integral component of the management of this patient, neither outpatient nor inpatient observation will address her issue adequately. Furthermore, a delay in diagnosis can lead to loss of the affected ovary and, thus, diminished reproductive capacity in this reproductive-aged woman.

Additional imaging modalities such as CT scan or magnetic resonance imaging can evaluate for potential intra-abdominal pathology and are particularly useful in diagnosing torsion in the second and third trimesters of pregnancy, when the ovaries are difficult to visualize by pelvic ultrasonography. However, CT or magnetic resonance imaging in this patient is unlikely to provide additional useful information. Although her symptoms of loss of appetite, elevated white blood cell count, and pain localized to the right lower quadrant are all potential symptoms of acute appendicitis, the abrupt onset of her symptoms and the finding of an enlarged or edematous ovary on ultrasonography make appendicitis a less likely cause for her pain. Thus, CT imaging is not warranted at this time.

Combination OCs are useful in decreasing the likelihood of developing subsequent functional ovarian cysts and may offer useful medical management for this patient in the future. However, combination OCs have no role in the acute management of ovarian cysts or adnexal torsion. Combination OCs would not be appropriate therapy for the acute management of the described patient.

Regardless of the presence of arterial or venous flow to the ovary, clinical suspicion for torsion warrants prompt surgical exploration; therefore, proceeding with laparoscopic evaluation would be the best next step in the management of this patient. Laparoscopic detorsion of the twisted adnexa is the mainstay of therapy for ovarian torsion, regardless of the condition of the ovary, and timely diagnosis with prompt surgical management will improve the likelihood of ovarian preservation. Furthermore, clinical appearance of the untwisted ovary does not correlate well with function, and residual ovarian function can be preserved even in ovaries that appear necrotic at the time of surgery. Therefore, untwisting rather than removal of the affected ovary is the appropriate course of action. Finally, laparoscopy would be useful to evaluate the patient for other etiologies if torsion is not found.

Amirbekian S, Hooley RJ. Ultrasound evaluation of pelvic pain. Radiol Clin North Am 2014;52:1215–35.

Vandermeer FQ, Wong-You-Cheong JJ. Imaging of acute pelvic pain. Clin Obstet Gynecol 2009;52:2–20.

Yildiz A, Erginel B, Akin M, Karadag CA, Sever N, Tanik C, et al. A retrospective review of the adnexal outcome after detorsion in premenarchal girls. Afr J Paediatr Surg 2014;11(4):304–7.

94

Late-term and postterm pregnancies

A 21-year-old nulligravid woman comes to your office for a routine prenatal visit at 40 5/7 weeks of gestation dated by last menstrual period and confirmed by 6-week ultrasonography. She has no significant medical history. To date, the pregnancy has been uncomplicated. Today, a vaginal examination is significant for a Bishop score of 2. Presentation is cephalic and estimated weight is 3,200 g, as determined by Leopold maneuvers. You offer her induction of labor at 41 weeks of gestation, and she declines. The most appropriate next step in management is to

(A) counsel her that the fetus is at great risk of stillbirth
(B) schedule an office visit in 1 week
* (C) perform fetal surveillance
(D) perform immediate delivery

Late-term pregnancy is defined as a pregnancy between 41 0/7 weeks and 41 6/7 weeks of gestation. Postterm pregnancy is one that extends beyond 42 0/7 weeks of gestation. In 2013, 8.5% of births in the United States were late-term pregnancies, and 5.5% were postterm pregnancies. Dating of a pregnancy is critical in the management of late-term and postterm pregnancies. A joint Committee Opinion published by the American College of Obstetricians and Gynecologists, the Society for Maternal–Fetal Medicine, and the American Institute of Ultrasound in Medicine provides guidelines on estimating due date (Table 94-1). Assigning an accurate estimated date of delivery by first-trimester ultrasonography has decreased the rate of postterm pregnancy to 1.5%. Using the date of the last menstrual period alone often leads to inaccurate dating.

Management of late-term and postterm pregnancies has been studied to determine the optimal strategy to minimize perinatal morbidity and mortality. Typically, management plans for late-term pregnancies have included antepartum fetal surveillance or induction of labor. In the described patient, initiating antepartum surveillance would be appropriate because she declines induction of labor.

Between 40 0/7 weeks and 40 6/7 weeks of gestation, stillbirth rates are approximately 1 per 1,000 pregnancies. This rate increases to 1.2 per 1,000 pregnancies at 41 0/7 weeks to 41 6/7 weeks of gestation. Between 42 0/7 weeks and 42 6/7 weeks of gestation, the rate of stillbirth is double the rate in term pregnancies, and after 43 0/7 weeks of gestation, this risk increases eightfold. The described patient should not be counseled that the fetus is at great risk of stillbirth because this risk does not increase significantly until after 42 0/7 weeks of gestation.

The best next step would be to initiate antenatal testing at 41 0/7 weeks of gestation. There are no randomized controlled trials that prove that antenatal testing leads to a decrease in perinatal mortality in late-term or postterm pregnancies. Despite this, antepartum fetal surveillance should begin at this time because observational data suggest an increased risk of complications after 41 0/7 weeks of gestation. Although frequency and type

TABLE 94-1. Guidelines for Redating Based on Ultrasonography

Gestational Age Range*	Method of Measurement	Discrepancy Between Ultrasound Dating and LMP Dating That Supports Redating
≤13 6/7 wk	CRL	
• ≤8 6/7 wk		More than 5 d
• 9 0/7 wk to 13 6/7 wk		More than 7 d
14 0/7 wk to 15 6/7 wk	BPD, HC, AC, FL	More than 7 d
16 0/7 wk to 21 6/7 wk	BPD, HC, AC, FL	More than 10 d
22 0/7 wk to 27 6/7 wk	BPD, HC, AC, FL	More than 14 d
28 0/7 wk and beyond†	BPD, HC, AC, FL	More than 21 d

Abbreviations: AC, abdominal circumference; BPD, biparietal diameter; CRL, crown–rump length; FL, femur length; HC, head circumference; LMP, last menstrual period.

*Based on LMP

†Because of the risk of redating a small fetus that may be growth restricted, management decisions based on third-trimester ultrasonography alone are especially problematic and need to be guided by careful consideration of the entire clinical picture and close surveillance.

Method for estimating due date. Committee Opinion No. 611. American College of Obstetricians and Gynecologists. Obstet Gynecol 2014;124:863–6.

of antenatal surveillance in late-term pregnancies have not been clearly defined, ultrasonographic assessment of amniotic fluid volume should be a component of testing. Oligohydramnios or nonreassuring fetal testing warrants induction of labor at that time. Cesarean delivery should be reserved for obstetric indications.

Scheduling an office visit in 1 week is reasonable; however, the patient should begin antenatal testing before this visit. Doppler studies are not indicated because the fetus is growing appropriately.

Reviewing the risks and benefits of continued expectant management after 41 0/7 weeks of gestation is recommended so that the patient has the opportunity to make an informed decision. Because there is not a significant increased risk of perinatal death at this gestational age, allowing the patient to decide on induction or continued expectant management follows the ethical principle of autonomy.

Heimstad R, Skogvoll E, Mattsson LA, Johansen OJ, Eik-Nes SH, Salvesen KA. Induction of labor or serial antenatal fetal monitoring in postterm pregnancy: a randomized controlled trial. Obstet Gynecol 2007;109:609–17.

Management of late-term and postterm pregnancies. Practice Bulletin No. 146. American College of Obstetricians and Gynecologists. Obstet Gynecol 2014;124:390–6.

Method for estimating due date. Committee Opinion No. 611. American College of Obstetricians and Gynecologists. Obstet Gynecol 2014;124:863–6.

95

Primary amenorrhea

A 14-year-old girl is referred to you by her pediatrician for absence of pubertal changes. She is otherwise healthy. She participates in a recreational soccer league on Sundays and eats a healthy diet with her family. Her mother and her older sister started their menses at age 13 years. She has Tanner stage I breasts and pubic hair, normal prepubescent female external genitalia, and the rest of her examination is unremarkable. She is 1.52 m (60 in.) tall (10th percentile for age) and weighs 54.4 kg (120 lb) (50–75th percentile for age), with a body mass index (calculated as weight in kilograms divided by height in meters squared [kg/m^2]) of 23 (50–75th percentile for age). She is developmentally normal for her age. The most appropriate next step is

(A) reassurance
* (B) follicle-stimulating hormone (FSH) level test
(C) testosterone level test
(D) transvaginal ultrasonography
(E) pelvic magnetic resonance imaging (MRI)

The median age at menarche in the United States is 12.4 years. This has remained stable across well-nourished populations in developed countries. Traditionally, primary amenorrhea is the absence of menarche by age 16 years. However, because 98% of females will have had menarche by age 15 years and many diagnosable and treatable disorders can and should be detected earlier, evaluation should be undertaken if there is no menarche by age 15 years, no menarche within 3 years of thelarche, or no thelarche by age 13 years. Thelarche is the onset of breast budding and usually precedes menarche by 2–3 years, with menarche typically occurring at Tanner stage IV breast development. A thorough history in patients with delayed puberty or primary amenorrhea includes inquiries regarding diet, exercise, medications, illicit drug use, psychiatric history, hirsutism, acne, and galactorrhea. Physical examination includes an assessment of Tanner staging, external genitalia, hirsutism, acne, and body mass index.

Causes of primary amenorrhea can be classified into those with and without breast development and those with elevated or low levels of FSH. In patients without breast development, such as the described patient, the FSH level should be measured. Patients with an elevated FSH level have gonadal dysgenesis and primary ovarian insufficiency. Gonadal failure can occur before the onset of puberty or at any time during the pubertal process. Patients with an elevated FSH level require an evaluation of their karyotype. When adolescents present with primary amenorrhea and no associated comorbidities, 50% are found to have an abnormal karyotype. The most common chromosome abnormality is Turner syndrome

(45,X karyotype) or a Turner mosaic variant. Patients who are diagnosed with Turner syndrome require evaluation for coexisting cardiovascular malformations, renal abnormalities, and hypertension. Much less common than Turner syndrome is Swyer syndrome, which is characterized by gonadal failure with a 46,XY karyotype. Such individuals are phenotypically female in spite of having a male genotype and have female internal genitalia and nonfunctioning gonads. When any Y chromosome material is identified, a prophylactic bilateral gonadectomy is indicated to avoid the increased risk of gonadal cancer, such as gonadoblastoma and dysgerminoma.

A patient with gonadal dysgenesis requires supplemental hormonal treatment to initiate or complete her pubertal development and enhance bone health. First, estrogen is given alone to stimulate breast development and uterine and external genitalia maturation. Once the patient experiences vaginal bleeding, progesterone is added to her hormonal regimen. The patient is treated with combination hormonal therapy until the normal age of menopause (approximately age 50 years).

Causes of primary amenorrhea with a low FSH level include constitutional delay, prolactinoma, Kallmann syndrome, other abnormalities and masses of the central nervous system, stress, weight loss, anorexia, congenital adrenal hyperplasia, and polycystic ovary syndrome.

Breast development is triggered by estrogen stimulation and is evidence of functioning gonads. Congenital abnormalities of the female reproductive organs account for approximately 20% of cases of primary amenorrhea. Secondary sex characteristics develop normally. Girls with outflow obstruction (imperforate hymen, a transverse vaginal septum, or vaginal agenesis with rudimentary uterus) may present with pelvic or lower abdominal pain. Müllerian agenesis, or Mayer–Rokitansky–Küster–Hauser syndrome, refers to congenital absence of the uterus and upper vagina. Ultrasonography or MRI can clarify the nature of müllerian agenesis and differentiate it from an imperforate hymen or transverse vaginal septum. Patients with müllerian agenesis require evaluation for associated congenital anomalies, especially of the urogenital system.

Androgen insensitivity syndrome (AIS) is a cause of amenorrhea in the setting of normal breast development that is much less common than müllerian agenesis. These conditions can be differentiated by measurement of a serum testosterone, which will be in the normal female range in patients with müllerian agenesis and in the normal male range for AIS. Androgen insensitivity syndrome is an X-linked recessive disorder in which 46,XY individuals are resistant to testosterone and do not develop male sexual characteristics. Testes may be palpable in the inguinal area or labia and the synthesis of müllerian-inhibiting substance causes regression of the fallopian tubes, uterus, and upper vagina. Breast development occurs at puberty, but areolae are pale and pubic and axillary hair is sparse. Historically, gonads have been removed after completion of puberty because of the increased risk of testicular cancer after age 25 years in patients with AIS. Patients should be involved fully in the process of shared decision making regarding timing of gonadectomy.

Reassurance is not an appropriate next step for the described patient. Patients who have not undergone thelarche by age 13 years require evaluation. Serum testosterone levels are indicated in patients with menstrual or pubertal abnormalities with hirsutism, acne, or virilization on physical examination or to differentiate between müllerian agenesis and AIS. Because this patient has none of those findings, serum testosterone testing would not be the most appropriate next step. Patients with delayed onset of puberty with or without primary amenorrhea may require imaging studies to assess the presence and development of müllerian structures as well as to assess ovarian follicular activity. However, transabdominal ultrasonography would be more appropriate than transvaginal ultrasonography as the initial imaging modality in a prepubertal 14-year-old patient. Pelvic MRI may be indicated to further evaluate müllerian structures if there is clinical concern about a congenital anomaly, but this would not be the most appropriate next step.

All patients with gonadal dysgenesis, müllerian agenesis, or AIS require psychosocial support to help them process the physical, sexual, and reproductive implications of the diagnosis. Special sensitivity should be given to their emotional and developmental maturity.

American College of Obstetricians and Gynecologists. Guidelines for women's health care: a resource manual. 4th ed. Washington, DC: American College of Obstetricians and Gynecologists; 2014.

Menstruation in girls and adolescents: using the menstrual cycle as a vital sign. ACOG Committee Opinion No. 349. American College of Obstetricians and Gynecologists. Obstet Gynecol 2006;108:1323–8.

Mullerian agenesis: diagnosis, management, and treatment. Committee Opinion No. 562. American College of Obstetricians and Gynecologists. Obstet Gynecol 2013;121:1134–7.

Primary ovarian insufficiency in adolescents and young women. Committee Opinion No. 605. American College of Obstetricians and Gynecologists. Obstet Gynecol 2014;124:193–7.

96
Obesity

A long-term patient visits your clinic to discuss her weight loss options. She is a 34-year-old woman, gravida 2, para 2, with a body mass index (BMI) (calculated as weight in kilograms divided by height in meters squared [kg/m^2]) of 48. She is otherwise healthy but has struggled with her weight for years. She currently is eating a Mediterranean diet and does at least 150 minutes per week of aerobic activity. She has been doing this for more than 1 year and has not experienced any significant weight loss. The option most likely to result in safe, maximal weight loss is

* (A) bariatric surgery
(B) increased physical activity
(C) phentermine hydrochloride
(D) orlistat
(E) dietary change

Unhealthy weight is increasingly common, with two thirds of U.S. adults classified as overweight or obese. Under current definitions, *obesity* is defined as a BMI of 30 or greater (Appendix H). At a personal and population level, this has numerous negative, long-term health consequences. Aside from being an independent risk factor for cardiovascular disease, obesity increases women's risk of numerous gynecologic problems. Within office practice, associated morbidities that are seen commonly include polycystic ovary syndrome, anovulation and resultant infertility, and estrogen-related malignancies such as endometrial cancer. Obesity also increases the risk of developing diabetes, which can lead to higher rates of surgical complications, including poor wound healing, wound infections, and thromboembolic events. Thus, obstetrician–gynecologists need to address weight-related health with patients in an unbiased and respectful manner to help them achieve maximal health while also maintaining their dignity.

For the described patient, a surgical procedure is most likely to result in maximal weight loss in a safe manner. Bariatric surgery is recommended for patients with a BMI greater than 40 (or more than 35 with obesity-related comorbidities) when other, less invasive management options (diet and lifestyle modifications, with or without medications) have not achieved the desired outcome. This patient has already attempted diet and lifestyle changes for more than 1 year and has not noticed any significant change in her weight. Given her class III obesity, surgical management is recommended at this point.

Numerous options for surgical management exist that fall into two general categories: 1) malabsorptive and 2) restrictive. Malabsorptive procedures, such as the Roux-en-Y gastric bypass and biliopancreatic diversion with duodenal switch, bypass parts of the gastrointestinal tract to decrease absorption of food. Restrictive procedures, such as sleeve gastrectomy, adjustable gastric banding, and vertical banded gastroplasty, decrease the size of the stomach, resulting in early satiety. Most of these procedures can be done as open or laparoscopic procedures. Surgical approaches are changing rapidly, with continued modifications. Although laparoscopic Roux-en-Y gastric bypass used to be considered the gold standard for surgical management of obesity, newer trials suggest that laparoscopic sleeve gastrectomy may offer similar or better efficacy in terms of weight loss, resolution of comorbidities, and safety. Although diet and lifestyle changes need to precede and follow surgical management, surgery has been shown to provide greater and more sustained weight loss, increased life expectancy, and resolution of obesity-associated comorbidities such as hypertension and diabetes mellitus. Because of these long-term health benefits, bariatric surgery is more cost-effective than diet and lifestyle interventions alone.

The described patient is taking an important first step in addressing her weight concerns by discussing with her physician how to get better results. Guidelines suggest that physicians should take an active role in this process, offering assistance to patients who would benefit from weight loss (ie, patients with a BMI of 30 or greater [obese] and those with a BMI of 25 or greater and one additional comorbidity or risk factor). When available, patients should be referred to intensive, multicomponent behavioral interventions. Generally, the initial goal of such programs is 5–10% weight loss, which often is enough to gain some health benefits. It is important that patients set realistic goals so that they will not be discouraged. Although such referrals are important, it is unclear how much benefit the described patient would get from this type of intervention because she is already following a healthy diet and doing the recommended amount of physical activity. Moreover, these programs are not as effective for long-term weight loss, with a 50% risk of regaining lost weight within 1–2 years, and high financial costs.

Pharmacotherapy also is a possibility for obesity management, with new formulations being explored. The medications that currently exist work by either decreasing fat absorption or suppressing appetite. Most are available only by prescription and have numerous adverse effects that complicate long-term use. Because obesity is a chronic condition, medical management is challenged by the need for ongoing treatment to maintain weight loss. Weight-loss medication has been shown to be an effective supplement to less intensive weight-loss programs but lacks evidence regarding long-term benefit and long-term risks. Thus, although orlistat or phentermine could benefit this patient, neither offers the same level of weight loss or long-term effect seen with bariatric surgery.

Bariatric surgery: an evidence-based analysis. Health Quality Ontario. Ont Health Technol Assess Ser 2005;5:1–148.

Colquitt JL, Pickett K, Loveman E, Frampton GK. Surgery for weight loss in adults. Cochrane Database of Systematic Reviews 2014, Issue 8. Art. No.: CD003641. DOI: 10.1002/14651858.CD003641.pub4.

Ethical issues in the care of the obese woman. Committee Opinion No. 600. American College of Obstetricians and Gynecologists. Obstet Gynecol 2014;123:1388–93.

Kushner RF, Ryan DH. Assessment and lifestyle management of patients with obesity: clinical recommendations from systematic reviews [published erratum appears in JAMA 2014;312:1593]. JAMA 2014;312:943–52.

Lee WJ, Almulaifi A. Recent advances in bariatric/metabolic surgery: appraisal of clinical evidence. J Biomed Res 2015;29:98–104.

97

Bloody nipple discharge

A 54-year-old menopausal woman comes to your office with a 2-week history of spontaneous bloody nipple discharge. On physical examination, you note no palpable masses. She has no tenderness, and you observe no retraction or dimpling of the breast. The nipple is in normal position, and no skin changes are present on the breast, areola, or nipple. You find no palpable axillary, clavicular, or neck nodes. Circumferential palpation around the areola elicits a bloody discharge from a single ductal orifice. Diagnostic mammography is negative for malignancy. The most likely diagnosis is

(A) ductal ectasia
* (B) intraductal papilloma
(C) ductal carcinoma
(D) Paget disease

The most common presenting breast concerns are breast masses, pain, and nipple discharge. Pathologic discharges include secretions that are clear, yellow, serosanguineous, and sanguineous. Such discharges tend to be unilateral, persistent, and spontaneous and can be expressed from a single mammary duct. Any discharge is more worrisome if it is associated with an underlying breast mass. Most of the time, however, discharge with the described patient's characteristics is not associated with malignancy. The characteristic discharge of fibrocystic changes is thick and greenish in color, and galactorrhea usually is bilateral with secretions that are clear or milky.

Intraductal papillomas are epithelial proliferations that frequently occur with bleeding. They are very rarely associated with malignancy, but excision is the only way to exclude atypia, ductal carcinoma in situ, or papillary carcinoma. Because intraductal papillomas usually are isolated lesions within a single ductal system, the bloody discharge will be expressed from a single ductal orifice. Therefore, careful, circumferential palpation in an hourly or clockwise fashion around the areola often will allow precise identification of which ductal system is involved.

Ductal ectasia occurs when a ductal wall becomes dilated and fills with inspissated inflammatory secretions. The discharge typically is very thick and sticky and either green or black in color but occasionally can become serosanguineous or bloody. Ductal ectasia is not associated with breast carcinoma, but the surrounding tissue may become fibrotic, causing a confusing palpable density. Ductal carcinoma is much more likely with a bloody discharge if there is an underlying palpable mass or imaging abnormality. With a bloody nipple discharge alone, the incidence of underlying cancer is 3–6%, but when it is accompanied by a palpable mass, the frequency increases to 27–61%.

Paget disease of the breast is an intraductal carcinoma, which presents as a scaly skin lesion similar to eczema appearing on the nipple and spreading to the areola. Ulceration can be present, and there may be a clear yellowish exudate with crusting. Patients commonly have pruritus, burning, pain, and, occasionally, bleeding. Paget disease accounts for only 1–3% of cases of breast cancer.

The described patient has a bloody discharge from a single nipple ductal orifice, no palpable mass, and normal mammography, all of which are typical of an intraductal papilloma. Evaluation of a patient with bloody nipple discharge should include a comprehensive history to help differentiate physiologic from pathologic discharge. Next, a complete breast and axillary examination is essential, in addition to an attempt to elicit the discharge and identify the individual duct involved. It is important to rule out skin lesions that could present as a discharge. A Hemoccult test can be used on a nonsanguineous discharge to exclude the presence of blood. Bilateral mammography should be the next step, with additional imaging as indicated by the mammographic examination result. For patients with intraductal papillomas, however, mammography will be normal in 85% of cases. Abnormal mammographic findings could include distended retroareolar ducts, asymmetry, architectural distortion, and periductal microcalcifications. Providing the clinical history of a new pathologic discharge on the mammography requisition is important to alert the radiologist to any changes from prior mammographic examinations and to look specifically for retroareolar changes, such as an isolated duct with ectasia.

Subareolar ultrasonography is a particularly useful adjunct to mammography in patients who have a pathologic discharge. One study of subareolar ultrasonography of patients who reported a bloody nipple discharge found a sensitivity of 97%, specificity of 60%, and positive predictive value of 95%. Doppler ultrasonographic examination may provide some additional benefit in detecting neoplastic intraductal masses. The ultrasonography is most useful if the result is positive. In this circumstance, ultrasonography-guided biopsy can provide a tissue diagnosis. If the biopsy is positive for carcinoma, then surgical planning with a single procedure is possible. If the biopsy is benign, however, it will not result in a cure of the patient's symptoms of pathologic discharge. The traditional approach to bloody nipple discharge was that all presenting patients should have a tissue diagnosis that explains the bloody nipple discharge, along with an excision that also results in control of the symptoms. Current recommendations, however, suggest that if mammography and subareolar ultrasonography are negative, then the patient can be counseled that the risk of a carcinoma is less than 3% and that she can make a choice about follow-up with heightened surveillance or definitive ductal excision. A useful clinical algorithm is shown in Figure 97-1. One study that employed this algorithm had 94 patients stratified to close clinical follow-up. In 20 of these patients, subsequent imaging led to ductal excision, with only one patient found to have ductal carcinoma in situ. Over 28 months of follow-up, 74 patients had no surgery and no carcinomas were identified; 81% of the patients had spontaneous resolution of their discharge.

Ashfaq A, Senior D, Pockaj BA, Wasif N, Pizzitola VJ, Giurescu ME, et al. Validation study of a modern treatment algorithm for nipple discharge. Am J Surg 2014;208:222–7.

Brookes MJ, Bourke AG. Radiological appearances of papillary breast lesions. Clin Radiol 2008;63:1265–73.

Gray RJ, Pockaj BA, Karstaedt PJ. Navigating murky waters: a modern treatment algorithm for nipple discharge. Am J Surg 2007;194:850–4; discussion 854–5.

Nelson RS, Hoehn JL. Twenty-year outcome following central duct resection for bloody nipple discharge. Ann Surg 2006;243:522–4.

Patel BK, Falcon S, Drukteinis J. Management of nipple discharge and the associated imaging findings. Am J Med 2015;128:353–60.

Vargas HI, Romero L, Chlebowski RT. Management of bloody nipple discharge. Curr Treat Options Oncol 2002;3:157–61.

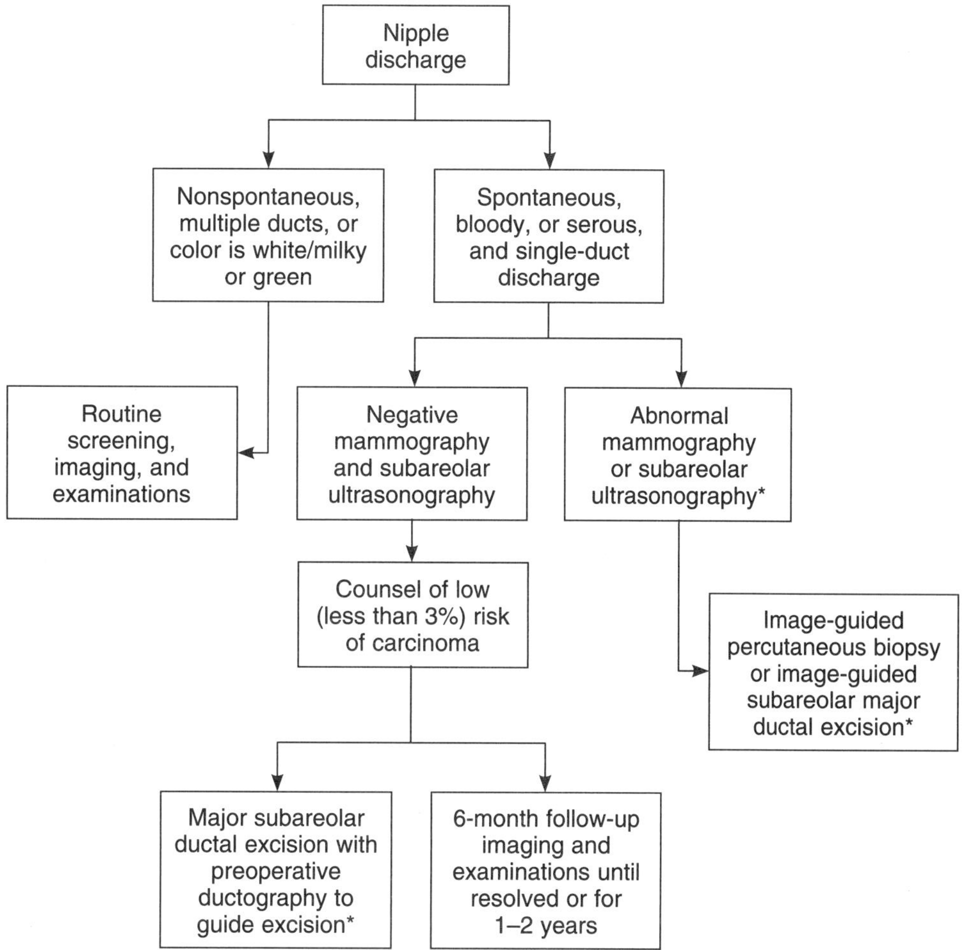

FIGURE 97-1. Algorithm for the treatment of nipple discharge. *If patient plans future breastfeeding, selective ductal excision is preferred over major ductal excision. (Reprinted from American Journal of Surgery. Gray RJ, Pockaj BA, Karstaedt PJ. Navigating murky waters: a modern treatment algorithm for nipple discharge. Am J Surg 2007;194: 850–4; discussion 854–5. Copyright 2007, with permission from Elsevier.)

98

Counseling for tubal sterilization

A 25-year-old woman, gravida 3, para 2, at 20 weeks of gestation requests information about permanent sterilization. She is obese, with a body mass index (calculated as weight in kilograms divided by height in meters squared [kg/m^2]) of 42, but has no other medical problems. Her spouse is aged 25 years and healthy. She and her spouse are planning on moving out of the country approximately 3 months after the birth of this baby to be closer to their family. The permanent sterilization option with the lowest risk for this couple is

(A) interval hysteroscopic sterilization
* (B) vasectomy
(C) immediate postpartum sterilization
(D) interval laparoscopic sterilization

Vasectomy is the best option for this couple because it exposes them to the lowest risk of permanent sterilization. Vasectomy is easier and safer than tubal ligation; it also is equally effective, with an overall pregnancy rate of approximately 1 in 2,000 for men who have documented postoperative azoospermia or rare nonmotile sperm. Most men are candidates for vasectomy because there are few contraindications (eg, coagulopathy, undescended testes, testicular tumor). Vasectomy is associated with shorter operative time and less morbidity than female sterilization techniques. The minimally invasive techniques used for vasectomy can be performed under local anesthesia and enables men to return to work more quickly than women can after undergoing postpartum or laparoscopic sterilization. Male sterilization is more cost-effective than female sterilization. Semen analysis is recommended 8–16 weeks after the procedure to ensure effectiveness. For the described couple, the procedure can be done before delivery or in the immediate postpartum period, giving the husband time to be tested before moving out of the country.

Because of the patient's degree of obesity, immediate postpartum and interval laparoscopic sterilization confer significant risk; therefore, neither is the best choice. Furthermore, national data show that up to 50% of women requesting postpartum sterilization do not undergo the procedure during hospitalization. Given her body mass index, postpartum and even interval laparoscopic sterilization may be technically challenging. Obesity also may be considered to be a relative contraindication to laparoscopy and immediate postpartum tubal ligation and is an independent risk factor for complications related to laparoscopic sterilization. Interval laparoscopic and immediate postpartum sterilization are associated with a greater risk of future ectopic pregnancy compared with hysteroscopic sterilization and vasectomy.

Interval hysteroscopic sterilization should be delayed until at least 6 weeks after delivery. Confirmatory hysterosalpingography is required 3 months after the procedure to document tubal occlusion. Lack of appropriate and recommended follow-up is a common factor among women who become pregnant after hysteroscopic sterilization. Obesity is not a contraindication to hysteroscopic sterilization; however, consideration must be given to the risk that obesity poses in terms of anesthesia or sedation. Hysteroscopic sterilization is less expensive than laparoscopic sterilization secondary to a shorter recovery period. Although hysteroscopic sterilization is appropriate for many obese patients, follow-up confirmation of tubal occlusion is imperative to ensure success. Therefore, hysteroscopic sterilization is not the best choice for this patient, who plans to move to a different country 3 months after giving birth.

Benefits and risks of sterilization. Practice Bulletin No. 133. American College of Obstetricians and Gynecologists. Obstet Gynecol 2013;121:392–404.

Chi I, Mumford SD, Laufe LE. Technical failures in tubal ring sterilization: incidence, perceived reasons, outcome, and risk factors. Am J Obstet Gynecol 1980;138:307–12.

Hysteroscopic tubal sterilization: a health economic literature review. Toronto Health Economic and Technology Assessment (THETA) Collaborative. Ont Health Technol Assess Ser 2013;13:1–25.

Jamieson DJ, Hillis SD, Duerr A, Marchbanks PA, Costello C, Peterson HB. Complications of interval laparoscopic tubal sterilization: findings from the United States Collaborative Review of Sterilization. Obstet Gynecol 2000;96:997–1002.

Sharlip ID, Belker AM, Honig S, Labrecque M, Marmar JL, Ross LS, et al. Vasectomy: AUA guideline. American Urological Association. Linthicum (MD): American Urological Association; 2012. Available at: https://www.auanet.org/common/pdf/education/clinical-guidance/Vasectomy.pdf. Retrieved June 17, 2016.

99

Coding for evaluation and management visit

A 36-year-old patient comes to your office for the first time in 2 years for her annual well-woman examination. Your now-retired partner was her regular obstetrician–gynecologist. She reports headaches and yellow nasal discharge for the past several days and thinks she might have had a mild fever. Her vital signs are normal. A thorough ear, nose, and throat examination reveals pain on palpation of her maxillary sinuses and fluid behind her left tympanic membrane, and you diagnose her with sinusitis. You prescribe an antibiotic, instruct the patient on how to use steam for the congestion, and recommend over-the-counter nonsteroidal antiinflammatory drugs for her discomfort. You document the problem-oriented component of her encounter and then proceed with her well-woman examination, which you document in detail. The correct way to code the encounter is

(A) annual visit only, new
(B) problem visit only, new
(C) problem visit only, established
(D) annual visit, new; and problem visit, new
* (E) annual visit, established; and problem visit, established

Professional services are face-to-face encounters provided by physicians and other qualified health care providers for patients and are reported using evaluation and management (E/M) *Current Procedural Terminology* (CPT) codes. These can be either problem-oriented visits or preventive health care visits. Distinction between new and established patient visits is important because the level of documentation in these two settings is different. *Current Procedural Terminology* defines a new patient as one who has not received any professional services within the past 3 years from the obstetrician–gynecologist or other qualified health care provider of the exact same specialty and subspecialty who belongs to the same group practice. Because the described patient has been seen by a physician within the same group during the past 3 years, she would be considered an established patient.

Correct coding for problem-oriented E/M services is based upon the clarity and completeness of documentation of the cognitive work provided by the physician or other health care provider in order to support code selection. The three key components required for E/M code selection are history, examination, and medical decision making. The history component includes history of present illness; review of systems and past, family, and social histories. The physical examination should be germane to the presenting issue; it can be either a full-body examination or a single-system examination, depending on the issue to be evaluated, and the examination should reflect the clinical relevance of the particular patient circumstances. Medical decision making refers to the complexity of establishing a diagnosis, selecting a management option, or both as measured by the following:

- The number of possible diagnoses or the number of management options that must be considered
- The amount or complexity of medical records, diagnostic tests, and other information that must be obtained, reviewed, and analyzed
- The risk of significant complications, morbidity, or mortality as well as comorbidities associated with the patient's presenting problems, the diagnostic procedure, or the possible management options

A problem-oriented visit must have a chief complaint and requires evaluation and documentation of all three of the key components for new patients and two out of three of the key components for established patients to determine the level of E/M service to report.

The amount of time spent in counseling must be explicitly stated. In addition, it must be clear what percentage of the encounter was dedicated to counseling. According to the CPT, when counseling or coordination of care dominates (ie, takes up more than 50%) of the physician encounter with the patient or family (ie, face-to-face time in the office or other outpatient setting or floor or unit time in the hospital or nursing facility), then time shall be considered the key or controlling factor to qualify for a particular level of E/M service(s). Counseling may include discussion of diagnostic results, prognosis, risks and benefits of treatment options, instructions for management and follow-up, the importance of adherence to chosen treatment options, risk reduction, and patient and family education.

A CPT preventive service code (code series 99384–99397) is reported for women who have no current symptoms or diagnosed illness and are presenting for a well-woman examination. These encounters include the following:

- Counseling, anticipatory guidance, and risk factor reduction interventions
- Age-appropriate comprehensive history (past medical history, past family and social histories, review of systems)
- Age-appropriate comprehensive examination, which typically includes the following:
  - — Gynecologic examination
  - — Breast examination
  - — Pap test, when indicated
- Discussions about the status of previously diagnosed stable conditions
- Ordering of appropriate laboratory tests for diagnostic procedures and immunizations

These preventive visit codes are divided by patient age and not by complexity of issues or time spent with the patient. There is no requirement for chief complaint, history of present illness, or medical decision-making documentation.

In some situations, the patient may have a concern that is significant and separately identifiable from the preventive health care visit. However, it is not appropriate to use any element of the history, examination, and medical decision making that occurred as part of the well-woman visit when determining the level of a separately identified problem-oriented visit. The problem-based services must be calculated independently of any work performed during the well-woman visit. The described patient's visit has a level of history, examination, and medical decision making that supports the level of service being reported as "above and beyond" the comprehensive preventive service. Therefore, it would be appropriate to code the visit as an established annual visit and established problem visit, which designates the additional, separately identified service on the same date. Modifier 25 is appended to the problem-oriented E/M code.

It is important to note that some payers do not pay for two E/M services provided on the same day. It is important to know what each specific payer requires. This is particularly important when providing a time-based E/M service in addition to a preventive service, because age-related, anticipatory guidance and risk factor reduction counseling are an included part of the preventive service code. Unlike other CPT E/M codes, preventive service codes do not have typical times because the time spent will vary based on the specific patient's requirements.

American Congress of Obstetricians and Gynecologists. 2016 ob/gyn coding manual: components of correct procedural coding. Washington, DC: American Congress of Obstetricians and Gynecologists; 2016.

American Medical Association. CPT: Current procedural terminology: 2016. Professional ed. Chicago (IL): AMA; 2016.

100

Pelvic inflammatory disease

A 21-year-old nulligravid woman comes to your office with abdominal pain and a fever of 38.4°C (101°F). On examination, she has cervical motion tenderness, and a purulent vaginal discharge is noted. She is given intramuscular ceftriaxone and oral doxycycline. She returns 3 days later and still has fever and pain. A computed tomography (CT) scan demonstrates 4-cm complex multiloculated masses involving the ovaries and fallopian tubes. The best next step in management is

(A) intramuscular cefoxitin and oral probenecid
(B) add metronidazole to current antibiotics
* (C) admit to the hospital to receive parenteral antibiotics
(D) consult with interventional radiology for drainage of the mass
(E) laparoscopy

A woman with pelvic inflammatory disease (PID) may be treated as an outpatient or admitted to the hospital for parenteral therapy. A large prospective study of women with mild-to-moderate PID showed no long-term differences in outcome when patients were randomized to inpatient or outpatient therapy. The decision of whether hospitalization is necessary should be based on the judgment of the obstetrician–gynecologist or other health care provider and whether the woman meets any of the suggested criteria in Box 100-1.

BOX 100-1

Suggested Criteria for Admission of Women With Pelvic Inflammatory Disease

Surgical emergency (eg, appendicitis)
Tubo-ovarian abscess
Pregnancy
Severe illness
Nausea and vomiting
High fever
Unable to follow or tolerate an outpatient oral regimen
No clinical response to oral antimicrobial therapy

Workowski KA, Bolan GA. Sexually transmitted diseases treatment guidelines, 2015. Centers for Disease Control and Prevention [published erratum appears in MMWR Recomm Rep 2015;64:924]. MMWR Recomm Rep 2015;64:78–82.

In patients with mild-to-moderate disease, outpatient antibiotic treatment is preferable if the woman is reliable for follow-up and is able to tolerate an outpatient oral regimen. Reexamination in 48–72 hours is recommended, and patients that have failed to show improvements with outpatient treatment should be admitted for parenteral antibiotics.

The described patient has not responded to outpatient management and has developed a tubo-ovarian abscess, an inflammatory phlegmon that encompasses the fallopian tubes and ovaries and may involve bowel and adjacent peritoneal surfaces. A tubo-ovarian abscess can be treated surgically or with antibiotics based on the size of the abscess. Rupture of a tubo-ovarian abscess is a surgical emergency, and mortality is high without prompt surgical intervention. Approximately 85% of abscesses that are 4 cm in size or smaller respond to parenteral broad-spectrum antibiotics, whereas only 40% of abscesses 10 cm in size or larger will respond to this treatment. Admission with administration of broad-spectrum antibiotics, including anaerobic coverage, is indicated. Women without improvement of symptoms after 48 hours or with increasing size of the abscess should have further treatment of the tubo-ovarian abscess. Drainage of a tubo-ovarian abscess can be performed with ultrasonography or with CT guidance. If an interventional approach is not available, the abscess can be drained surgically with laparotomy or through a minimally invasive approach; removal of the infected tube is typical, and hysterectomy is rarely required.

The Centers for Disease Control and Prevention has provided multiple options for the treatment of PID. The described patient was initially treated with ceftriaxone and doxycycline; her clinical condition has worsened, and selecting an alternative outpatient antibiotic (cefoxitin and probenecid) would be inappropriate.

Anaerobic coverage with metronidazole may be combined with outpatient therapy, and when bacterial vaginosis is present, it is likely to be advantageous. Anaerobic antimicrobial coverage should be part of the initial antibiotic coverage of a tubo-ovarian abscess; it is inappropriate to simply add metronidazole to the ongoing outpatient treatment.

Drainage of a tubo-ovarian abscess by means of radiologic guidance may be done in select cases. Radiologic imaging can use ultrasonography, CT, or magnetic resonance imaging modalities and route of drainage can be transabdominal, transgluteal, or transvaginal. Complications include rupture of the abscess or damage to adjacent vessels or organs. Such radiologically guided drainage requires an experienced interventional radiologist. Some abscesses are inaccessible or undrainable because of their location or the proximity of adjacent structures. In addition, the success of percutaneous abscess drainage depends on the consistency of the contents within a collection. In the described patient, parenteral antibiotic therapy is the best option and is very likely to be successful because of the smaller size of the abscesses.

The diagnosis of PID is made using clinical criteria. The described patient had the minimal clinical criteria for diagnosis as well as several supportive signs. In cases where the diagnosis is uncertain, endometrial biopsy, ultrasonography, or diagnostic laparoscopy may be indicated. In this case, ultrasonography has confirmed the diagnosis of tubo-ovarian abscess, so confirmation with diagnostic laparoscopy is unwarranted.

American College of Obstetricians and Gynecologists. Guidelines for women's health care: a resource manual. 4th edition. Washington, DC: American College of Obstetricians and Gynecologists; 2014. p. 406–12.

Soper DE. Infections of the female pelvis. In: Mandell G, Bennett J, Dolin R, editors. Mandell, Douglas, and Bennett's principles and practice of infectious diseases. 8th edition. Philadelphia (PA): Elsevier Saunders; 2015. p. 1372–80.

Workowski KA, Bolan GA. Sexually transmitted diseases treatment guidelines, 2015. Centers for Disease Control and Prevention [published erratum appears in MMWR Recomm Rep 2015;64:924]. MMWR Recomm Rep 2015;64:1–137.

101

Cough in a nonpregnant patient

A 59-year-old nulligravid obese woman comes to your office and tells you that she has had a cough for the past 8 weeks. She has a body mass index (calculated as weight in kilograms divided by height in meters squared [kg/m^2]) of 45. Her medical history is notable for type 2 diabetes mellitus and hypertension that is well controlled with metoprolol. She has a 30-pack-per-year history of smoking and reports generalized fatigue, excessive daytime sleepiness, and poor productivity at work. Of particular concern to the patient and her husband is her newly developed nocturnal cough that has become more troublesome than her typical loud snoring. Based on her history and symptomatology, the intervention most likely to lead to the correct diagnosis is

(A) upper endoscopy
(B) smoking cessation
(C) pulmonary function testing
* (D) nocturnal oximetry study

Cough is a common problem worldwide and affects approximately 9–33% of the adult population. In the United States, cough is one of the most common symptoms for which patients seek medical attention. Based on duration of symptoms, cough often is divided into three categories: 1) acute, 2) subacute, and 3) chronic. Acute and subacute cough typically are caused by viral upper respiratory infections, and patients will present to primary care physicians. Conversely, chronic cough lasts for longer than 8 weeks and can be caused by a wide array of conditions. Regardless of the cause, cough can result in significant disturbances in quality of life because of absences from work and social embarrassment with adverse events such as urinary incontinence. The evaluation and management of chronic cough should include a broad differential and often requires a multidisciplinary approach. Diagnoses to consider initially include gastroesophageal reflux disease (GERD), asthma, rhinosinusitis, chronic obstructive pulmonary disease, postnasal drip syndrome, atopic cough, medication adverse effect, or unknown etiology.

Along with asthma and postnasal drip syndrome, GERD represents one of the most common causes of chronic cough and accounts for up to 41% of cases (Appendix E). Common symptoms of GERD include heartburn and acid regurgitation. Symptoms such as laryngitis, bronchospasm, halitosis, and cough are seen less commonly and tend to occur when gastric contents enter the oral cavity. The diagnosis of GERD can be made reliably in the presence of clinical symptoms and response to a trial of acid suppression therapy. Although the described patient does not have the typical symptoms of GERD, her cough could reflect an atypical presentation. However, upper endoscopy would not be the first-line investigative step for a patient who may have GERD and would not be the approach most likely to lead to the correct diagnosis in this patient. In general, upper endoscopy with biopsies should be reserved for cases that are refractory to medical management or for patients in whom the diagnosis remains unclear.

According to the U.S. Preventive Services Task Force, tobacco screening and counseling regarding smoking cessation are rated among the three most effective and efficacious preventive health actions that can be undertaken in a clinical setting. Additionally, tobacco use is the leading cause of death in women in the United States and remains the single greatest modifiable risk factor for cardiovascular disease. Obstetrician–gynecologists are in a unique position to counsel patients regarding the adverse health risks of smoking. Although this patient should be counseled on the importance of smoking cessation, this intervention will not aid in determining the diagnosis.

Asthma can present at any age; however, new-onset asthma in older adults is quite uncommon. The classic symptoms of asthma include shortness of breath, difficulty breathing, and wheezing in addition to coughing, which tends to be worse at night. Given this patient's smoking history, chronic obstructive pulmonary disease is a more likely diagnosis; however, in the absence of shortness of breath and a productive cough, this diagnosis is unlikely. Chronic cough often occurs in nonsmokers with normal chest X-rays and pulmonary function testing. Pulmonary function testing would not be indicated at this stage of the patient's evaluation.

An additional and less commonly considered cause of chronic cough is obstructive sleep apnea (OSA). In fact, cough can be the sole presenting symptom of OSA. The prevalence of OSA increases with age and body mass index. Obesity and OSA have been shown to increase airway inflammation. Symptoms concerning for OSA include chronic nighttime cough, snoring, obesity, and the presence of GERD. The described patient has multiple risk factors and symptoms that are concerning for OSA. Although daytime somnolence is not always present, her excessive daytime sleepiness probably is a result of poor sleep quality in the setting of OSA. Therefore, the intervention most likely to lead to the correct diagnosis in this patient is a nocturnal oximetry study. If her overnight oximetry study is abnormal, the intervention that is likely to alleviate her symptoms would be continuous positive airway pressure during sleep.

Birring SS, Kavanagh J, Lai K, Chang AB. Adult and paediatric cough guidelines: ready for an overhaul? Pulm Pharmacol Ther 2015 Dec;35:137–44.

Chan K, Ing A, Birring SS. Cough in obstructive sleep apnoea. Pulm Pharmacol Ther 2015 Dec;35:129–31.

Iyer VN, Lim KG. Chronic cough: an update. Mayo Clin Proc 2013; 88:1115–26.

Sundar KM, Daly SE. Chronic cough and OSA: a new association? J Clin Sleep Med 2011;7:669–77.

Tobacco use and women's health. Committee Opinion No. 503. American College of Obstetricians and Gynecologists. Obstet Gynecol 2011;118:746–50.

102

Nonsteroidal antiinflammatory drug use in the elderly

A 72-year-old woman, gravida 2, para 2, comes to your office worried about decreased urinary output and a dark tinge to her urine. She has otherwise been feeling well, although she is fatigued and has aching joints. She takes ibuprofen as needed for sore muscles and osteoarthritis, which have been bothering her a lot after a week-long walking tour. She has been taking lisinopril for hypertension and atorvastatin for elevated cholesterol for the past 2 years. Recently, she has been taking diphenhydramine or trazodone to help her sleep. While completing her workup, the first medication you should advise her to discontinue is

* (A) ibuprofen
(B) lisinopril
(C) atorvastatin
(D) diphenhydramine
(E) trazodone

The U.S. Administration of Aging predicts that by 2030, there will be 72 million people older than 65 years in the United States, almost double the number that there were in 2000. This is in part because of improvements in management of chronic conditions, as well as general demographic trends in the country. This shift will have a large effect on the health care system because the elderly access care more frequently and have more medication use. More than 90% of people older than 75 years take medication on a regular basis. Polypharmacy also is quite common in this group, with one half of Medicare beneficiaries taking five or more medications. Polypharmacy is associated with elevated levels of drug-associated adverse events, hospital admissions, and worsened functional status. This, in large part, is because of the pathophysiologic process that happens with aging, including declines in organ function, especially renal and hepatic function. Because these two organ systems are critical in medication metabolism and excretion, drug-associated complications are much more common in the elderly. Declining cognitive function also influences drug-related adverse events because dosage or medication errors become more common.

Aspirin and nonsteroidal antiinflammatory drugs (NSAIDs) are among the most commonly prescribed drugs in this age group because they are effective against numerous conditions typically seen in this population, such as osteoarthritis. In certain populations, approximately 40% of older women use prescription-strength NSAIDs. These drugs have a well-documented association with numerous adverse effects, most notably gastrointestinal and renal problems. Although much of the focus around NSAID use in the elderly has been on the gastrointestinal effects—mainly bleeding—the renal effects can cause complications that also need to be recognized and treated quickly. Community-acquired acute kidney injury is as common as hospital-acquired acute kidney injury and has equally poor long-term outcomes.

Because NSAIDs decrease prostaglandin synthesis by inhibition of the cyclooxygenase (COX) enzyme, they work as effective reducers of inflammation and fever.

However, as with all medications, there are known adverse drug interactions that limit their use. There is C-level evidence to suggest the need for monitoring creatinine levels after initiation of NSAID therapy in women at risk of renal failure or in women who are taking certain antihypertensive medications, such as angiotensin-converting enzyme inhibitors and angiotensin receptor blockers. Such monitoring is needed because the renal system is dependent on vasodilation from prostaglandins, mainly COX-2. This dependence is greater in patients who are sensitive to volume status (ie, patients with renal disease, congestive heart failure, or liver cirrhosis). Thus, all NSAIDs, whether they are COX-2 selective or not, can lead to volume-dependent renal dysfunction by vasoconstriction. Although this vasoconstriction usually is temporary, extended duration or higher dosage can have an adverse effect.

The described patient has numerous risk factors for renal dysfunction, including age, hypertension, use of an angiotensin-converting enzyme inhibitor, and increased ibuprofen use because of muscle and joint aches. Thus, decreased urine output and darkened urine probably are due to acute kidney injury secondary to her ibuprofen use. Ibuprofen should be stopped immediately. Up to 2% of older patients taking NSAIDs stop using them because of development of renal complications similar to those experienced by the described patient.

After stopping the patient's use of ibuprofen, a urinalysis and laboratory evaluation of kidney function (ie, creatinine, creatinine clearance, glomerular filtration rate) should be initiated. She also should be referred to her primary care doctor or a specialist who manages polypharmacy and the associated comorbidities more frequently. After she stops taking ibuprofen, the vasoconstriction that likely led to acute kidney injury should resolve. The other medications she is taking—lisinopril, atorvastatin, diphenhydramine, and trazodone—are unlikely to be the main cause of her renal dysfunction. Although lisinopril also is associated with renal dysfunction in the setting of low renal blood flow, discontinuing the ibuprofen will address more directly the most immediate cause of the renal dysfunction. Angiotensin-converting enzyme inhibitors and angiotensin receptor blockers generally are thought to be renal protective, but overly restrictive blood pressure control combined with NSAID use can lead to complications, especially in older patients. This patient has been taking her antihypertensive medication for 2 years, suggesting the etiology of the sudden change is secondary to an acute increase in ibuprofen use. However, this incident suggests the need to reassess her blood pressure control and her need for multiple agents. The gynecologist's role in this setting is to recognize the signs of renal impairment, stop the offending agent (primarily ibuprofen), and initiate the workup as she is referred to her primary care provider.

Franco Palacios CR, Haugen EN, Rasmussen RW, Thompson AM. Avoidance of polypharmacy and excessive blood pressure control is associated with improved renal function in older patients. Ren Fail 2015;37:961–5.

Risser A, Donovan D, Heintzman J, Page T. NSAID prescribing precautions. Am Fam Physician 2009;80:1371–8.

Taylor R Jr, Lemtouni S, Weiss K, Pergolizzi JV Jr. Pain management in the elderly: an FDA Safe Use Initiative Expert Panel's view on preventable harm associated with NSAID therapy. Curr Gerontol Geriatr Res 2012:196159.

103

Indications for hepatitis B vaccination

A 29-year-old primigravid woman comes to your office at 10 weeks of gestation. She was diagnosed with human immunodeficiency virus (HIV) 1 year ago and is being treated at a community HIV clinic. She is asymptomatic and was started on antiretroviral therapy. She received the 3-dose series of hepatitis B virus (HBV) vaccine as an adolescent. Her test results for hepatitis B surface antigen (HBsAg) and anti-hepatitis B (anti-HB) surface antigen, also commonly known as antibody to the hepatitis B surface, are negative. Based on these results, the best next step in management is

(A) postexposure prophylaxis with HBV immune globulin
(B) repeat the 3-dose series
* (C) single booster dose of the HBV vaccine
(D) repeat HBV vaccination postpartum

Hepatitis B virus is a DNA virus transmitted by percutaneous or mucosal exposure to infected blood or body fluids. It also can be transmitted vertically from infected women to their infants. Chronic infection increases an individual's risk of cirrhosis and hepatocellular carcinoma. Strategies to eliminate HBV transmission in the United States include the following four steps:

1. Universal vaccination of infants at birth (first recommended in 1991)
2. Prevention of perinatal transmission by screening pregnant women for HBsAg and administration of immunoprophylaxis to infants born to HBsAg-positive women and to infants born to women with unknown HBsAg status
3. Vaccination of children and adolescents not immunized previously
4. Immunization of adults who are at risk of HBV infection (Box 103-1)

Vaccination is the most effective measure to prevent HBV infection and its sequelae. The vaccine is administered in 3 doses at 0 months, 1 month, and 6 months. The third dose offers the maximum level of seroprotection and acts as a booster to provide long-term immunity. There currently is no recommendation for routine repeat vaccination or administration of a booster dose. Pregnancy is not a contraindication to HBV vaccination because it contains the recombinant form of HBsAg and is not infectious. Pregnant women with a high risk of infection should be vaccinated in any trimester.

Determination of anti-HB surface antigen status for patients with a prior history of HBV immunization is not recommended routinely except for high-risk individuals. If the anti-HB surface antigen level is 10 international units/L or higher, the patient is considered immune. The described patient is at high risk of HBV infection because of her HIV-positive status. She has no measurable immunity from her prior vaccination and, therefore, should be given a single booster dose to protect her and her fetus. The patient should then be retested 1 month later to determine her anti-HB surface antigen level. If her level is lower than 10 international units/L, the other two doses of the vaccine should be administered again per the normal schedule. There are a few individuals with persistent anti-HB surface antigen levels lower than 10 international units/L even after two series of three vaccinations (ie, six vaccinations total). Such individuals are referred to as nonresponders. These patients require postexposure prophylaxis with hepatitis B immune globulin within 12 hours of an exposure and a second dose 1 month later. Contraindications to HBV vaccine are life-threatening allergy to yeast, history of life-threatening allergic reaction to a previous dose of HBV vaccine, and being acutely ill.

BOX 103-1

Adults Recommended to Receive Hepatitis B Virus Vaccination

Individuals at risk of infection by sexual exposure

- Sex partners of HBsAg-positive individuals
- Sexually active individuals who are not in a long-term, mutually monogamous relationship (eg, individuals with more than one sex partner during the previous 6 months)
- Individuals seeking evaluation or treatment for a sexually transmitted infection
- Men who have sex with men

Individuals at risk of infection by percutaneous or mucosal exposure to blood

- Current or recent injection-drug users
- Household contacts of HBsAg-positive individuals
- Residents and staff of facilities for developmentally disabled individuals
- Health care and public safety workers with reasonably anticipated risk of exposure to blood or blood-contaminated body fluids
- Individuals with end-stage renal disease, including predialysis, hemodialysis, peritoneal dialysis, and home dialysis patients

Others

- International travelers to regions with high or intermediate levels (HBsAg prevalence 2% or more) of endemic HBV infection
- Individuals with chronic liver disease
- Individuals with HIV infection
- All other individuals seeking protection from HBV infection

Abbreviations: HBV, hepatitis B virus; HIV, human immunodeficiency virus; HBsAg, hepatitis B surface antigen.

Mast EE, Margolis HS, Fiore AE, Brink EW, Goldstein ST, Wang SA, et al. A comprehensive immunization strategy to eliminate transmission of hepatitis B virus infection in the United States: recommendations of the Advisory Committee on Immunization Practices (ACIP) part 1: immunization of infants, children, and adolescents. Advisory Committee on Immunization Practices [published errata appear in MMWR Morb Mortal Wkly Rep 2006;55:158-9.] MMWR Morb Mortal Wkly Rep 2007;56:1267]. MMWR Recomm Rep 2005;54:1–31.

Centers for Disease Control and Prevention. Who should NOT get vaccinated with these vaccines? Atlanta (GA): CDC; 2015. Available at: http://www.cdc.gov/vaccines/vpd-vac/should-not-vacc.htm. Retrieved June 16, 2016.

Mast EE, Margolis HS, Fiore AE, Brink EW, Goldstein ST, Wang SA, et al. A comprehensive immunization strategy to eliminate transmission of hepatitis B virus infection in the United States: recommendations of the Advisory Committee on Immunization Practices (ACIP) part 1: immunization of infants, children, and adolescents. Advisory Committee on Immunization Practices [published errata appear in MMWR Morb Mortal Wkly Rep 2006;55:158–9. MMWR Morb Mortal Wkly Rep 2007;56:1267]. MMWR Recomm Rep 2005;54:1–31.

Schillie S, Murphy TV, Sawyer M, Ly K, Hughes E, Jiles R, et al. CDC guidance for evaluating health-care personnel for hepatitis B virus protection and for administering postexposure management. Centers for Disease Control and Prevention. MMWR Recomm Rep 2013;62:1–19.

104

Screening for Down syndrome

A 32-year-old nulligravid woman comes to your office for initiation of prenatal care at 11 weeks of gestation. She wishes to discuss options for aneuploidy screening. She has no significant medical history other than being a carrier of a balanced 14;21 robertsonian translocation. Given this history, her best option for screening for Down syndrome is

(A) quadruple screening
(B) first-trimester screening
(C) integrated screening
(D) sequential screening
* (E) cell-free DNA screening

Aneuploidy is the most common genetic cause of miscarriage and congenital anomalies. The American College of Obstetricians and Gynecologists (the College) recommends that all pregnant women, regardless of maternal age, be offered an evaluation for aneuploidy by screening or invasive diagnostic testing.

Traditionally, nondiagnostic testing has been in the form of maternal serum markers with or without the use of a fetal nuchal translucency measurement. More recently, the analysis of cell-free DNA contained within maternal plasma has become available to evaluate the risk of fetal aneuploidy. This is the most appropriate screening modality for the described patient. A balanced 14;21 robertsonian translocation is an indication to use cell-free DNA testing. Female carriers of this translocation have a 10–15% risk of Down syndrome with each pregnancy. Patients with elevated risk may be offered diagnostic testing.

Cell-free DNA is DNA that is no longer contained within a cell nucleus and takes the form of small, fragmented pieces. A pregnant woman's plasma contains cell-free DNA from her fetus and the placenta. The cell-free DNA technology capitalizes on this phenomenon to provide risk information for trisomy 21 (Down syndrome) and some other aneuploidies. Cell-free DNA is reliably detectable before the end of the first trimester, with commercial laboratories making this screening available by 10 weeks of gestation.

For high-risk women, cell-free DNA screening has been established as the screening modality with the highest detection rate (approximately 99%) and the lowest false-positive rate (less than 0.5%) for Down syndrome. The College and the Society for Maternal–Fetal Medicine have published a joint Committee Opinion (*Cell-free DNA Screening for Fetal Aneuploidy*) in support of cell-free DNA screening for high-risk women. Women meeting the following criteria are considered to be at high risk of aneuploidy:

- Maternal age 35 years or older at delivery
- Fetal ultrasonographic findings suggestive of an increased risk of aneuploidy
- History of a prior pregnancy with a trisomy
- Increased risk of aneuploidy on traditional maternal serum screening
- Maternal or paternal balanced robertsonian translocation involving chromosome 21 or chromosome 13

At this time, the College, the Society for Maternal–Fetal Medicine, the American College of Medical Genetics and Genomics, and the National Society of Genetic Counselors recommend that cell-free DNA screening not be used for low-risk women. Although the sensitivity and specificity of cell-free DNA screening is similar for all populations of women, the cost-effectiveness of offering this test universally has not been studied extensively.

It is important to understand that although cell-free DNA screening is an advanced screening tool, it is not a diagnostic test. Women who receive a high-risk cell-free DNA screening result should be offered confirmatory diagnostic testing by chorionic villus sampling or amniocentesis. For women with a high-risk test result who decline invasive testing, obtaining a postnatal karyotype would be appropriate.

Although cell-free DNA screening is thought to be the superior screening test for the high-risk population, it has limitations. Unlike traditional maternal serum screening, cell-free DNA screening poses a risk of test failure. If an insufficient amount of cell-free DNA is present, the test will not give a result, a scenario that has been associated with increased aneuploidy risk. Obesity has been correlated with increased rates of low fetal fraction and cell-free DNA screening failure. Therefore, this screening may not be the best option for obese women in the high-risk category.

Traditional maternal serum screening will provide aneuploidy risk information for high-risk women but with decreased detection rates and increased false-positive rates compared with cell-free DNA screening. Because cell-free DNA screening is not recommended for low-risk women, traditional screening is the standard of care in this population. Several traditional screening options exist and are dependent on the gestational age of the fetus and whether specialized ultrasonography is available.

The quadruple screen is performed in the second trimester and measures free β-hCG, alpha fetoprotein, estriol, and inhibin A. The quadruple screen carries an 81% detection rate for Down syndrome with a 5% false-positive rate. First-trimester screening, which combines the serum markers human chorionic gonadotropin and pregnancy-associated plasma protein A with a nuchal translucency measurement, has an 87% detection rate for Down syndrome with a 5% false-positive rate.

When considering traditional screening, the highest detection rates for Down syndrome are obtained through combined screening in the first and second trimesters. Fully integrated screening combines pregnancy-associated plasma protein A and nuchal translucency measurement in the first trimester with the markers of the quadruple screen in the second trimester. This offers a detection rate for Down syndrome of 96%, with a 5% false-positive rate. In integrated screening, a result is produced only after both portions of the screening have been completed. Alternatively, sequential screening, which results in a detection rate for Down syndrome of slightly less than that of integrated screening, reports a first-trimester result as well as a second-trimester result. In this way, patients may pursue diagnostic testing after the first results are obtained instead of waiting until the second trimester for the cumulative result.

Cell-free DNA screening for fetal aneuploidy. Committee Opinion No. 640. American College of Obstetricians and Gynecologists. Obstet Gynecol 2015;126:e31–7.

Malone FD, Canick JA, Ball RH, Nyberg DA, Comstock CH, Bukowski R, et al. First-trimester or second-trimester screening, or both, for Down's syndrome. N Engl J Med 2005;353:2001–11.

Prenatal aneuploidy screening using cell-free DNA. #36. Society for Maternal-Fetal Medicine. Am J Obstet Gynecol 2015;212:711–6.

Swanson A, Sehnert AJ, Bhatt S. Non-invasive prenatal testing: technologies, clinical assays and implementation strategies for women's healthcare practitioners. Curr Genet Med Rep 2013;1:113–21.

105

Adnexal cyst in a postmenopausal woman

A 74-year-old woman who is otherwise healthy is being evaluated for pelvic pain. On examination, an adnexal mass is palpated. The result of the ultrasonography is shown in Figure 105-1 (see color plate). The most appropriate next step in this patient's management is

(A) serum CA 125 level test
(B) magnetic resonance imaging (MRI)
(C) computed tomography (CT) scan
(D) follow-up ultrasonography in 6 months
* (E) referral to gynecologic oncologist

Figure 105-1 shows several features that raise suspicion for ovarian malignancy, including solid components, increased vascularity, ascites, septations, and irregular contours. When suspicion for malignancy is high, the patient will benefit from surgical treatment by a gynecologic oncologist. Studies show higher rates of optimal debulking when the surgery is performed by a gynecologic oncologist, which is positively associated with prolonged survival. If a pelvic mass is detected on examination or with imaging, the presence of elevated CA 125, ascites, nodularity, fixation to the pelvic sidewall or surrounding structures, or evidence of metastasis should lead to a referral to an oncology specialist.

Serum CA 125 is elevated in approximately 80% of cases of ovarian malignancy, so measurement is most useful in monitoring patients after treatment. Its role in screening asymptomatic patients is less defined, and it generally is not recommended for this purpose, given the poor specificity for ovarian malignancy. Even if the CA 125 level is normal in the described patient, referral to a gynecologic oncologist is still appropriate because of the suspicion for malignancy based on the characteristics shown on ultrasonography.

Adnexal cysts that can be managed safely in an expectant fashion include those that display benign characteristics (eg, unilocular, smaller than 10 cm, no ascites). Studies have demonstrated that such adnexal cysts are rarely malignant and do not require surgical management. Ultrasonography is virtually always the imaging modality of choice in characterizing adnexal lesions because of its availability, low cost, and lack of radiation.

Data from large-scale ovarian screening trials demonstrate that ovarian cysts or enlargements are common in postmenopausal women. In the Prostate, Lung, Colorectal, and Ovarian Cancer Screening Trial, the prevalence of adnexal cysts in this age group was 14%, and if initial screening ultrasonography was negative, the incidence of new adnexal cysts detected on subsequent examination was 8%. Even with some complex features, more than one half of ovarian masses will resolve spontaneously within 2 months.

Additional imaging modalities in the evaluation of pelvic pathology include MRI and CT scans, although such imaging scans are rarely necessary to establish a diagnosis. In the identification of nodal metastases or diaphragmatic involvement, CT scans can be helpful and may offer some predictive value in assessing the likelihood of suboptimal debulking of ovarian malignancies. Frequently, a CT scan is the imaging test first obtained in a symptomatic patient with abdominal or pelvic pain and with findings reported as suspicious for malignancy. Pelvic ultrasonography then is performed to provide clearer imaging of the mass. Ovarian cancer is staged surgically, so neither a CT nor an MRI scan is required for staging. However, gynecologic oncologists frequently order CT or MRI scans for surgical planning in patients with suspected ovarian malignancy.

The MRI scan provides some advantages over the CT scan in the evaluation of ultrasonographically indeterminate tumors. Tissue characteristics that can be differentiated with MRI can help clarify whether a tumor possesses features associated with being benign. This is especially true in premenopausal women, who are at significantly lower risk of ovarian malignancy than postmenopausal women. An MRI scan also can be helpful in the evaluation of predominantly or completely solid tumors. The chief benefit of MRI is its improved specificity compared with ultrasonography. Additionally, MRI may be helpful in visualizing a normal ovary that may not be seen with ultrasonography secondary to overlying bowel or other adnexal pathology. Because of its expense, MRI should be reserved for the unusual cases of indeterminate ultrasonographic findings.

Iyer VR, Lee SI. MRI, CT, and PET/CT for ovarian cancer detection and adnexal lesion characterization. AJR Am J Roentgenol 2010;194: 311–21.

Rauh-Hain JA, Melamed A, Buskwofie A, Schorge JO. Adnexal mass in the postmenopausal patient. Clin Obstet Gynecol 2015;58:53–65.

The role of the obstetrician-gynecologist in the early detection of epithelial ovarian cancer. Committee Opinion No. 477. American College of Obstetricians and Gynecologists. Obstet Gynecol 2011;117:742–6.

106

Gestational hypertension

A 19-year-old nulligravid woman at 34 weeks of gestation comes to your clinic for a prenatal visit. Her blood pressure (BP) to this point has been in the range of 100–110 mm Hg (systolic) over 60–70 mm Hg (diastolic). She is experiencing normal fetal movements and reports no health issues; her BP at this visit is 146/93 mm Hg. Physical examination is otherwise unremarkable. Fetal heart rate is 140 beats per minute. Urine dipstick is negative for protein. Estimated fetal weight is 2,288 g (43rd percentile). She returns 3 days later for another prenatal visit, at which time her BP is 150/92 mm Hg. A 24-hour urine collection result shows 100 mg of protein in the urine. Platelets are 202,000/mm^3. Serum alanine aminotransferase is 20 units/L. Serum aspartate aminotransferase is 23 units/L. The most appropriate next step in management is

(A) corticosteroids
(B) magnesium sulfate
(C) oral labetalol
* (D) continued expectant management

Hypertensive disorders affect 5–10% of all pregnancies in the United States. Worldwide, 60,000 maternal deaths are attributed to preeclampsia. Despite improvements in obstetric care, the incidence of preeclampsia in the United States has increased by 25% during the past two decades. The etiology of preeclampsia is still unknown, as is a means of preventing the condition. In 2013, the American College of Obstetricians and Gynecologists published *Hypertension in Pregnancy*, which classified hypertension during pregnancy into four categories: 1) preeclampsia–eclampsia, 2) chronic hypertension (of any cause), 3) chronic hypertension with superimposed preeclampsia, and 4) gestational hypertension.

Hypertension is defined as either a systolic BP of 140 mm Hg or more or a diastolic BP of 90 mm Hg or more. In order to diagnose hypertension, these BP values should be present on two separate occasions at least 4 hours apart. Blood pressure reaches the severe range when the systolic BP is 160 mm Hg or more or the diastolic BP is 110 mm Hg or more. If the BP increases to these values, the diagnosis of hypertension can be confirmed within a shorter interval to facilitate timely antihypertensive therapy. Women with severe hypertension require antihypertensive therapy. Intravenous labetalol and hydralazine are first-line medications in this situation. If a woman does not have intravenous access, oral nifedipine may be used.

Preeclampsia–eclampsia is defined as hypertensive disease that is specific to pregnancy. Almost always, it occurs after 20 weeks of gestation. Preeclampsia is defined by new-onset hypertension with new-onset proteinuria. Alternatively, if proteinuria is absent, preeclampsia is diagnosed if any of the following is noted: thrombocytopenia (platelets less than 100,000/microliter), liver transaminases that are twice the normal limit, serum creatinine greater than 1.1 mg/dL or a doubling of serum creatinine, pulmonary edema, or new-onset cerebral symptoms such as blurred vision or severe headache (Box 106-1). Preeclampsia may be classified as either preeclampsia without severe features or preeclampsia with severe features.

Chronic hypertension is defined as elevated BP noted either before pregnancy or before 20 weeks of gestation. Because most women who become pregnant are young and relatively healthy, they may not have had a recent physical examination, and hypertension may have gone undetected for some time. Therefore, if elevated BP is appreciated early in pregnancy, chronic hypertension should be diagnosed, and the risks of superimposed preeclampsia should be discussed thoroughly with the patient. Women with chronic hypertension have a fourfold increased risk of preeclampsia. Because of preexisting hypertension, diagnosing preeclampsia in these patients tends to be more difficult. In a patient with chronic hypertension, superimposed preeclampsia is likely to be the diagnosis if one of the following occurs: a sudden exacerbation of hypertension; a sudden onset of symptoms such as severe headache, visual changes, or epigastric pain; thrombocytopenia, pulmonary edema, or new-onset renal insufficiency; or marked increases in proteinuria. The BP goal for a pregnant woman who has chronic hypertension is 120–160 mm Hg over 80–105 mm Hg. Labetalol, nifedipine, or methyldopa are appropriate first-line agents used to maintain BP within these parameters.

Gestational hypertension is defined as elevated BP that occurs after 20 weeks of gestation in the absence of proteinuria. *Proteinuria* is defined as the presence of protein in the urine measuring 300 mg/dL or greater over

BOX 106-1

Severe Features of Preeclampsia (Any of These Findings)

- Systolic blood pressure of 160 mm Hg or higher or diastolic blood pressure of 110 mm Hg or higher on two occasions at least 4 hours apart while the patient is on bed rest (unless antihypertensive therapy is initiated before this time)
- Thrombocytopenia (platelet count less than 100,000/microliter)
- Impaired liver function as indicated by abnormally elevated blood concentrations of liver enzymes (to twice normal concentration), severe persistent right upper quadrant or epigastric pain unresponsive to medication and not accounted for by alternative diagnoses, or both
- Progressive renal insufficiency (serum creatinine concentration greater than 1.1 mg/dL or a doubling of the serum creatinine concentration in the absence of other renal disease)
- Pulmonary edema
- New-onset cerebral or visual disturbances

Hypertension in pregnancy. Report of the American College of Obstetricians and Gynecologists' Task Force on Hypertension in Pregnancy. Obstet Gynecol 2013; 122:1122–31.

a 24-hour period. Recently, the protein-to-creatinine ratio has been used as an alternative method of diagnosing proteinuria. The advantage of this test is that it requires only a single random specimen. The protein-to-creatinine ratio is consistent with proteinuria if it is 0.3 or more. Typically, gestational hypertension occurs near term. The described patient was normotensive until 34 weeks of gestation. Because of her elevated BP and a lack of proteinuria or other findings that would lead to a diagnosis of preeclampsia, her clinical presentation is consistent with gestational hypertension. For management of gestational hypertension, antihypertensive therapy should not be administered. No evidence exists that antihypertensive therapy decreases the risk of progression to preeclampsia or improves overall maternal or neonatal outcomes. Treatment with antihypertensive medications for nonsevere gestational hypertension may compromise blood flow to the fetoplacental unit and lead to intrauterine growth restriction. Furthermore, treatment with antihypertensive medication for gestational hypertension may delay recognition of preeclampsia.

Corticosteroids may be administered in a patient at less than 34 weeks of gestation who is likely to deliver within the next 7 days. Because the described patient is beyond this gestational age, corticosteroids are not indicated. Magnesium sulfate is only administered to patients who have preeclampsia with severe features. Because this patient has gestational hypertension, continued expectant management is appropriate with close surveillance for the progression to preeclampsia. This includes at least weekly prenatal visits, testing for proteinuria, education on preeclampsia symptoms, and weekly antenatal testing. Women with mild gestational hypertension should give birth at 37 weeks of gestation.

Abalos E, Duley L, Steyn DW. Antihypertensive drug therapy for mild to moderate hypertension during pregnancy. Cochrane Database of Systematic Reviews 2014, Issue 2. Art. No.: CD002252. DOI: 10.1002/14651858.CD002252.pub3.

Brown CM, Garovic VD. Mechanisms and management of hypertension in pregnant women. Curr Hypertens Rep 2011;13:338–46.

Emergent therapy for acute-onset, severe hypertension during pregnancy and the postpartum period. Committee Opinion No. 623. American College of Obstetricians and Gynecologists. Obstet Gynecol 2015;125:521–5.

Hypertension in pregnancy. Report of the American College of Obstetricians and Gynecologists' Task Force on Hypertension in Pregnancy. Obstet Gynecol 2013;122:1122–31.

Redman CW. Hypertension in pregnancy: the NICE guidelines. Heart 2011;97:1967–9.

107

Hirsutism in a patient with polycystic ovary syndrome

A 26-year-old nulligravid woman comes to your office for her annual well-woman examination. She requests your advice on bothersome hair growth on her lip and chin that she has been waxing for several years. She does not feel that the hair growth is getting worse but says the waxing is aggravating her acne. She is sexually active and occasionally uses condoms. She menstruates spontaneously every 60–90 days and does not experience bothersome symptoms. She is 1.68 m (66 in.) tall and weighs 89 kg (198 lb); her body mass index (calculated as weight in kilograms divided by height in meters squared [kg/m^2]) is 32. On examination, she has moderate acne and a Ferriman–Gallwey score of 5. Breast and pelvic examination are unremarkable. Her thyroid-stimulating hormone level is 2.0 mIU/L, prolactin level is 10 ng/mL, morning 17α-hydroxyprogesterone level is 1 ng/mL, and total testosterone level is 100 ng/dL. For initial management, you recommend

(A) reassurance
(B) metformin hydrochloride
(C) finasteride
* (D) combination hormonal contraceptive
(E) spironolactone

Polycystic ovary syndrome (PCOS) is a constellation of disorders that includes hyperandrogenism, ovulatory dysfunction, and polycystic ovaries. Clinical manifestations of PCOS include menstrual irregularities, infertility, hirsutism, and acne. The condition is associated with metabolic disorders, including diabetes mellitus and cardiovascular disease. It is a clinical diagnosis, and various criteria have been proposed. The most broadly recognized diagnostic scheme for PCOS is the Rotterdam criteria, which requires that at least two of the three criteria of androgen excess, ovulatory dysfunction, and polycystic ovaries are present on ultrasound evaluation and that other endocrine disorders are excluded (Appendix C).

Hirsutism is observed in 5–15% of the general population, and PCOS is the most common cause. It is present in 65–75% of patients with PCOS. It is less common in Asian populations and tends to be more severe in patients with central obesity. Presence of hirsutism does not fully predict ovulatory dysfunction but may be predictive of metabolic comorbidities or infertility. The described patient meets the criteria for PCOS based on a menstrual history suggestive of ovulatory dysfunction and clinical hyperandrogenism.

Combination hormonal contraception, in oral, transdermal, or vaginal ring form, is recommended by the American College of Obstetricians and Gynecologists and the Endocrine Society for first-line management of menstrual abnormalities and hirsutism or acne in patients who have been diagnosed with PCOS, assuming no contraindications to hormonal contraception. Progestins in hormonal contraceptives suppress luteinizing hormone levels and, thus, ovarian androgen production, whereas estrogen increases sex hormone–binding globulin, thereby reducing bioavailable androgen. Some progestins have antiandrogenic properties, but there are no randomized controlled trials to support the superiority of one hormonal contraceptive formulation over another, nor of oral versus parenteral delivery, in patients with PCOS.

Reassurance is not appropriate for this patient because she reports that her hirsutism is bothersome. The Ferriman–Gallwey score is an objective scoring system for hirsutism. However, its clinical use is limited because most patients use some form of cosmetic hair removal before seeking medical treatment for hirsutism and because it does not account for ethnic differences. Treatment should be offered based on the degree to which the hirsutism bothers the patient rather than based on the Ferriman–Gallwey score or other objective measures.

Women with PCOS are at increased risk of impaired glucose tolerance and type 2 diabetes mellitus. Metformin is recommended as second-line therapy in women with PCOS and type 2 diabetes or impaired glucose tolerance for whom lifestyle modifications are insufficient and for women with menstrual irregularities who cannot take hormonal contraceptives. Insulin-lowering drugs such as metformin and thiazolidinediones can decrease hyperandrogenemia. However, their place in treating hirsutism in the absence of menstrual or metabolic disorders is controversial.

Antiandrogen therapy is not appropriate for the described patient because she is not using reliable contraception and there is the potential for teratogenic feminization of a male fetus. Antiandrogens may be added to hormonal contraceptives in patients with a suboptimal response after 6 months. It takes 6 months to see a clinical response to pharmacologic treatment of hirsutism because that is the life cycle of the terminal hair follicles. In the meantime, although new hair growth may be halted by treatment, current growth must be managed by hair removal methods. Antiandrogens may be used as monotherapy only in patients who use another reliable form of contraception. Spironolactone is an aldosterone antagonist and exhibits dose-dependent competitive inhibition of androgen receptors as well as inhibition of 5α-reductase. It is well tolerated and has been shown in placebo-controlled trials to decrease hirsutism as measured by Ferriman–Gallwey scores. Adverse effects include menstrual irregularities, hyperkalemia, diuresis, and postural hypotension. Finasteride is a 5α-reductase inhibitor that also has shown efficacy in treatment of hirsutism, but it is not first-line therapy and needs to be used with reliable contraception. Combination therapy with hormonal contraceptives and finasteride or spironolactone may be more effective than monotherapy with hormonal contraceptives.

Legro RS, Arslanian SA, Ehrmann DA, Hoeger KM, Murad MH, Pasquali R, et al. Diagnosis and treatment of polycystic ovary syndrome: an Endocrine Society clinical practice guideline. Endocrine Society. J Clin Endocrinol Metab 2013;98:4565–92.

Martin KA, Chang RJ, Ehrmann DA, Ibanez L, Lobo RA, Rosenfield RL, et al. Evaluation and treatment of hirsutism in premenopausal women: an endocrine society clinical practice guideline. J Clin Endocrinol Metab 2008;93:1105–20.

Polycystic ovary syndrome. ACOG Practice Bulletin No. 108. American College of Obstetricians and Gynecologists. Obstet Gynecol 2009;114:936–49.

Swiglo BA, Cosma M, Flynn DN, Kurtz DM, Labella ML, Mullan RJ, et al. Clinical review: Antiandrogens for the treatment of hirsutism: a systematic review and metaanalyses of randomized controlled trials. J Clin Endocrinol Metab 2008;93:1153–60.

108

Painful bladder syndrome

A 43-year-old woman visits your office with a 3-month history of suprapubic pain and pressure symptoms, which she relates to bladder filling. She also has symptoms of urgency, which usually are relieved with bladder emptying. She has frequency up to 10 times a day but has neither dysuria nor incontinence. She has experienced several episodes of exacerbated symptoms lasting 2–3 days that have precluded her from being able to go to work. She has not noticed any correlation of these episodes to her menstrual cycles. The diagnostic test that is most important in the initial evaluation of this patient is

(A) pelvic ultrasonography
* (B) urinalysis with culture
(C) potassium sensitivity test
(D) cystoscopy
(E) urodynamic testing

The symptoms in the described patient are most consistent with painful bladder syndrome (also known as interstitial cystitis), which is a chronic and often debilitating condition characterized by chronic bladder pain. With an unknown etiology and symptoms that are nonspecific, painful bladder syndrome is often a diagnosis of exclusion (Box 108-1).

Painful bladder syndrome is more common in patients aged 40 years and older. It can manifest as a single symptom (eg, urgency, frequency, pain, pressure, dysuria, nocturia) or a constellation of lower urinary tract symptoms, which can intensify or flare up for several hours, days, or weeks. The hallmark symptom is pain (pressure) in the suprapubic or pelvic region that increases with bladder filling. The pain can extend to the lower abdomen, back, and pelvic floor muscles and frequently is lessened with bladder emptying.

Because approximately two thirds of patients who have painful bladder syndrome report dyspareunia and approximately one third experience an exacerbation of pain either premenstrually or with menses, it is important to consider endometriosis of the bladder. Pain may be aggravated by specific foods or drinks, such as caffeine, alcohol, or citrus foods. For this reason, a food and drink diary can

BOX 108-1

Conditions That Are Important to Exclude When Considering a Diagnosis of Painful Bladder Syndrome

Urinary tract infection
Endometriosis
Adnexal masses
Pelvic organ prolapse
Suburethral diverticulum
Sexually transmitted infections
Carcinoma or carcinoma in situ of bladder wall
Tuberculosis
Renal/bladder stones

be helpful. The pain can be debilitating and result in loss of work, sleep deprivation, sexual dysfunction, and depression, along with an overall poor quality of life. Patients with prior pelvic surgery (eg, hysterectomy) or pelvic trauma have a higher incidence of painful bladder syndrome. The syndrome affects more than 1 million U.S. women and frequently coexists with other conditions such as fibromyalgia, irritable bowel syndrome, chronic fatigue syndrome, vulvodynia, depression, and anxiety.

The American Urological Association published clinical guidelines in 2014 for the diagnosis and treatment of painful bladder syndrome. One of the main components of patient evaluation is to exclude other conditions or causes of pain (Box 108-1). A history documenting symptoms for at least 6 weeks and exploration of triggers and alleviators is important, as is a physical examination of the abdomen and pelvis. Pain during palpation of the bladder or the pelvic floor muscles may be present.

An initial evaluation with negative urine dipstick, normal microscopic analysis, and urine culture with documented negative bacterial growth is the first diagnostic step to eliminate acute or chronic infection as an etiology. Cytology should be considered if hematuria is present or if the patient has risk factors for carcinoma, such as smoking. Cystoscopy and pelvic ultrasonography are considered when an alternative diagnosis is suspected but are not necessary for diagnosis in women with uncomplicated presentations. Urodynamic testing may be helpful for presentations complicated by incontinence, pelvic organ prolapse, or other medical conditions that might predispose patients to neurologic disorders. The potassium sensitivity test is not diagnostic, causes pain, and does not alter the management plan.

After assessment and exclusion of other conditions, management depends on severity, symptoms, and patient quality of life (Fig. 108-1). Conservative therapy, such as dietary adjustment, pelvic floor relaxation techniques, bladder retraining, stress reduction, and over-the-counter analgesics are considered first-line therapy.

Inadequate symptom control may require oral or intravesical treatments and further evaluation. Cystoscopy under anesthesia may reveal Hunner ulcers, and hydrodistention may demonstrate petechiae, glomerulations, or terminal hematuria. Oral pentosan polysulfate sodium is approved by the U.S. Food and Drug Administration for painful bladder syndrome, but symptom control takes months, and this drug is only helpful in approximately one third of patients. There is less evidence to support use of nonsteroidal analgesics, antihistamines, amitriptyline, and anticholinergics. One other treatment that has been approved by the U.S. Food and Drug Administration is the intravesical instillation of dimethyl sulfoxide.

Referral to a specialist is important if the symptoms do not improve. Studies are ongoing for treatment with percutaneous nerve stimulation, sacral neuromodulation, and botulinum toxin. Surgery is reserved for patients who have inadequate improvement after standard management.

Hanno PM, Erickson D, Moldwin R, Faraday MM. Diagnosis and treatment of interstitial cystitis/bladder pain syndrome: AUA guideline amendment. American Urological Association. J Urol 2015;193: 1545–53.

Lentz GM, Fialkow MF. Lower urinary tract disorders: update [online only]. Clin Update Womens Health Care 2014;1–15.

Lentz GM, Fialkow MF. Lower urinary tract disorders. Clin Update Womens Health Care 2008;VII (4):1–65.

Quillin RB, Erickson DR. Management of interstitial cystitis/bladder pain syndrome: a urology perspective. Urol Clin North Am 2012; 39:389–96.

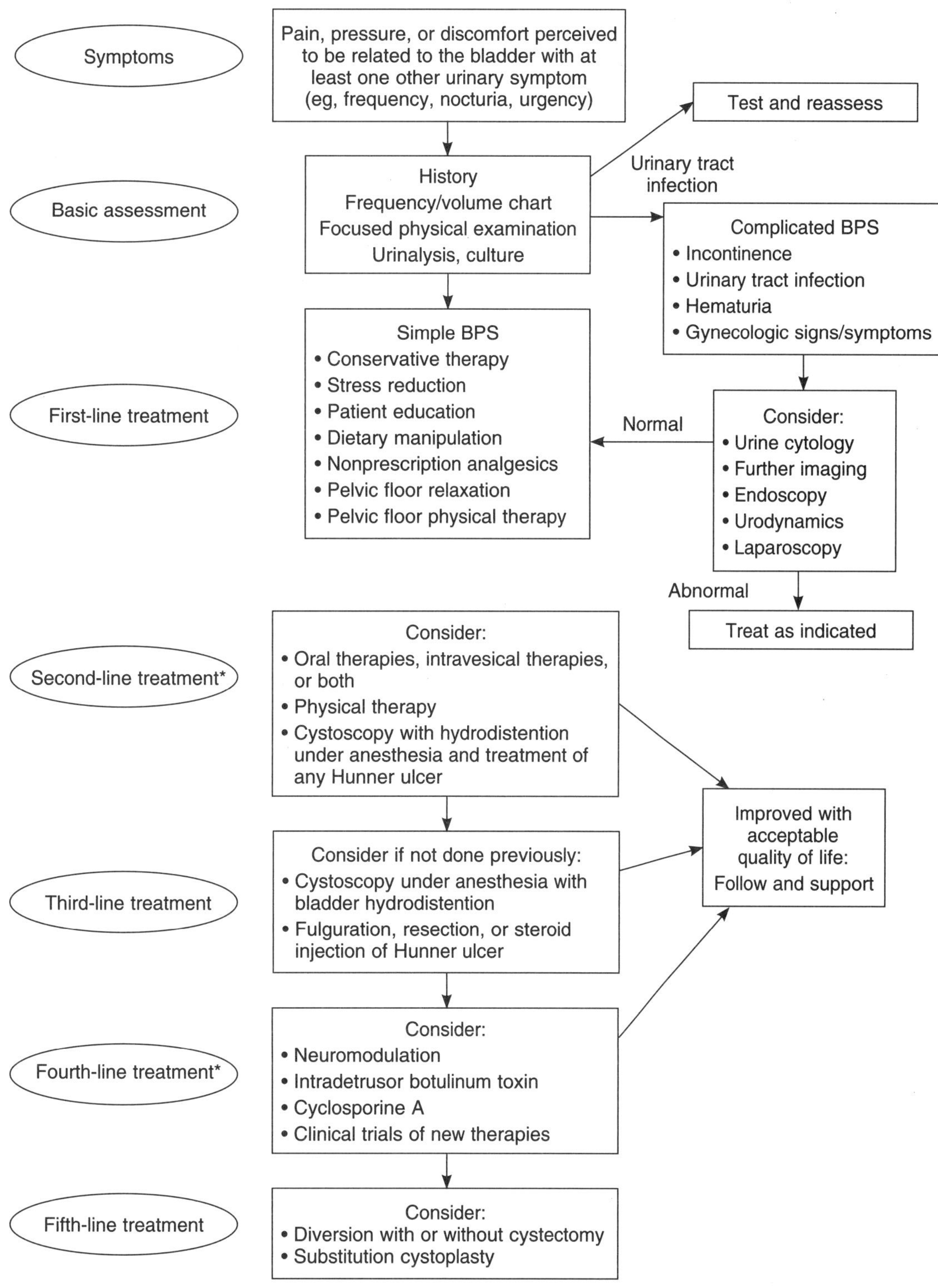

FIGURE 108-1. Bladder pain syndrome. Abbreviation: BPS, bladder pain syndrome. *No hierarchy implied for these treatments. Pain management is a primary consideration at every step of algorithm. Patient enrollment in appropriate research trial is reasonable option at any point. Evidence supporting neuromodulation, cyclosporine A, and botulinum toxin for painful bladder syndrome indication is limited. These interventions are appropriate only for practitioners with experience treating painful bladder syndrome and willing to provide long-term care postintervention. Algorithm is courtesy of the International Consultation on Incontinence committee members and the International Consultation on Urologic Disease. (Hanno P, Dinis P, Lin A, Nickel C, Nording J, van Ophoven A, et al. Algorithm for Diagnosis and Treatment of Bladder Pain Syndrome; International Consultation on Incontinence [2012], p. 133–4.)

109

Maternal grieving after stillbirth

A 37-year-old woman, gravida 1, is seen in the obstetric triage unit at your hospital for decreased fetal movements, and she is diagnosed with an intrauterine fetal demise at 37 weeks of gestation. She is admitted to the labor floor and undergoes labor induction; she has a vaginal delivery 18 hours later without complications. You discharge her home from the hospital with a plan for follow-up in your office in 3–4 weeks. She returns to your office in 1 week and reports feeling emotionally flat, not crying, and being preoccupied with thoughts of the baby. She states that she sometimes hears the baby cry in the nursery. The most appropriate diagnosis is

(A) adjustment disorder
(B) postpartum depression
* (C) normal grief
(D) unipolar depression
(E) psychotic depression

Stillbirth complicates 1 in 160 deliveries in the United States. High levels of distress are part of the normal grieving process after a fetal death; the cyclical nature of grief may be compounded by feelings of guilt, blame, and fear of recurrence. Perinatal grief after stillbirth can be as intense as other kinds of grief, including the loss of first-degree relatives. Some parents may develop mental health problems, but most will not. Support given to grieving parents is variable across institutions and obstetrician–gynecologists or other health care providers. Interventions such as referral to peer support groups, bereavement counselors, psychologic counseling, and short-term medication use are common, but there is little high-quality evidence about the most effective interventions to support parents in the period after a perinatal loss.

Grief can be seen as a normal response to an abnormal event, and the process of accepting the loss takes time. Grief symptoms tend to peak in the first 6–12 months, although they may last as long as 2 years. Normal grief response can include temporary impairment of day-to-day function, retreat from social activities, intrusive thoughts, and feelings of yearning and numbness. The persistence of those symptoms and prolonged dysfunction are indicative of complicated or traumatic grief that requires intervention. Obstetrician–gynecologists and other health care providers need to counsel the patient and her family about what to expect in the weeks and months after a stillbirth.

Adjustment disorder is a short-term condition in which an individual has a more severe response than would be expected after a stressful event. This disorder, also called stress response syndrome, occurs within 3 months of the triggering event. The emotional or behavioral symptoms cannot be considered normal bereavement, and the patient cannot meet the diagnostic criteria of major depression or generalized anxiety disorder. The diagnosis of adjustment disorder is made based on a patient's functioning rather than her symptoms, which may vary in severity over time. The described patient's symptoms are within the range of expected responses after perinatal loss, so she does not fit the criteria for adjustment disorder.

The *Diagnostic and Statistical Manual of Mental Disorders*, Fifth Edition, defines the *postpartum period* as the first 4 weeks after giving birth, although other definitions range from 3 months to 12 months. Features of postpartum depression are similar to those of major depressive disorder and include changes in sleep, energy, appetite, and weight; anxiety and panic attacks; irritability and anger; and feelings of inadequacy, being overwhelmed, shame, and guilt. These symptoms need to be interpreted within the context of what is normal in the immediate postpartum period when caring for an infant, although stillbirth and neonatal death are known risk factors for development of postpartum depression. Although the described patient is at risk of developing postpartum depression, she is still in the acute phase of grief and bereavement, and her symptoms do not warrant the clinical diagnosis of depression. Commonly used instruments to screen for postpartum depression, such as the Edinburgh Postnatal Depression Scale, have not been validated in the first 2 weeks postpartum or in women experiencing pregnancy loss (see Appendix B).

The diagnosis of unipolar depression, also called major depressive disorder or clinical depression, is made by the presence of five or more symptoms over at least a 2-week period that cause clinically significant stress or impairment in daily functioning. These symptoms can include depressed mood; diminished interest in or pleasure from daily activities; significant weight change; sleep disturbances; fatigue; feelings of worthlessness or guilt; diminished ability to concentrate or indecisiveness; and recurrent thoughts of death or suicide. Response to a significant loss such as bereavement may include many of these symptoms, or a major depressive episode may coexist with normal bereavement. Given that this patient's symptoms have been present for 1 week, she does not meet the criteria for unipolar depression at this time.

Unipolar major depression with psychotic features, or psychotic depression, is a severe subtype marked by the presence of delusions, hallucinations (usually auditory), or both that are consistent with the depressive features of guilt and worthlessness. The described patient is aware that what she is feeling and hearing is not normal; in fact, it is common after pregnancy loss to hear the sounds of a baby crying. Because the patient's symptoms are within the expected experiences in the time after an acute loss, they do not warrant a diagnosis of depression with psychotic features. The most appropriate diagnosis is, therefore, that she is experiencing normal grief.

American Psychiatric Association. Diagnostic and statistical manual of mental disorders: DSM-5. 5th ed. Washington, DC: APA; 2013.

Flenady V, Boyle F, Koopmans L, Wilson T, Stones W, Cacciatore J. Meeting the needs of parents after a stillbirth or neonatal death. BJOG 2014;121(suppl):137–40.

Kersting A, Wagner B. Complicated grief after perinatal loss. Dialogues Clin Neurosci 2012;14:187–94.

Management of stillbirth. ACOG Practice Bulletin No. 102. American College of Obstetricians and Gynecologists. Obstet Gynecol 2009;113:748–61.

Robinson GE. Pregnancy loss. Best Pract Res Clin Obstet Gynaecol 2014;28:169–78.

110

Abnormal uterine bleeding

A 32-year-old woman, gravida 2, para 2, has a 6-month history of heavy but regular menstrual bleeding. She is healthy and takes no medications. She and her spouse use condoms and wish to attempt pregnancy next year. Her body mass index (calculated as weight in kilograms divided by height in meters squared [kg/m^2]) is 24. She has a normal-appearing parous cervix; a 9-week-sized mobile, multinodular, nontender uterus; and no adnexal masses on examination. Her hemoglobin level is 10.1 g/dL, and a urine pregnancy test is negative. Cervical cytology and human papillomavirus test results are negative. The best next step to evaluate her bleeding is

(A) pelvic ultrasonography
(B) endometrial biopsy
(C) hysteroscopy
* (D) sonohysterography

The subjective concern of heavy menstrual bleeding results from a perception of increased volume, duration of menstrual flow, or both. Quantification of blood loss by pad or tampon count or duration of flow is imprecise. Structural lesions, such as adenomyosis, uterine polyps, endometrial hyperplasia, and submucosal leiomyomas, are the most common causes of abnormal uterine bleeding in nonpregnant women.

Intracavitary uterine pathology is identified in as many as 40% of nonpregnant women with abnormal uterine bleeding. Coagulopathy, ovulatory dysfunction, and medication or botanical exposure are examples of nonstructural lesions that may be associated with heavy cyclic vaginal bleeding. The finding of a multinodular uterus on examination should lead to a consideration of leiomyomas as a cause of heavy bleeding in this patient.

Pelvic ultrasonography is the recommended imaging study for women with abnormal uterine bleeding and abnormal physical findings. Although standard transvaginal ultrasonography detects most leiomyomas, the uterine distention by sterile saline during sonohysterography provides more accurate information regarding the size, location, and characteristics of all types of intracavitary lesions than pelvic ultrasonography. Studies have shown sonohysterography to have similar or improved diagnostic accuracy compared with hysteroscopy. Furthermore, sonohysterography facilitates the visualization of leiomyoma characteristics, such as size, location, depth, and width (Fig. 110-1).

Submucosal leiomyomas are associated with decreased pregnancy rates, and their removal has been shown to improve fertility. The identification and classification of potential submucosal leiomyomas are important considerations in this patient because she desires fertility. Data obtained from sonohysterography may be used for surgical planning. The test is easy to perform in the

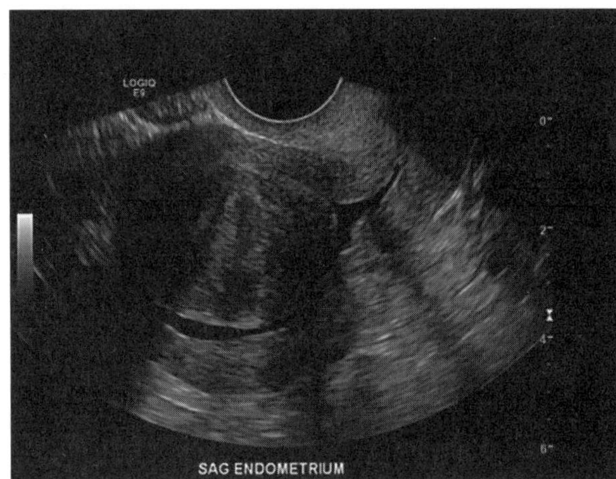

FIGURE 110-1. Transverse endometrium. Courtesy of Laurie Swaim, MD.

ambulatory setting and requires no special preparation. Sonohysterography provides an opportunity to directly biopsy a suspicious lesion if one is identified. Office hysteroscopy is costly, requires the use of specialized instruments, and has been associated with more pain than sonohysterography. Important information regarding leiomyoma depth cannot be determined reliably with office hysteroscopy.

An endometrial biopsy is not indicated for this patient, who is at low risk of endometrial hyperplasia and carcinoma. Sonohysterography is the most efficient diagnostic modality for determining the cause of heavy bleeding in the described patient.

Alborzi S, Parsanezhad ME, Mahmoodian N, Alborzi S, Alborzi M. Sonohysterography versus transvaginal sonography for screening of patients with abnormal uterine bleeding. Int J Gynaecol Obstet 2007;96:20–3.

Kelekci S, Kaya E, Alan M, Alan Y, Bilge U, Mollamahmutoglu L. Comparison of transvaginal sonography, saline infusion sonography, and office hysteroscopy in reproductive-aged women with or without abnormal uterine bleeding. Fertil Steril 2005;84:682–6.

Livingstone M, Fraser IS. Mechanisms of abnormal uterine bleeding. Hum Reprod Update 2002;8:60–7.

Ludwin A, Ludwin I, Banas T, Knafel A, Miedzyblocki M, Basta A. Diagnostic accuracy of sonohysterography, hysterosalpingography and diagnostic hysteroscopy in diagnosis of arcuate, septate and bicornuate uterus. J Obstet Gynaecol Res 2011;37:178–86.

Management of acute abnormal uterine bleeding in nonpregnant reproductive-aged women. Committee Opinion No. 557. American College of Obstetricians and Gynecologists. Obstet Gynecol 2013;121: 891–6.

van Dongen H, de Kroon CD, Jacobi CE, Trimbos JB, Jansen FW. Diagnostic hysteroscopy in abnormal uterine bleeding: a systematic review and meta-analysis. BJOG 2007;114:664–75.

111

Chronic bronchitis

A 43-year-old woman, gravida 2, para 2, with no history of prior lung disease or medical problems, presents with a history of dyspnea on exertion, wheezing, and intermittent cough productive of yellow sputum. Her symptoms have been present for the past 3 months, and she reports similar symptoms every winter. She has not traveled or had sick contacts recently, nor has she experienced any fever or constitutional symptoms. Her medical history is notable for a 20-pack-per-year smoking history. Her only medication is a multivitamin. On examination, she appears well, with a temperature of 37°C (98.6°F), pulse of 72 beats per minute, and respiratory rate of 18 breaths per minute; oxygen saturation is 98% on room air. On auscultation of the lungs, you hear no crackles or rales but appreciate scattered wheezes throughout the lung fields bilaterally. The most appropriate intervention for her at this time is

(A) smoking cessation
* (B) β_2-agonist
(C) antibiotic
(D) cough suppressant
(E) corticosteroid

Cough is one of the most common presenting concerns for which patients in the United States seek medical care and can be further categorized as acute or chronic based on duration of symptoms. Acute bronchitis is a clinical term that describes the self-limited inflammation of the large airways of the lung and is characterized by cough without associated pneumonia. Cough related to acute bronchitis typically persists for 10–20 days but can last for 4 weeks or more. This is in contrast to *chronic bronchitis*, which is defined by the presence of a cough productive of sputum on most days of the month for at least 3 months in duration in each of 2 consecutive years and in the absence of other cardiac or pulmonary etiologies.

Approximately 8.7 million adults are diagnosed with chronic bronchitis each year. The condition is characterized by chronic inflammation of the bronchial airways that results in excessive mucous production and subsequent cough with no requirement of airflow obstruction. Although airway obstruction is not a clinical feature of chronic bronchitis, if left untreated, chronic bronchitis can evolve into chronic obstructive bronchitis, which is characterized by progressive and irreversible airway obstruction.

Chronic obstructive pulmonary disease (COPD) is defined as a common preventable and treatable disease characterized by airflow limitation that often is progressive and associated with a heightened chronic inflammatory response in the lungs and airways after exposure to noxious stimuli. Earlier definitions of COPD have emphasized the different clinical variants of chronic bronchitis, asthma, and emphysema. Asthma typically differs significantly from COPD in its pathogenic and therapeutic response; however, some patients exhibit poor reversibility of symptoms and cannot easily be distinguished from patients with COPD. *Emphysema* is defined pathologically as the presence of permanently enlarged airspaces distal to the terminal bronchioles and is accompanied by destruction of the bronchial walls without obvious fibrosis. Although current definitions of COPD no longer include these clinical distinctions, it is important to note that patients can have symptoms that progress across the clinical spectrum, and there often is significant overlap between each individual clinical entity.

The described patient has symptoms consistent with chronic bronchitis. Smoking cessation is the intervention that has the greatest ability to influence the natural history of COPD and is appropriately a central component of the treatment of chronic bronchitis. Elimination of smoking will result in resolution of cough for 50% of patients within the first month of therapy and almost 100% of patients in the first year after smoking cessation. Although smoking cessation should be recommended for this patient, given her current symptoms of dyspnea and the presence of audible wheezes on examination, smoking cessation alone will not address her symptoms adequately.

The Centers for Disease Control and Prevention and the American College of Clinical Pharmacy recommend macrolide antibiotics as first-line therapy for cough related to pertussis and for pneumonia caused by *Mycoplasma pneumoniae*. However, the primary role of antibiotic therapy in the treatment of COPD and its clinical variants remains unclear. Although antibiotic therapy with azithromycin may reduce COPD exacerbation rates, there is an unfavorable balance between benefits and adverse effects. Additionally, concern remains regarding the growing rates of antibiotic resistance due to widespread overuse. Presently, the routine use of antibiotic therapy for chronic bronchitis or other exacerbations of COPD is not recommended unless a bacterial infection is suspected. The described patient has no signs or symptoms concerning for a bacterial infection; thus, primary treatment with azithromycin is not indicated at this time.

Cough suppressants are effective for short-term therapy and are a useful adjunct to smoking cessation, but their role as a primary treatment modality has not been well studied. The described patient probably would benefit from antitussive therapy; however, a cough suppressant alone, such as dextromethorphan, would not address her wheezing or dyspnea adequately. Pharmacologic therapy for COPD is useful for symptom reduction, decreasing the frequency and severity of exacerbations, and to improve overall health status and exercise tolerance.

Available evidence suggests that inhaled corticosteroids decrease exacerbations and progression of respiratory symptoms seen in COPD but do not appear to significantly improve lung function and mortality. Additionally, inhaled corticosteroid use is indicated as part of a combined regimen and should not be used as sole therapy without a long-acting bronchodilator. The described patient currently is not using bronchodilator therapy, so primary use of an inhaled corticosteroid is not indicated.

The most appropriate intervention for this patient with chronic bronchitis would be a short-acting bronchodilator such as a β_2-agonist. β_2-agonists have been shown to improve symptoms as well as overall lung function and would adequately address the patient's symptoms of dyspnea and wheezing. Additionally, the short-term use of bronchodilator therapy will decrease bronchospasm and assist in alleviation of her cough.

Anderson B, Brown H, Bruhl E, Bryant K, Burres H, Conner K, et al. Diagnosis and management of chronic obstructive pulmonary disease (COPD): Health care guideline. 10th ed. Bloomington (MN): Institute for Clinical Systems Improvement; 2016. Available at: https://www.icsi.org/_asset/yw83gh/COPD.pdf. Retrieved June 20, 2016.

Balkissoon R, Lommatzsch S, Carolan B, Make B. Chronic obstructive pulmonary disease: a concise overview. Med Clin N Am 2011;95:1125–41.

Barnes PJ. Chronic obstructive pulmonary disease. N Engl J Med 2000;343:269–80.

Braman SS. Chronic cough due to acute bronchitis. ACCP evidence-based clinical practice guidelines. CHEST 2006;129:958–1038.

Global Initiative for Chronic Obstructive Lung Disease. Global strategy for the diagnosis, management, and prevention of chronic obstructive pulmonary disease. Global Initiative for Chronic Obstructive Lung Disease: 2016. Available at: http://goldcopd.org/. Retrieved June 20, 2016.

Kim V, Criner GJ. The chronic bronchitis phenotype in chronic obstructive pulmonary disease: features and implications. Curr Opin Pulm Med 2015;21:133–41.

112

Opioid overuse and abuse

A 33-year-old woman, gravida 2, para 2, comes to your office for a 1-week postoperative visit after a laparoscopic tubal ligation. The procedure was uncomplicated. Per your routine, you sent her home with high-dose ibuprofen and 20 narcotic tablets. However, she reports ongoing pain and has called your office to request refills. You request that she come into your office to be seen. She reports no bleeding or fever, and on physical examination all of your findings are reassuring. As you review her electronic chart, you see that her primary care provider gave her a prescription for narcotics less than 1 month ago for back pain after a fall and the orthopedist who repaired a finger fracture filled the same prescription 2 weeks earlier. After using electronic resources to investigate all possible prescription sources, the most appropriate next step is to

(A) refer her to a pain specialist
(B) refill her narcotic prescription
(C) prescribe a stronger narcotic
* (D) counsel her regarding narcotic abuse
(E) offer a benzodiazepine

Use of prescription pain medications has increased significantly over the past decade, with sales of opioid pain relievers quadrupling between 1990 and 2010. The number of deaths from prescription drug overdoses continues to rise (Fig. 112-1). Although people report getting prescription pain medication from friends and relatives (given, sold, and stolen), drug dealers, and the Internet, 18% of opioid pain relievers diverted for nonmedical use were obtained directly from a physician. This growing and excessive nonmedical use of prescription pain medication resulted in more than 1 million emergency department visits in 2009, a 98% increase from 2004.

This increased overuse of prescription pain medication overlaps with another public health problem that gynecologists frequently encounter: chronic pain. Chronic pain is a major public health problem that is estimated to affect up to 75 million Americans with significant economic, social, and medical costs. Severe physical pain can affect all aspects of a person's life, impairing his or her ability to function successfully at work, as a member of a family, or even with daily life activities. Such impairment can lead to secondary problems such as depression, social isolation, and low self-esteem. The office gynecologist is challenged with managing chronic pelvic pain safely and appropriately and with being mindful of the increasing epidemic of nonmedical use of prescription pain medication.

The described patient does not have a clear indication for ongoing narcotic use. She underwent a simple procedure over 1 week ago for which most patients do not require narcotics. She has had numerous prescription pain relievers filled over the past month, suggesting medication misuse or abuse or an undiagnosed chronic pain condition. Thus, the most beneficial intervention at this time would be to talk with her regarding your concerns about her pain medication abuse. Before having this conversation, it also may be beneficial to access a state prescription drug monitoring program, if available. Prescription drug monitoring programs are statewide electronic databases that collect data on all substances dispensed in the state. They are operated at the state level, outside of the federal Drug Enforcement Agency but often with interstate sharing of information, with the goal of providing information about prescription drug abuse, addiction, and diversion. Accessing these records before a conversation with the patient can give additional information regarding the scope of her problem.

Prescribing anything at this point—whether it is a refill of the medication she is currently taking, a stronger medication, or a different class of medication—will not address the issue at hand. She needs to hear that an obstetrician–gynecologist or other health care provider is concerned about her medication use. Some studies suggest that only one half of patients with substance abuse report their physicians ever discussing the issue with them. Although the U.S. Preventive Services Task Force has found insufficient evidence to recommend routine screening for substance abuse (besides tobacco and alcohol), addressing signs of medication abuse when they present is imperative. Pregnancy presents a high-risk time when routine screening is recommended and appropriate.

Although referral to a pain specialist may benefit this patient, the first step should be a frank conversation. However, if it is determined that she has a pain condition that merits ongoing management with medication, other adjunctive measures, such a referral,

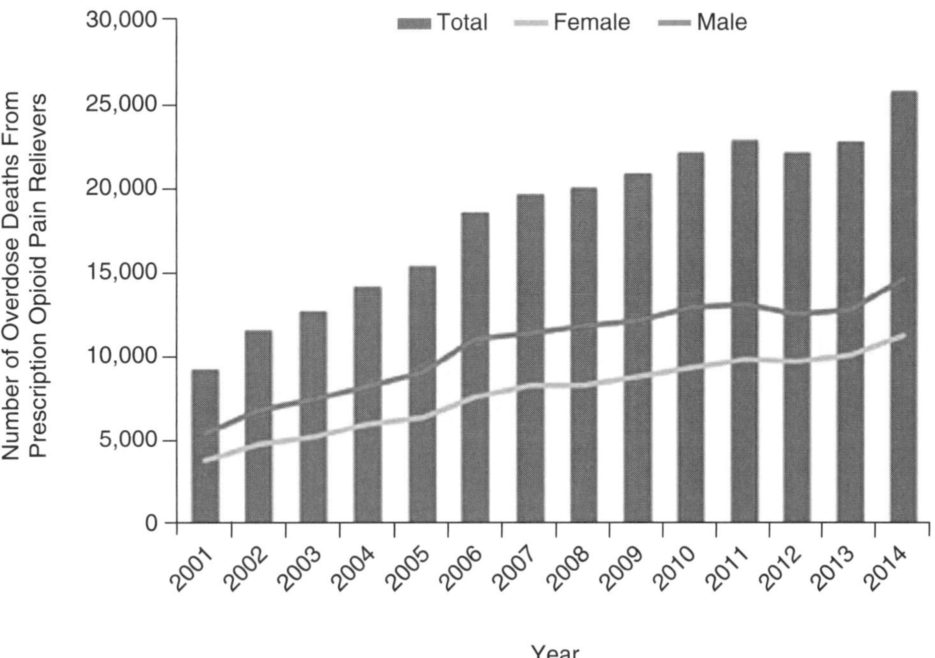

FIGURE 112-1. National overdose deaths—number of deaths from prescription opioid pain relievers. The bar chart shows the total number of U.S. overdose deaths involving opioid pain relievers from 2001 to 2014. The chart is overlayed by a line graph showing the number of deaths by females and males. From 2001 to 2014 there was a 3.4-fold increase in the total number of deaths. (National Institute on Drug Abuse. Overdose death rates. Bethesda (MD): NIDA; 2015. Available at: https://www.drugabuse.gov/related-topics/trends-statistics/overdose-death-rates. Retrieved June 16, 2016.)

may be useful. Many primary care providers, including obstetrician–gynecologists, do not feel skilled in managing chronic pain conditions or the associated medication use. Pain specialists often are more skilled than the general practitioner in understanding the different modalities aside from narcotics (eg, acupuncture, relaxation training, and physical therapy) that exist for managing chronic pain. However, primary care providers often serve the role as care coordinators for patients with complex pain syndromes and may be designated as the prescriber of narcotics to minimize the chance of medication abuse and interactions. Thus, all gynecologists need to have a general understanding of the signs of prescription pain medication misuse and abuse and the resources that exist for them and their patients.

Manubay JM, Muchow C, Sullivan MA. Prescription drug abuse: epidemiology, regulatory issues, chronic pain management with narcotic analgesics. Prim Care 2011;38:71,90, vi.

Opioid abuse, dependence, and addiction in pregnancy. Committee Opinion No. 524. American College of Obstetricians and Gynecologists. Obstet Gynecol 2012;119:1070–6.

Shapiro B, Coffa D, McCance-Katz EF. A primary care approach to substance misuse. Am Fam Physician 2013;88:113–21.

113

Mammography in the elderly patient

A 76-year-old woman comes to your office because of burning with urination. She is otherwise in good health, and her only medication is a low-dose antihypertensive agent. She reports no abnormal Pap test results. All of her mammographic and colon screening results have been negative. Her last mammography was 2 years ago. In addition to evaluating her urinary concern, you also counsel her about breast screening. Your recommendation for breast surveillance for this patient should be

* (A) annual mammography
(B) twice annual clinical breast examination
(C) monthly breast self-examination
(D) breast ultrasonography
(E) discontinue breast surveillance

There is no universal consensus about the role of mammography in elderly women. No mammographic screening trials and few treatment trials enrolled women older than 74 years. Therefore, the decision about screening for a woman in this age group should be based on informed discussion between the patient and her physician. Relevant statistics include the fact that for women younger than 65 years, the incidence of breast cancer is approximately 83 per 100,000, and for those aged 65 years or older, the incidence is 421 per 100,000. Mortality from breast cancer is 11 per 100,000 in women younger than 65 years and 99 per 100,000 in women 65 years and older.

Points that deserve consideration include life expectancy for the patient, risk of a false-positive mammography result, and risk of identifying cancer that would otherwise not be lethal to the patient. As in younger women, the most meaningful measure in making a decision about the benefits of mammography is whether this continued screening will lower the risk of breast cancer mortality. The American College of Obstetricians and Gynecologists, the National Comprehensive Cancer Network, and the American Cancer Society each espouse individualizing the decision to continue mammographic screening past age 75 years. The U.S. Preventive Services Task Force offers no recommendation for continuing or stopping screening in this age group but does note that the harm associated with mammography increases dramatically after age 75 years.

The risk of developing breast cancer is higher in every decile of life through the eighth decade and peaks between ages 75 years and 79 years. Most breast cancer risk models (eg, the Gail model) are not designed for women in this age group and demonstrate little predictive ability. Reduced life expectancy because of aging lowers the likelihood of dying from asymptomatic screen-detected breast cancer. Many classic risk factors for developing breast cancer are more relevant in younger age groups. Current use of hormone therapy (estrogen plus progestin) increases the incidence of breast cancer in this age group, but the effect decreases after cessation of therapy. Most women in their 70s do not use hormone therapy.

Despite these caveats, it is reasonable to offer the option of continued mammographic screening to women in whom life expectancy is believed to be 10 years or more. Medicare continues to pay for annual mammography with no defined age-related endpoint. Some observational studies show survival of breast cancer in this age cohort is longer with screen-detected cancer than with clinically detected cancer. Statistical modeling has demonstrated that mammographic screening after age 70 years probably would result in 2 per 1,000 fewer deaths from breast cancer. Cost-effectiveness also has been predicted with biennial mammography if life expectancy is 9.5 years or more. In the United States, 50% of women aged 80 years are expected to live an additional 10 years or more.

Data from the Surveillance, Epidemiology, and End Results Program reveal that most elderly women who are diagnosed with breast cancer were not being screened with mammography. Less than one half of women older than 70 years who were diagnosed with breast cancer were current on mammography, and approximately one quarter of them had not had mammography in the preceding 5 years.

There is no evidence to support increased clinical examination as a method for early breast cancer detection in this age group. Although the cost of such an examination is less than that of mammography, studies in younger women demonstrate a higher false-positive rate, leading to more biopsies than mammography alone.

Ultrasonography is not recommended as a breast cancer screening tool in women of any age group. Its utility is in assisting with guided biopsies or to clarify findings from other imaging. There also is a trend to move away from teaching breast self-examination across all populations.

For the otherwise healthy woman older than 70 years, continued annual mammographic screening appears justified if predicted life expectancy is at least another 10 years and if the patient is counseled about the caveats of detecting non-life-threatening disease.

Breast cancer screening. Practice Bulletin No. 122. American College of Obstetricians Gynecologists. Obstet Gynecol 2011;118:372–82.

Vacek PM, Skelly JM. A prospective study of the use and effects of screening mammography in women aged 70 and older. J Am Geriatr Soc 2015;63:1–7.

Vyas A, Madhavan S, Sambamoorthi U. Association between persistence with mammography screening and stage at diagnosis among elderly women diagnosed with breast cancer. Breast Cancer Res Treat 2014;148:645–54.

Walter LC, Schonberg MA. Screening mammography in older women: a review. JAMA 2014;311:1336–47.

114

Early pregnancy loss

A 24-year-old woman, gravida 1, para 0, visits your office after ultrasonography revealed an intrauterine fetal demise at 8 weeks of gestation. After options counseling, she elects for medical management. You prescribe vaginal misoprostol. She returns to your office in 1 week and reports heavy bleeding with passage of tissue after misoprostol use. Her bleeding is now mild to moderate, and her cramping has abated. On vaginal examination, her cervix is closed and her uterus is the size of a 7-week gestation and is nontender. Transvaginal ultrasonography shows an endometrial stripe measuring 22 mm and absence of a gestational sac. The best next step in management is to

(A) perform a suction curettage
(B) schedule repeat ultrasonography
* (C) continue to observe
(D) repeat the dose of misoprostol
(E) order a serum β-hCG test

Early pregnancy loss occurs in approximately 10–15% of clinically recognized pregnancies and will affect one in four women during their lifetime. *Early pregnancy loss* is defined as a nonviable, intrauterine pregnancy with either an empty gestational sac (anembryonic gestation) or with a fetal pole with no heartbeat before 13 weeks of gestation. Women who experience early pregnancy loss should be counseled that serious complications are rare for any form of management, whether expectant, medical, or surgical.

Benefits of medical management of early pregnancy loss include the ability to avoid surgery and anesthesia, the perception that medical treatment is a more natural process, the ability of patients to assume more control, and additional privacy. It is superior to expectant management in avoidance of a suction curettage and is about 85% effective overall. Studies have repeatedly shown high patient acceptability of medical management. Patients need to be counseled that adverse effects such as nausea, vomiting, diarrhea, and fever are common and self-limited. Vaginal bleeding may be initially heavy and last up to 2 weeks, and cramping may require analgesics for the first 2–3 days after misoprostol administration.

Completion of the procedure frequently is defined by ultrasonography, patient symptoms, or both. Although there is no consensus, the most commonly used method is ultrasonography performed 7–14 days after misoprostol; a complete abortion is confirmed by findings of an absent gestational sac and an endometrial thickness measuring less than 30 mm. There is no evidence that morbidity is increased if a thicker lining is present in asymptomatic women, so surgical intervention is not required in asymptomatic women with a thickened endometrial stripe. For the described patient, there is no need for a suction curettage because she has no signs or symptoms of an incomplete abortion. Similarly, because ultrasonography confirms passage of the gestational sac, there is no need for repeat ultrasonography.

The largest randomized trial conducted in the United States of women with early pregnancy loss showed complete expulsion by day 3 in 71% of women after a single dose of vaginal misoprostol. The success rate increased to 84% after a second dose of misoprostol was administered if needed. Because the described patient is asymptomatic and passed a gestational sac, there is no need to repeat the misoprostol dose. If she had persistent heavy bleeding or pelvic pain or had ultrasonographic evidence of a retained gestational sac, a repeat dose could be an acceptable alternative to suction curettage.

Follow-up approaches with urine pregnancy testing or serial β-hCG testing have not been well studied but may be useful if ultrasonography is not available to confirm complete uterine evacuation. There is no role for routine β-hCG testing in the follow-up of early pregnancy loss if an intrauterine pregnancy had been confirmed previously. The β-hCG level should return to normal in the 4–8 weeks after a pregnancy loss, but there are no guidelines correlating the rate of decrease with the success of uterine evacuation. Even a negative β-hCG test result does not rule out retained products of conception, which may not be hormone producing.

The described patient has symptoms, signs, and findings consistent with a complete abortion. There is no indication for further intervention; observation is sufficient. She can be counseled that she can begin contraception if desired, or she may try to become pregnant. No evidence indicates that patients need to delay pregnancy after an uncomplicated first-trimester pregnancy loss.

Dempsey A, Davis A. Medical management of early pregnancy failure: how to treat and what to expect. Semin Reprod Med 2008;26:401–10.

Early pregnancy loss. Practice Bulletin No. 150. American College of Obstetricians and Gynecologists. Obstet Gynecol 2015;125:1258–67.

Neilson JP, Gyte GM, Hickey M, Vazquez JC, Dou L. Medical treatments for incomplete miscarriage (less than 24 weeks). Cochrane Database of Systematic Reviews 2013, Issue 3. Art. No.:CD007223. DOI: 10.1002/14651858.CD007223.pub2.

115

Eating disorders in pregnancy

A 25-year-old nulligravid woman at 9 weeks of gestation comes to your office for her first prenatal visit. She has a history of anxiety and depression, though she has never been prescribed psychiatric medications. She has a body mass index (calculated as weight in kilograms divided by height in meters squared [kg/m^2]) of 16. She reports no other medical problems, and her mood is appropriate. She has never had suicidal or homicidal ideation. On physical examination, her blood pressure is 80/58 mm Hg, pulse is 54 beats per minute, and her temperature is 36.1°C (97.0°F). Her skin is very dry with lanugo hair, and there are calluses on her knuckles (Russell sign). The initial step in management to achieve optimal weight is

(A) antidepressant medication
* (B) nutritional rehabilitation
(C) aversion therapy
(D) progesterone
(E) whey protein supplementation

Eating disorders affect 1% of women in the United States and include anorexia nervosa, bulimia nervosa, and binge-eating disorder. Such eating disorders are most prevalent in adolescent and young adult women and may be diagnosed during pregnancy because weight gain and dietary habits are closely monitored during this time. Box 115-1 lists gynecologic and other presentations of eating disorders. In addition, the American Psychiatric Association's *Diagnostic and Statistical Manual of Mental Disorders*, Fifth Edition, presents a thorough discussion of criteria for diagnoses of anorexia nervosa (severe caloric restriction resulting in low body weight), bulimia nervosa (binge-eating accompanied by compulsive behaviors, including vomiting, taking laxatives, and fasting, to compensate for the high caloric intake), and binge-eating disorder (recurrent binge-eating episodes for at least 3 months).

The described patient's diagnosis is most consistent with anorexia, given that she has an abnormally low body weight along with typical physical findings of hypotension, bradycardia, and dry skin with lanugo hair. The calluses on her knuckles are due to repeated self-induced vomiting, which may be seen in either anorexia or bulimia. Because women with either anorexia or bulimia may binge eat and purge, it is critical to make the correct diagnosis because management of these eating disorders differs. The main difference between anorexia and bulimia is that women with anorexia are always underweight (body mass index less than 18.5), whereas women with bulimia

BOX 115-1

Common Presentations of Eating Disorders

Gynecologic presentations

- Amenorrhea
- Menstrual irregularity
- Constipation or abdominal pain
- Sexually transmitted infections
- Contraceptive needs
- Pelvic pain
- Atrophic vaginitis
- Breast atrophy

Other presentations

- Depression
- Weakness
- Sports injuries and fractures
- Mouth sores
- Pharyngeal trauma
- Dental caries
- Heartburn
- Chest pain
- Muscle cramps
- Bloody diarrhea
- Bleeding or easy bruising
- Fainting
- Routine medical care

American College of Obstetricians and Gynecologists. Guidelines for women's health care: a resource manual. 4th ed. Washington, DC: American College of Obstetricians and Gynecologists; 2014.

may be of normal weight. Women with anorexia nervosa may have endocrine, cardiovascular, reproductive, or gastrointestinal complications. Patients who become pregnant have a higher rate of complications, including hyperemesis, preeclampsia, and low birth weight. Standard treatment of anorexia nervosa centers on nutritional rehabilitation and counseling. The goal is gradual weight gain and normalization of eating habits. This consists of an appropriate diet to achieve ideal body weight and can be a long-term process. A multidisciplinary team consisting of an obstetrician, a psychiatrist, and a dietitian is important in providing these patients with the best possible pregnancy outcome.

Antidepressants do not constitute first-line treatment for a woman with anorexia but can be considered if the patient does not respond to nutritional rehabilitation. Pharmacotherapy has been associated with an increased risk of adverse effects caused by poor drug absorption, toxicity, and the patient's refusal to take medication. Psychiatric illnesses, specifically mood and anxiety disorders, are encountered more frequently in women who have eating disorders. Along with initial treatment to restore weight and nutrition, treatment of the psychiatric disorder is indicated for acutely ill patients. Because the described patient has never required antidepressant medication and is not experiencing acute depression, antidepressant medication is not necessary at this time.

Aversion therapy simultaneously exposes a patient to a behavior and an unpleasant stimulus. The goal is to associate the behavior and the unpleasant stimulus, which ultimately will stop the untoward behavior. Indications for aversion therapy include alcoholism, drug addiction, and excessive gambling. Aversion therapy is not effective in treating anorexia nervosa.

Progesterone is a steroid hormone that can be used to treat endometrial hyperplasia, dysfunctional uterine bleeding, and progesterone deficiency. It also is used as prophylaxis to reduce the risk of recurrent preterm birth. Anorexia nervosa is not an indication for progesterone therapy.

Whey is composed of albumin, lactose, and various minerals. Whey protein may be used to improve muscle strength, improve athletic performance, supplement a normal diet, provide an alternative to milk, and reverse weight loss. Whey protein is a nutritional supplement and, therefore, does not replace the benefits of whole food. Whey would not be appropriate first-line therapy for the described patient.

American College of Obstetricians and Gynecologists. Eating disorders in adolescents. In: Guidelines for adolescent health care [CD-ROM]. 2nd Ed. Washington, DC: American College of Obstetricians and Gynecologists; 2011. p. 134–47.

American Psychiatric Association. Diagnostic and statistical manual of mental disorders: DSM-5. 5th ed. Washington, DC: APA; 2013.

Attia E, Walsh BT. Behavioral management for anorexia nervosa. N Engl J Med 2009;360:500–6.

Bulik CM, Berkman ND, Brownley KA, Sedway JA, Lohr KN. Anorexia nervosa treatment: a systematic review of randomized controlled trials. Int J Eat Disord 2007;40:310–20.

Koubaa S, Hallstrom T, Lindholm C, Hirschberg AL. Pregnancy and neonatal outcomes in women with eating disorders [published erratum appears in Obstet Gynecol 2008;111:1217]. Obstet Gynecol 2005;105:255–60.

Marshall K. Therapeutic applications of whey protein. Altern Med Rev 2004;9:136–56.

Meehan KG, Loeb KL, Roberto CA, Attia E. Mood change during weight restoration in patients with anorexia nervosa. Int J Eat Disord 2006;39:587–9.

116
Vulvar pain

A 26-year-old woman, gravida 0, visits your office for vulvar pain. She has been sexually active with one male partner for the past 6 months and reports burning pain with intercourse. She has had episodes of painful intercourse with her previous two partners, but the pain has worsened so that it now occurs with every act of intercourse. Her medical history is significant for attention deficit disorder, which is managed with methylphenidate. She has a history of a low-grade squamous intraepithelial lesion, has had a positive test result for human papillomavirus (HPV), and was treated for chlamydial infection as an adolescent. She is using a low-dose combination hormonal oral contraceptive (OC) for birth control. She is frustrated that lubricants have not helped with the pain and is uncertain of what to try next. You counsel her that her pain may be related to her

(A) HPV infection
(B) history of chlamydial infection
* (C) use of combination OCs
(D) use of methylphenidate

Vulvar pain syndromes are classified into two categories: 1) vulvar pain related to a specific disorder or vulvodynia—burning pain, occurring in the absence of relevant visible findings—and 2) a specific, clinically identifiable neurologic disorder. By definition, the etiology and progression of vulvodynia are unknown, and often a series of treatments alone or in combination are required for treatment.

Some vulvovaginal infections may cause vulvar pain. Herpes lesions are associated with acute pain during an outbreak and with postherpetic neuralgia. Frequent candidiasis infections have been implicated in the development of vulvar pain. Infection with low-risk HPV can lead to genital warts. No relationship has been found between high-risk HPV infection and vulvar pain.

Other pelvic diseases may be associated with pelvic pain. Endometriosis is a common cause of deep dyspareunia. Pelvic inflammatory disease is a common sequela of gonorrhea and chlamydial infections. Chlamydial infection alone, however, is not associated with vulvodynia or insertional dyspareunia.

Tricyclic antidepressants and anticonvulsants often are used for treatment of vulvodynia; these medications, as well as medications for comorbid conditions, may lead to their own adverse effects. Both classes of medications may lead to constipation, drowsiness, and stomach pain. However, with the use of methylphenidate, there is no reported association with vulvar pain.

The medication that has shown a possible association with vulvodynia is combination OCs. There is biologic plausibility for this relationship—estrogen may affect sensory discrimination and pain sensitivity as well as alter innervation of estrogen-responsive tissues. Progestin effects on the vaginal epithelium also may contribute to pain. For a patient with vulvodynia who is using OCs, stopping the contraceptive for 3–6 months and assessing for a change in symptoms may be beneficial; if the patient is sexually active, she will need another contraceptive method in the interim.

Arnold LD, Bachmann GA, Rosen R, Kelly S, Rhoads GG. Vulvodynia: characteristics and associations with comorbidities and quality of life. Obstet Gynecol 2006;107:617–24.

Leo RJ. A systematic review of the utility of anticonvulsant pharmacotherapy in the treatment of vulvodynia pain. J Sex Med 2013;10: 2000–8.

Leo RJ, Dewani S. A systematic review of the utility of antidepressant pharmacotherapy in the treatment of vulvodynia pain. J Sex Med 2013;10:2497–505.

Stockdale CK, Lawson HW. 2013 Vulvodynia Guideline update. J Lower Genital Tract Disease 2014;18:93–100.

Vulvodynia. ACOG Committee Opinion No. 345. American College of Obstetricians and Gynecologists. Obstet Gynecol 2006;108:1049–52.

117

Risks of surgery in an obese patient

A 48-year-old woman with uterine leiomyomas has decided to undergo hysterectomy for heavy menstrual bleeding that is unresponsive to medical management. Her body mass index (BMI) (calculated as weight in kilograms divided by height in meters squared [kg/m^2]) is 38.8. She is not hypertensive, is a nonsmoker, and does not have any chronic medical problems. Preoperative complete blood count showed a hemoglobin level of 10.3 g/dL and a serum glucose level of 90 mg/dL. In addition to preoperative antibiotics, the most important intervention to reduce perioperative and postoperative morbidity for this patient is

(A) β-blockers
(B) bowel preparation
* (C) venous thromboembolism prophylaxis
(D) respiratory treatment

The described patient is classified as obese based on her BMI, and as such, she is at increased risk of certain surgical complications compared with normal-weight women (Appendix H). *Obesity* typically is defined as having a BMI greater than 30. There are further classifications of obesity, and this patient is categorized as class II. Despite health risks associated with obesity, most women with less than morbid obesity (class III) will not suffer major surgical or postsurgical complications. Notably, most women who fall into the class I obesity weight category (BMI of 30–34.9) suffer fewer postoperative complications than other women (known as the obesity paradox).

However, obesity at any level has been associated with increased rates of venous thromboembolism in many studies. In a study using data from the National Surgical Quality Improvement Program, the mean BMI was 32 for women who had venous thromboembolism, compared with a BMI of 30 for women who had no venous thromboembolism. The described patient is more likely to experience venous thromboembolism than either cardiac or respiratory morbidities. In addition to thromboprophylaxis, choosing the least invasive surgical approach is associated with a reduction in risk of venous thromboembolism. For this patient with leiomyomas, vaginal hysterectomy may not be feasible, but a laparoscopic approach likely would provide a larger safety margin than would abdominal hysterectomy. Although absence of comorbidities helps reduce the incidence of other surgical complications, venous thromboembolism risk is not eliminated. It is unclear why obesity is an additional risk factor for venous thromboembolism, but it may relate to reduced mobility and venous stagnation.

The most important intervention for this patient, in addition to antibiotics, is venous thromboembolism prophylaxis. The American College of Obstetricians and Gynecologists recommends routine venous thromboembolism prophylaxis using one of several regimens, stratifying the interventions based on the preoperative risk level (Appendix G). Such interventions include sequential compression devices, unfractionated heparin or low-molecular-weight heparin, or both. Preoperative planning for these interventions and counseling the patient about their use should be a standard part of the preoperative visit. Evidence to support when to administer venous thromboembolism prophylaxis is less abundant. Many surgeons are reluctant to start anticoagulation preoperatively because of concerns about intraoperative bleeding. No randomized trials exist in gynecologic patients to determine whether preoperative therapy (at least 2 hours before surgery) or therapy soon after surgery (6 hours postoperatively) is preferable. Until such studies exist, either approach is considered acceptable.

Preoperative treatment with a β-blocker within 1 day or more of surgery has been done in the past because of early studies demonstrating reduction in major cardiac complications. When considering noncardiac surgery, more recent evidence has shown higher rates of overall mortality when β-blockers are used, particularly if started within 1 day of surgery. A large systematic review prepared by the American Heart Association concluded that although there were lower rates of nonfatal myocardial infarction in the treated groups, there were higher rates of stroke, death, hypotension, and bradycardia. The American Heart Association therefore advises against such β-blocker therapy, although it does not make a recommendation regarding β-blockers initiated more than 1 day before surgery. It also should be noted that the types of surgery included in these trials were varied, and only a small percentage were gynecologic.

Mechanical bowel preparation has been used commonly in preoperative intervention for gynecologic surgery, but recent evidence does not support its use. Several randomized trials have been performed examining the role of preoperative bowel preparation in gynecologic and nongynecologic surgery, and the overwhelming preponderance of evidence is against its use. Not only is there poor patient acceptance, but most surgeons indicated that there were no advantages of bowel preparation in terms of clear operative field or reduced surgical infections. Such findings were confirmed specifically in laparoscopic procedures as well as vaginal prolapse surgery.

Respiratory treatment with a β-agonist preoperatively is recommended for individuals with reactive airway disease to reduce postoperative pulmonary infection. Because the described patient has no history of underlying respiratory disease, such an intervention is not indicated.

Arnold A, Aitchison LP, Abbott J. Preoperative mechanical bowel preparation for abdominal, laparoscopic, and vaginal surgery: a systematic review. J Minim Invasive Gynecol 2015;22:737–52.

Barber EL, Neubauer NL, Gossett DR. Risk of venous thromboembolism in abdominal versus minimally invasive hysterectomy for benign conditions. Am J Obstet Gynecol 2015;212:609.e–7.

Chung F, Yegneswaran B, Liao P, Chung SA, Vairavanathan S, Islam S, et al. STOP questionnaire: a tool to screen patients for obstructive sleep apnea. Anesthesiology 2008;108:812–21.

Clarke-Pearson DL, Abaid LN. Prevention of venous thromboembolic events after gynecologic surgery [published erratum appears in Obstet Gynecol 2012;119:872]. Obstet Gynecol 2012;119:155–67.

Gynecologic surgery in the obese woman. Committee Opinion No. 619. American College of Obstetricians and Gynecologists. Obstet Gynecol 2015;125:274–8.

Wijeysundera DN, Duncan D, Nkonde-Price C, Virani SS, Washam JB, Fleischmann KE, et al. Perioperative beta blockade in noncardiac surgery: a systematic review for the 2014 ACC/AHA guideline on perioperative cardiovascular evaluation and management of patients undergoing noncardiac surgery: a report of the American College of Cardiology/American Heart Association Task Force on Practice Guidelines. ACC/AHA Task Force Members. Circulation 2014;130:2246–64.

118

Vaccination in early pregnancy

A 24-year-old woman at 9 weeks of gestation comes to the emergency department with a penetrating injury to the hand that she received from a rusty metal object. She reports that she received all of her required childhood immunizations but does not recall having any "shots" since leaving for college at age 18 years. The emergency department physician has managed the wound but consults you about how to proceed with preventing possible tetanus infection this early in pregnancy. The most appropriate recommendation is

(A) diphtheria and tetanus toxoids and acellular pertussis (DTaP) vaccine
(B) tetanus and diphtheria toxoids (TD) vaccine
* (C) tetanus toxoid, reduced diphtheria toxoid, and acellular pertussis (Tdap) vaccine
(D) tetanus immune globulin

Tetanus toxoid-containing vaccines (eg, TD, Tdap) are recommended for acute wound management if 5 years or more have elapsed since the patient received a tetanus vaccination. The described patient should receive the Tdap vaccine because it will serve not only as her tetanus booster for the new wound but also will provide her and her fetus with protection from pertussis. If Tdap is given for acute wound management early in pregnancy, the patient should not receive an additional dose at 27–36 weeks of gestation. Although several small studies have not demonstrated serious adverse events related to the receipt of Tdap shortly after TD, there is the possibility of a higher chance of a more intense local reaction. It is, therefore, more prudent to give the Tdap vaccine early in gestation than to repeat the TD vaccine at 27 weeks of gestation just to provide the additional protection from pertussis.

Pertussis infection (whooping cough) in newborns younger than 3 months of age is a significant cause of morbidity and mortality. Although infants receive the vaccine starting at 2 months of age, newborns are vulnerable to infection from parents, other family members, caregivers, and any person in direct contact with the newborn. Because of increasing outbreaks of pertussis in the United States and studies that demonstrate a significant waning of immunity with time after immunization, the Advisory Committee on Immunization Practices recommended in 2005 that all adults receive a single adult dose of Tdap, in lieu of a TD booster, every 10 years. Additionally, in an effort to minimize the burden of pertussis disease in newborns, the committee recommended in 2013 that Tdap be administered during each pregnancy, regardless of prior immunization history.

Optimal timing for the Tdap vaccine is between 27 weeks and 36 weeks of gestation, which allows for maximum maternal antibody response and passive antibody transfer to the fetus. Tdap is an inactivated vaccine and has demonstrated safety and efficacy at any time during pregnancy. If not administered during pregnancy, the Tdap vaccine should be given to the woman immediately postpartum in an effort to reduce the risk of transmission to the newborn. Family members and caregivers with planned direct contact with the newborn also should receive the Tdap vaccine at least 2 weeks before contact. This effort, termed "cocooning," provides a protective cocoon of immunity among all those who might have contact with the infant. In spite of this, infants still are vulnerable from birth if exposed to the nonimmunized public and until they acquire immunity when they receive the first series of immunizations.

The difference between the DTaP and Tdap vaccines should be noted: DTaP is the vaccine given to infants and children younger than 7 years and has considerably higher antigen concentration. Therefore, if an adult were to mistakenly receive the DTaP vaccine instead of Tdap, there is a much higher chance of a significant local reaction. This is particularly important in clinics that care for adults and children.

The administration of the inactivated vaccine during pregnancy has proven benefits with no evidence of adverse fetal sequelae. Obstetrician–gynecologists and other health care providers can use a variety of techniques to promote immunization in the office setting (Box 118-1). Tetanus immune globulin is indicated as prophylaxis after injury in a patient whose immunization is incomplete or uncertain. Because this patient reports that she has undergone all required immunizations, she would not be a candidate for tetanus immune globulin.

BOX 118-1

Summary of Techniques Used for Promotion of Immunization in Office Settings

Advocate. Recommend indicated immunizations.

Identify. Use prompts, alerts (paper or electronic), and staff reminders to identify patients with indications.

Educate and Vaccinate. Educate office staff, delegate a vaccine coordinator in the office, use appropriate vaccine information statements, and immunize office obstetrician–gynecologists and other health care providers and staff.

Integrate. Institute standing orders for vaccines, document recommendations, education, and patient choice.

Modified from Integrating immunizations into practice. Committee Opinion No. 661. American College of Obstetricians and Gynecologists. Obstet Gynecol 2016;127:e104–7.

Integrating immunizations into practice. Committee Opinion No. 661. American College of Obstetricians and Gynecologists. Obstet Gynecol 2016;127:e104–7.

Update on immunization and pregnancy: tetanus, diphtheria, and pertussis vaccination. Committee Opinion No. 566. American College of Obstetricians and Gynecologists. Obstet Gynecol 2013;121:1411–4.

Updated recommendations for use of tetanus toxoid, reduced diphtheria toxoid, and acellular pertussis (Tdap) vaccine in adults aged 65 years and older—Advisory Committee on Immunization Practices (ACIP), 2012. Centers for Disease Control and Prevention [published erratum appears in MMWR Morb Mortal Wkly Rep 2012;61:515]. MMWR Morb Mortal Wkly Rep 2012;61:468–70.

Updated recommendations for use of tetanus toxoid, reduced diphtheria toxoid and acellular pertussis (Tdap) vaccine from the Advisory Committee on Immunization Practices, 2010. Centers for Disease Control and Prevention. MMWR Morb Mortal Wkly Rep 2011;60:13–5.

119
Rhinosinusitis

A 21-year-old woman, gravida 1, para 1, experienced the onset of a fever and runny nose 3 days ago. She presents with a temperature of 37.9°C (100.2°F), controlled with acetaminophen. She had associated symptoms of fatigue, headache, postnasal drip, and maxillary pressure that gets worse when she leans over. She has no history of asthma or seasonal allergies. The best next step in management is to

* (A) continue antipyretics and decongestants
(B) obtain a plain film X-ray of the sinuses
(C) obtain a computed tomography (CT) scan of the sinuses
(D) prescribe a course of antibiotics

Acute rhinosinusitis is the infection of the nasal passages and paranasal sinuses. It is a major cause of lost work, a frequent concern in medical offices, and one of the most common diagnoses that prompts a prescription of antibiotics. Most cases of rhinosinusitis are caused by a viral infection, and only approximately 0.5–2% of cases will develop into a bacterial infection. Despite bacterial infection being an uncommon cause of sinusitis, antibiotics are prescribed in approximately 80% of all cases.

The symptoms of viral rhinosinusitis are similar to the symptoms of the common cold and include nasal congestion, purulent nasal discharge, cough, facial pain, pressure exacerbated by leaning forward, headache, fever, and malaise. The nature of the nasal secretions is not discriminatory. During a typical viral infection, the nasal discharge will begin as clear and watery and will become thicker, more mucoid, and purulent after several days, until reverting to clear discharge or simply resolving. The diagnosis of rhinosinusitis typically is made on clinical grounds. Radiologically, acute rhinosinusitis is defined by the complete opacification of the sinuses, by air–fluid levels, or by marked mucosal thickening. Both viral and bacterial sinusitis will demonstrate these findings on plain radiography. Imaging studies (plain film X-ray and CT scan) are nonspecific and do not distinguish between bacterial or viral rhinosinusitis and, therefore, should not be ordered. Imaging may be helpful for recurrent cases of rhinosinusitis, if there is antibiotic failure, or when there is a suspicion of alternative diagnoses (such as malignancy or soft tissue infection); in such cases, a CT scan is the preferred imaging modality. The symptoms of viral rhinosinusitis typically will peak by days 3–5 and resolve in 7–10 days. The addition of antibiotics will not affect the outcome because treatment with antibiotic or placebo similarly result in improvement in 50% of patients by 1 week and 74% at 2 weeks.

The goals of initial therapy are the relief of symptoms through the restoration of normal mucosal environment by humidification, mucolytics, and control of local swelling. Topical decongestants typically are avoided because rebound symptoms after discontinuation are common. Most cases of acute rhinosinusitis are due to viral infections, and antibiotic therapy should be reserved for bacterial sinusitis.

The most common causes of acute bacterial sinusitis are *Streptococcus pneumoniae* and *Haemophilus influenzae*. In some parts of the United States, there is significant bacterial resistance to antibiotics. Signs and symptoms that would suggest a bacterial cause are

- persistence of symptoms beyond 10 days
- severe symptoms (high fever of at least 39°C [102°F], purulent nasal discharge, or facial pain lasting for at least 3–4 consecutive days from the beginning of the illness)
- worsening of symptoms with new onset of fever, headache, or increased discharge initiated by a typical upper respiratory infection that was improving in the initial 5–6 days ("double sickening")

Because of resistance patterns, amoxicillin–clavulanate is the recommended first-line treatment. The fluoroquinolones (levofloxacin and moxifloxacin) have no advantage over the β-lactam antibiotics but may be an appropriate choice for a patient who has a penicillin allergy. Although commonly prescribed, the macrolides (clarithromycin and azithromycin) are not recommended for initial therapy because of high rates of resistance to *S pneumoniae*.

Chow AW, Benninger MS, Brook I, Brozek JL, Goldstein EJ, Hicks LA, et al. IDSA clinical practice guideline for acute bacterial rhinosinusitis in children and adults. Infectious Diseases Society of America. Clin Infect Dis 2012;54:e72–112.

Lemiengre MB, van Driel ML, Merenstein D, Young J, De Sutter AIM. Antibiotics for clinically diagnosed acute rhinosinusitis in adults. Cochrane Database of Systematic Reviews 2012, Issue 10. Art. No.: CD006089. DOI: 10.1002/14651858.CD006089.pub4.

Piccirillo JF. Clinical practice. Acute bacterial sinusitis. N Engl J Med 2004;351:902–10.

120

Safety of breastfeeding in a patient with hepatitis C

A 23-year-old woman, gravida 1, comes to your office for prenatal care at 20 weeks of gestation. She reports a recent history of intravenous (IV) heroin use. She tests positive for the hepatitis C virus (HCV) antibody. Tests for the hepatitis B virus, human immunodeficiency virus (HIV), and syphilis are negative. You counsel her that the greatest risk factor for perinatal transmission of HCV to her offspring would be

* (A) elevated viral load of HCV
(B) HCV genotype 4
(C) the use of a fetal scalp electrode
(D) vaginal birth
(E) breastfeeding

The main risk factors for acquisition of HCV are IV drug use and history of a blood transfusion. With improved screening of blood donors for HCV, the rates of transfusion-related hepatitis have decreased to 1 in 2 million, and the relative number of patients who acquire HCV through IV drug use has increased. The leading cause of childhood HCV is vertical transmission. The rate of HCV seropositivity among pregnant women ranges from 0.6% to 6%, with vertical transmission ranging from 2% to 10%. The greatest risk factors for transmission of HCV are coinfection with HIV and maternal viremia.

Because the described patient is HIV negative, her biggest risk factor for vertical transmission would be an elevated viral load. Elevated alanine aminotransferase is a hallmark of high viral replication and has been demonstrated to be associated with an increased risk of vertical transmission. Hepatitis C genotype has not been shown to influence the risk of vertical transmission. In contrast to hepatitis B virus or HIV, no immunologic or pharmaceutical intervention has been found to decrease the risk of vertical transmission of HCV. New antiviral medications that are under development may affect this risk.

Maternal coinfection with HIV increases the risk of vertical transmission of HCV twofold to fourfold, with transmission rates as high as 44%. One study found increased risk when maternal HCV viral load was above 6 log international units/mL with an odds ratio of 8.3, but the association did not persist with viral load below this level. Many experts recommend cesarean delivery when there is coinfection with HIV and HCV. Risk of vertical transmission of HCV is negligible in the absence of maternal viremia. A number of studies have demonstrated that increased maternal viral load is associated with an increase in the risk of vertical transmission. Viral load of hepatitis C has been shown to peak in the third trimester.

The influence of various obstetric management practices on vertical transmission of HCV has been investigated but to date, no type of management has been shown to reduce transmission. One study showed an increased risk of vertical transmission with the use of internal monitors, whereas a larger study failed to find such an association. Two cohort studies found an association between longer duration of ruptured membranes and increased risk of vertical transmission, with one study finding an odds ratio of 9.3 with greater than 6 hours between rupture of membranes and delivery. In spite of longer duration of membrane rupture with vaginal birth than with scheduled cesarean delivery, the route of delivery has not been shown to affect vertical transmission rates. Therefore, in women who have HCV, cesarean delivery is recommended only for obstetric indications.

Although HCV has been found in breast milk, breastfeeding has not been shown to increase vertical transmission of HCV. A recent in vitro study found that lipases in human milk generate free fatty acids that damage the viral envelope structure, providing a potential mechanism for the lack of transmission of HCV through breastfeeding in spite of its presence in the breast milk.

The absence of a specific intervention to decrease vertical transmission can be used as an argument against prenatal screening. The Centers for Disease Control and Prevention has identified risk factors for which screening for HCV is recommended (Box 120-1). Screening of high-risk individuals during pregnancy can offer the opportunity for counseling and for referral for treatment after delivery.

BOX 120-1

Centers for Disease Control and Prevention Recommendations for Hepatitis C Virus Screening

HCV testing is recommended in an individual who

- was born in 1945–1965
- is currently injecting drugs
- has ever injected drugs, even once
- received clotting factor precipitates produced before 1987
- was ever on long-term hemodialysis
- has a persistently abnormal alanine aminotransferase
- has HIV
- was a prior recipient of a blood transfusion or organ transplant, including a person who was notified that he or she received blood from a donor who later tested positive for HCV or received a transfusion of blood, blood components, or an organ transplant before July 1992
- is a health care, emergency medical, or public safety worker working with needle sticks or sharps or has had mucosal exposures to HCV-positive blood
- was born to an HCV-positive woman

HCV testing is of uncertain benefit in an individual who

- was a recipient of transplanted tissue (corneal, musculoskeletal, skin, ova, sperm)
- used cocaine or other noninjectable illegal drugs
- has a history of tattoos or body piercing
- has a history of multiple sexual partners or sexually transmitted infections
- has long-term sexual partners who are HCV positive

HCV testing is not recommended (in the absence of other risk factors) in

- health care, emergency medical, or public safety workers
- pregnant women
- household contacts of HCV-positive individuals
- the general population

Abbreviations: HCV, hepatitis C virus; HIV, human immunodeficiency virus.

Centers for Disease Control and Prevention. Viral hepatitis - hepatitis C information. Atlanta (GA): CDC; 2015. Available at: http://www.cdc.gov/hepatitis/HCV/guidelinesC.htm. Retrieved June 13, 2016.

Centers for Disease Control and Prevention. Viral hepatitis - hepatitis C information. Atlanta (GA): CDC; 2015. Available at: http://www.cdc.gov/hepatitis/HCV/guidelinesC.htm. Retrieved June 13, 2016.

Cottrell EB, Chou R, Wasson N, Rahman B, Guise JM. Reducing risk for mother-to-infant transmission of hepatitis C virus: a systematic review for the U.S. Preventive Services Task Force. Ann Intern Med 2013;158:109–13.

Pfaender S, Heyden J, Friesland M, Ciesek S, Ejaz A, Steinmann J, et al. Inactivation of hepatitis C virus infectivity by human breast milk. J Infect Dis 2013;208:1943–52.

Tosone G, Maraolo AE, Mascolo S, Palmiero G, Tambaro O, Orlando R. Vertical hepatitis C virus transmission: main questions and answers. World J Hepatol 2014;6:538–48.

Viral hepatitis in pregnancy. ACOG Practice Bulletin No. 86. American College of Obstetricians and Gynecologists. Obstet Gynecol 2007;110:941–56.

Yeung CY, Lee HC, Chan WT, Jiang CB, Chang SW, Chuang CK. Vertical transmission of hepatitis C virus: current knowledge and perspectives. World J Hepatol 2014;6:643–51.

121

Family history of intellectual and developmental disabilities

A 24-year-old nulligravid woman comes to your office for prepregnancy counseling. She reports a brother with developmental delay and a congenital heart malformation, who at age 1 year received a diagnosis of Smith–Lemli–Opitz syndrome, an autosomal recessive condition. No other familial disorders have been reported. You counsel her that her chance of being a carrier of Smith–Lemli–Opitz syndrome is

(A) 25%
(B) 33%
(C) 50%
* (D) 67%
(E) 100%

This patient's family has a member with Smith–Lemli–Opitz syndrome, which is due to deficiency of 7-dehydrocholesterol reductase (*DHCR7*), preventing final conversion of 7-dehydrocholesterol to cholesterol. Although it is a relatively rare disorder, it is one of the most common single-gene disorders leading to intellectual disability and is a condition that is screened for in the California maternal serum screening program. Birth incidence is reported at approximately 1 in 20,000, and the carrier frequency in the general population is 1 in 70.

Because of the described patient's family history, she is at significantly increased risk of being a carrier of Smith–Lemli–Opitz syndrome. Because the condition is autosomal recessive, both of her parents are obligate heterozygotes. If the normal gene is *S* and the mutated gene is *s*, the patient is not affected by Smith–Lemli–Opitz syndrome because it is fully penetrant, meaning all affected individuals have some manifestations (eg, structural anomalies or intellectual disabilities). Therefore, her genotype cannot be *ss*. The other gamete combinations representing unaffected individuals are *SS, Ss*, and *sS*. Thus, the patient has a 2 in 3 chance of being a carrier. This is the carrier risk in any unaffected sibling of an individual with an autosomal recessive condition.

Molecular testing for this disorder is straightforward and readily available. Ideally, the DNA mutations in the affected individual (or carrier parents) are known, which simplifies carrier testing for the described patient. Carrier screening for Smith–Lemli–Opitz syndrome is on many of the expanded carrier screening panels being used clinically. The described patient's partner also has the option of carrier testing. When mutation status is known, prenatal diagnostic testing is available in the form of chorionic villus sampling or amniocentesis. In population screening for Smith–Lemli–Opitz syndrome carriers, the detection rate has been reported as approximately 70% when screening for the most common mutations. If the described patient receives a negative test result for the familial mutation, there is no need to pursue testing of the fetus or of the father. Should the patient be a carrier, the partner's status should be determined, either by mutation screening or sequencing of the *DHCR7* gene.

In many families, a history of developmental delay in some relative may be reported but with no specific disorder known. In such situations, consultation with a genetics professional may be helpful to assess risk stratification. If the affected family members are only or predominantly males, it is appropriate to screen the patient for fragile X syndrome. Fragile X syndrome is an X-linked disorder and, thus, is more likely to be expressed in males, although some females also can be affected. Carrier screening for fragile X syndrome is done by DNA analysis.

Counseling a woman about fragile X carrier testing is more complex than with most other mendelian disorders because of the nature of its inheritance. Fragile X syndrome is a "triplet repeat" disorder, which means the DNA alteration responsible for this condition is an expansion of repeated CGG trinucleotide in the gene. As the number of repeats increases during meiosis across generations, the size may change from a premutation, which is 55–200 repeats, to a full mutation size (more than 200 repeats). When full mutation size is reached, function of the *FMR1* gene is shut down, leading to full fragile X syndrome in males (who have no compensatory second normal X). Females with a full fragile X mutation may have milder but similar manifestations of fragile X syndrome. Women who are premutation carriers also have adverse health effects. Approximately 15–20% of women with a fragile X premutation will have premature ovarian insufficiency. They also may develop a tremor/ataxia syndrome, but it is usually of milder severity than in men with a fragile X premutation. Thus, counseling about determining carrier state carries reproductive and general health considerations.

Other neurologic disorders do not have such clear-cut mendelian inheritance patterns. Additionally, because neurocognitive impairment can be the result of infectious etiologies, prematurity, and other nongenetic causes, providing an accurate counseling figure to other family members about their individual risk is difficult.

Nowaczyk MJ, Irons MB. Smith-Lemli-Opitz syndrome: phenotype, natural history, and epidemiology. Am J Med Genet C Semin Med Genet 2012;160C:250–62.

Willemsen R, Levenga J, Oostra BA. CGG repeat in the *FMR1* gene: size matters. Clin Genet 2011;80:214–25.

122
Skin cancer

You are seeing a 68-year-old white woman who just moved to the area and wants to establish gynecologic care. She reassures you that her health care maintenance screening is all up to date and normal, but you do not have any of her records yet. She is a smoker with no personal or family history of gynecologic or other malignancies. She appears thin and healthy with numerous moles on her face and hands. She reports she is doing well and has no specific concerns. The most important screening assessment you should perform is

* (A) whole-body skin examination
(B) Pap test
(C) fecal occult blood test
(D) thyroid-stimulating hormone level
(E) pelvic examination

Skin cancer is the most common cancer diagnosis in the United States. Most of these cases of skin cancer are basal cell or squamous cell cancer rather than melanoma. Melanoma is the sixth most common type of cancer among white women. The incidence of all types of skin cancer has been growing over the past several decades. Although mortality from other common types of cancer (eg, colorectal, breast, cervical) has decreased over the past several decades, melanoma mortality rates rose throughout that time and have just begun to stabilize.

Prevention strategies for skin cancer include whole-body skin examination; avoiding outdoor exposures during the peak ultraviolet hours of the day (10:00 AM to 3:00 PM); and using sunblock, protective clothing, or both. Reducing rates of sunburn, whether through avoidance of peak ultraviolet hours or through using protective measures, is of prime importance. Sunblock use varies widely in studies, with reports ranging from 7% to 90%. Women are more likely to use sunblock than men, as are those who perceive themselves to be at higher risk of getting skin cancer, such as fair-skinned women and women with blonde or red hair. However, patients who use sunblock may not be doing so effectively, as evidenced by their higher vitamin D levels compared with those who use sun avoidance or protective clothing. These preventive strategies are especially important for those at high risk of skin cancer—ie, patients who are older or fair-skinned or who have atypical moles, a strong family history of melanoma, multiple prior sunburn episodes, or a history of tanning bed use. There are data to support targeted screening for patients at increased risk of melanoma. Given the described patient's numerous risk factors (older than 65 years, fair skin, and numerous moles), she is considered to be at high risk and should undergo a whole-body skin examination. On examination, obstetrician–gynecologists or other health care providers should look at the number and distribution of moles and other pigmented lesions, with focused attention to sun-exposed areas. Lesions can be evaluated using the "ABCDE" approach (Box 122-1). Different characteristics help to distinguish normal moles (nevi) from premalignant (actinic keratosis) and malignant (squamous cell carcinoma, basal cell carcinoma, melanoma) lesions (Fig. 122-1, Fig. 122-2, Fig. 122-3, and Fig. 122-4; see color plates).

The U.S. Preventive Services Task Force found insufficient evidence to recommend for or against routine screening of all patients for skin cancer by using whole-body skin examination to detect skin cancer of any kind. This assessment was based mainly on the lack of data

BOX 122-1

ABCDE Approach to Evaluating Moles

- **A**symmetry: One half of the mole does not match the other half.
- **B**order: The border or edges of the mole are ragged, blurred, or irregular.
- **C**olor: The mole has different colors or it has shades of tan, brown, black, blue, white, or red.
- **D**iameter: The diameter of the mole is larger than the eraser of a pencil.
- **E**volving: The mole appears different from others or is changing in size, color, or shape.

National Institute on Aging. Skin care and aging. Available at: https://www.nia.nih.gov/health/publication/skin-care-and-aging. Retrieved June 16, 2016.

directly linking screening to better health outcomes and on the minimal information regarding primary care providers' ability to perform these examinations adequately. However, since the U.S. Preventive Services Task Force report was issued, some new studies have suggested a potential benefit of screening, especially for melanoma. Thus, this high-risk patient could benefit from a thorough examination.

None of the other screening tests are the most appropriate single test to perform at this time. Cervical cytology screening is not recommended after age 65 years. However, it is reasonable to wait to receive and review her outside records. In-office fecal occult blood testing is no longer recommended for screening. Colonoscopy is the recommended screening tool and should have started at age 50 years in this patient and be repeated every 10 years if results are normal. This patient has no worrisome family history and reports that her screening tests are all up to date. Elderly patients are at increased risk of thyroid dysfunction. However, current recommendations do not support screening of asymptomatic patients. Although many patients expect an annual pelvic examination from their gynecologist, there is increasing, although highly controversial, evidence questioning its benefit in asymptomatic patients. The American College of Obstetricians and Gynecologists endorses an annual pelvic examination. However, if only one screening test can be performed today for this asymptomatic patient with no family history of ovarian cancer, the one from which she would most likely benefit is the whole-body skin examination.

Curiel-Lewandrowski C, Chen SC, Swetter SM. Screening and prevention measures for melanoma: is there a survival advantage? Melanoma Prevention Working Group-Pigmented Skin Lesion Sub-Committee. Curr Oncol Rep 2012;14:458–67.

Habif, TP, editor. Clinical dermatology: a color guide to diagnosis and therapy. 5th ed. London: Elsevier Health Sciences; 2009.

Well-woman visit. Committee Opinion No. 534. American College of Obstetricians and Gynecologists. Obstet Gynecol 2012;120:421–4.

Wolff T, Tai E, Miller T. Screening for skin cancer: an update of the evidence for the U.S. Preventive Services Task Force. Ann Intern Med 2009;150:194–8.

123

Premenstrual disorder

A 21-year-old nulligravid woman visits your office for contraceptive counseling. She is in college and plans to go to graduate school. She tells you that she desires a highly effective method of birth control. She started intermittent fluoxetine 3 months ago for premenstrual symptoms, which has helped her mood lability. She continues to report pelvic cramping, bloating, and fatigue beginning before her menses. The most effective contraceptive method that also will address her physical symptoms is

* (A) continuous combination hormonal contraception
(B) copper intrauterine device (IUD)
(C) depot medroxyprogesterone acetate (DMPA)
(D) contraceptive implant
(E) levonorgestrel IUD

Premenstrual syndrome (PMS) is defined as recurrent moderate psychologic or physical symptoms that occur only during the luteal phase of menses and resolve with menstruation. Up to one third of premenopausal women experience PMS. In premenstrual dysphoric disorder, symptoms are more severe and debilitating and consistently involve affective symptoms that affect the patient's relationships and functioning, socially and at school or work. The American College of Obstetricians and Gynecologists recommends diagnosing PMS based on prospective symptom diaries to confirm that the symptoms occur during the luteal phase. The goal of treatment is symptom relief and often begins with dietary changes, exercise, and stress reduction.

Selective serotonin reuptake inhibitors, taken daily or only during the luteal phase of menstruation, constitute first-line medical therapy for severe PMS or premenstrual dysphoric disorder. Common adverse effects of these medications include nausea, insomnia, headache, and decreased libido. It has been observed that selective serotonin reuptake inhibitors are more effective against the affective symptoms of PMS, and often another medication is indicated for the physical symptoms if nonmedication therapies fail. Nonsteroidal antiinflammatory drugs are effective for dysmenorrhea but not for the treatment of bloating. Conversely, low-dose diuretic agents will treat bloating symptoms but not pain.

The copper IUD is a highly effective, long-acting method of contraception that provides more than 99% protection against pregnancy for up to 10–12 years. Because the copper IUD is a nonhormonal method of birth control, it does not affect the physical symptoms of PMS. However, given that increased cramping is a common adverse effect of the copper IUD, it may worsen the described patient's dysmenorrhea. For these reasons, a copper IUD would not be the first-line contraceptive choice for her.

Depot medroxyprogesterone acetate is another highly effective contraceptive method that does not require frequent adherence by the user. Injections last up to 13 weeks and provide 94% efficacy with typical use. Users of DMPA have up to a 50% chance of amenorrhea after 1 year of use and may experience fewer menstrual cramps. Common adverse effects of DMPA, as with other progestin-only methods of birth control, include headache, bloating, mood changes, and mastalgia. Because DMPA will not address the described patient's current symptoms, it is not the best choice for her.

The contraceptive implant is another long-acting method that is more than 99% effective. The implant is effective for 3 years, and implant users report improvement of dysmenorrhea. There are no specific studies of the effects on PMS symptoms with implant use. The implant works through ovulation suppression, so theoretically it would have some benefit; however, it does not appear to be effective for the nonpain symptoms of PMS, so it would not the best choice for this patient.

The levonorgestrel IUD, like the copper IUD, is a highly effective, long-acting method of contraception. It works locally in the uterus to thicken cervical mucus, inhibit fertilization, and thin the endometrium; the levonorgestrel IUD does not provide consistent ovulation suppression. The levonorgestrel IUD has been shown to improve dysmenorrhea, but it has not been well studied for the other symptoms of PMS. The levonorgestrel IUD may have a role for endometrial protection in conjunction with estrogen patch therapy for PMS. Although the levonorgestrel IUD will provide excellent contraception for the described patient, it may not address her other symptoms.

For this patient with premenstrual pain and bloating, her best choice for contraception is a combination hormonal method, as long as she has no contraindication to estrogen. Ovarian suppression is key for maximum symptom control, and it is best achieved by use of an estrogen–progestin oral contraceptive (OC) or the vaginal ring used in a continuous fashion (without the traditional hormone-free week each month). Two randomized trials have shown that OCs with drospirenone have an indication for treatment of PMS and premenstrual dysphoric disorder, but all combination OCs should help mitigate pelvic pain and possibly bloating. The contraceptive ring was equivalent to an OC in one study for the treatment of physical symptoms of PMS. There are few data on the effectiveness of the contraceptive patch for this purpose.

Allen LM, Lam AC. Premenstrual syndrome and dysmenorrhea in adolescents. Adolesc Med State Art Rev 2012;23:139–63.

Biggs WS, Demuth RH. Premenstrual syndrome and premenstrual dysphoric disorder. Am Fam Physician 2011;84:918–24.

Lopez LM, Kaptein AA, Helmerhorst FM. Oral contraceptives containing drospirenone for premenstrual syndrome. Cochrane Database of Systematic Reviews 2012; Issue 2. Art. No.: CD006586. DOI: 10.1002/14651858.CD006586.pub4.

Noncontraceptive uses of hormonal contraceptives. ACOG Practice Bulletin No. 110. American College of Obstetricians and Gynecologists. Obstet Gynecol 2010;115:206–18.

O'Brien S, Rapkin A, Dennerstein L, Nevatte T. Diagnosis and management of premenstrual disorders. BMJ 2011;342:d2994.

Rapkin AJ, Mikacich JA. Premenstrual dysphoric disorder and severe premenstrual syndrome in adolescents. Paediatr Drugs 2013;15(3): 191–202.

124
Oral health during pregnancy

A 20-year-old nulligravid woman visits your office for her annual well-woman examination. It has been 3 years since she last saw her dentist for a dental cleaning and examination. She rarely brushes her teeth and does not use dental floss. Oral examination is significant for severe inflammation of the gum tissue, halitosis, and tooth mobility. The gingiva is a deep red color, swollen, and bleeds easily, and hard calculus deposits are visible on her teeth (Fig. 124-1; see color plate). She intends to become pregnant this year. You counsel her on the importance of treating her underlying oral health problems before pregnancy because they have been associated with an increase in

(A) hyperemesis gravidarum
* (B) preterm birth
(C) fetal anomalies
(D) spontaneous abortion

The U.S. Surgeon General's report on oral health stressed the importance of maintaining good dental hygiene throughout life. This is especially important for the overall health of reproductive-aged women because poor oral health may have significant effects during pregnancy and could affect the obstetric outcome. The Centers for Disease Control and Prevention's Pregnancy Risk Assessment Monitoring System reports that only 23–43% of pregnant women receive dental care during pregnancy.

Because of the hormonal effects of pregnancy, numerous physiologic changes in the oral cavity can occur. Pregnancy gingivitis is an inflammatory reaction that causes the gingivae to swell and become friable. Bleeding during toothbrushing is common as a result of this inflammation. Pregnancy gingivitis is noted most commonly in the third trimester. A benign gingival lesion such as a pyogenic granuloma is seen in approximately 5% of pregnancies. This is a hyperplastic and vascularized lesion, typically less than 2 cm in size, that results from an inflammatory response to oral pathogens. These benign tumors generally recede in the postpartum period. Occasionally, they need to be removed if they interfere with mastication. Teeth may become more mobile during pregnancy, even in the absence of gum disease, because the increase in estrogen and progesterone causes a loosening of the ligaments and bone (periodontium) that support the teeth. Tooth enamel may become eroded because of increased exposure to gastric acid from vomiting and gastroesophageal reflux. Dental caries is commonly seen during pregnancy for several reasons, including increased acidity of the oral cavity pH, increased intake of sugary snacks and drinks because of cravings, and compromised routine oral health maintenance. If gingivitis is untreated, it can progress to periodontitis. This inflammatory reaction releases bacterial toxins, which destroy gums and lead to bone loss in the jaw. As a result, bacteremia may occur. Approximately 40% of pregnant women have some level of periodontal disease. Risk factors for periodontal disease include African American ethnicity and use of public assistance programs and tobacco.

Because of severe inflammation of the gums, evidence of plaque, calculus, and tooth mobility, the described patient has significant periodontal disease. A study in 1996 demonstrated an association between periodontal disease and preterm birth. Several other studies since then have confirmed this finding. Although the mechanism leading to preterm birth still is being researched, it is postulated that the gram-negative anaerobic bacteria in the periodontal pockets cause bacteremia that indirectly triggers the hepatic acute phase response. This results in production of cytokines, prostaglandins, and interleukins (inflammatory mediators), which can be transported to the placental tissues as well as the uterus and cervix, which may in turn precipitate preterm labor. Elevated levels of such inflammatory markers have been found in the amniotic fluid of women who have periodontitis and preterm birth who were compared with healthy control patients.

Treatment of periodontal disease during pregnancy may not prevent the potential adverse effects to the woman and infant triggered by the bacteremia. Therefore, it is essential that the described patient is counseled on the importance of treating her dental disease before becoming pregnant. Counseling also should include educating women that oral diseases such as dental caries may be transmitted from the woman to her to child by contact with saliva. *Streptococcus mutans* is the bacteria associated with dental caries and may be noted in high levels among women with poor oral health. Transmission typically occurs during normal parenting behavior, such as sharing utensils and drinking cups. Thus, the children of women with significant oral disease are at greater risk of developing dental caries. No consistent evidence exists that periodontal disease increases the risk of hyperemesis gravidarum, fetal anomalies, or spontaneous abortion.

Boggess KA. Maternal oral health in pregnancy. Society for Maternal-Fetal Medicine Publications Committee. Obstet Gynecol 2008;111: 976–86.

Kumar J, Samelson R. Oral health care during pregnancy recommendations for oral health professionals. N Y State Dent J 2009;75:29–33.

Oral health care during pregnancy and through the lifespan. Committee Opinion No. 569. American College of Obstetricians and Gynecologists. Obstet Gynecol 2013;122:417–22.

Silk H, Douglass AB, Douglass JM, Silk L. Oral health during pregnancy. Am Fam Physician 2008;77:1139–44.

125
Primary ovarian insufficiency

A 23-year-old nulligravid woman visits your office with 3 months of amenorrhea. She underwent menarche at age 12 years and had regular menstrual periods until age 18 years, when they became unpredictable. She has no significant past medical history but notes that her mother had early menopause at age 30 years and that her brother has severe intellectual disability. On physical examination, she has normal secondary sexual characteristics, and her pelvic examination is normal. An office urine pregnancy test is negative, and thyroid-stimulating hormone and prolactin levels are normal. Her follicle-stimulating hormone (FSH) level is 98 international units/L. One month later, her repeat FSH level is 92 international units/L, her serum estradiol level is 27 pg/mL, and her karyotype is 46,XX. The most likely etiology of her primary ovarian insufficiency is

(A) Turner mosaic
(B) adrenal antibodies
* (C) fragile X premutation carrier
(D) FSH receptor mutation
(E) Swyer syndrome

Primary ovarian insufficiency is the cessation of menses before age 40 years secondary to the absence of estrogen production by the ovary in the presence of high gonadotropin production by the pituitary gland. Therefore, it is appropriately termed hypergonadotropic hypogonadism and is identical to the physiologic state of menopause but occurs prematurely. In the past, this syndrome was commonly referred to as premature ovarian failure; however, up to 5–10% of women with this diagnosis can spontaneously or intermittently ovulate or else become pregnant, so it is more appropriate to think of the condition as a state of endocrine insufficiency or diminished ovarian reserve. Among all women who have secondary amenorrhea, only 2–10% will be found to have primary ovarian insufficiency.

The described patient has secondary amenorrhea, and the workup appropriately includes medical history and physical examination, a pregnancy test, assessment of thyroid function, and prolactin level. If a progestin withdrawal challenge had been done, the described patient would not have had any bleeding because of her estrogen deficiency state. Her FSH level was assessed and found to be in the postmenopausal range, which confers the diagnosis of hypergonadotropic hypogonadism. Along with repeat FSH level, her serum estradiol is confirmed to be low, and a karyotype was ordered because a common etiology of primary ovarian insufficiency is gonadal dysgenesis. In fact, gonadal dysgenesis, including mosaicism for Turner syndrome, will be found in up to 50% of adolescent women who have primary ovarian insufficiency and in 13% of women younger than 30 years who have a similar presentation. The normal karyotype in the described patient, however, excludes gonadal dysgenesis, including Swyer syndrome, which has a 46,XY karyotype. Other common etiologies for primary ovarian insufficiency are listed in Box 125-1.

At this point in the patient's workup, the most important step is to screen her for a fragile X premutation. After exclusion of gonadal dysgenesis, the next most common genetic abnormality is fragile X syndrome, which is found in up to 6% of women who have primary ovarian insufficiency and a normal karyotype. Fragile X syndrome is the most common cause of hereditary intellectual disability and may be the explanation for her brother's disability. Screening is done with a fragile X permutation (*FMR1*) panel using DNA-based molecular testing. Prenatal and preimplantation genetic diagnosis should be offered to patients who are diagnosed with fragile X syndrome.

In patients who do not have a fragile X premutation, screening should be undertaken for a multiple endocrinopathy. Even though primary ovarian insufficiency may be the result of an autoimmune ovarian process, there is no clinical value to testing for ovarian autoantibodies. Likewise, testing for antimüllerian hormone and inhibin B has not been shown to be clinically useful. It is important, however, to exclude other associated endocrinopathies, the most common of which is autoimmune thyroiditis. Testing with thyroid peroxide antibodies should be done at least every 1–2 years. Adrenal autoantibody levels also should be tested because if positive there is a 50% chance of developing clinical adrenal

BOX 125-1

Common Etiologies for Primary Ovarian Insufficiency

Idiopathic
Chromosomal abnormalities
- Gonadal dysgenesis with or without Turner syndrome
- Premutation in the fragile X mental retardation 1 (*FMR1*) gene for fragile X
- 46,XY karyotype (Swyer syndrome, complete gonadal dysgenesis)
- Trisomy X

Damage from chemotherapy or radiation therapy
Autoimmune multiple endocrinopathies, including ovarian autoantibodies
- Thyroid
- Adrenal
- Parathyroid

Infiltrative or infectious ovarian process
Pelvic surgery
Enzyme deficiencies
Defects in reproductive hormones or their receptors

Modified from Rebar RW. Premature ovarian failure. Obstet Gynecol 2009;113:1355–63.

insufficiency. Other disorders associated with primary ovarian insufficiency include diabetes mellitus, pernicious anemia, myasthenia gravis, rheumatoid arthritis, systemic lupus erythematosus, and dry eye syndrome.

Treatment for this patient should be directed toward restoration of reproductive-age estrogen levels, not just resolution of estrogen deficiency vasomotor symptoms. This is best accomplished with the transdermal delivery of estradiol, which avoids the higher risk of thromboembolic complications associated with oral estrogens. The described patient also would need continuous or cyclical progestin therapy to prevent endometrial neoplasia. Because the ethinyl estradiol in combination oral contraceptives (OCs) is much more potent than estradiol, OCs would not constitute first-line management. Alternatively, OCs would be appropriate if contraception is the goal to preclude a pregnancy in the event that the patient has a spontaneous ovulatory event, which is observed in 5–10% of patients with primary ovarian insufficiency.

It also is important to be cognizant of and address the potential psychologic and social effects of primary ovarian insufficiency not only for the patient but also for her partner (or partners) and family members. Referral to a reproductive endocrinologist should be offered and is essential if the patient wants to explore reproductive potential, which most likely will be by in vitro fertilization with donor oocytes.

Carrier screening for fragile X syndrome. Committee Opinion No. 469. American College of Obstetricians and Gynecologists. Obstet Gynecol 2010;116:1008–10.

Primary ovarian insufficiency in adolescents and young women. Committee Opinion No. 605. American College of Obstetricians and Gynecologists. Obstet Gynecol 2014;124:193–7.

Rebar RW. Premature ovarian failure. Obstet Gynecol 2009;113:1355–63.

126

Transcervical hysteroscopic sterilization

A healthy 35-year-old woman underwent uncomplicated hysteroscopic sterilization 3 months ago. Follow-up hysterosalpingography (HSG) reveals right tubal occlusion and left tubal patency. Both coils are visualized in the anticipated anatomic location. In addition to continuing her current contraceptive method, the best next step in management is

* (A) repeat HSG in 3 months
(B) diagnostic laparoscopy
(C) ultrasonography
(D) hysteroscopy
(E) pelvic magnetic resonance imaging (MRI)

Hysteroscopic sterilization involves the transcervical placement of tubal microinserts. The procedure is quick and effective and may be performed in the ambulatory setting or the traditional operating room. The success of the procedure for the prevention of pregnancy is dependent on fibrosis and resultant occlusion of the fallopian tube. The U.S. Food and Drug Administration recommends postprocedure HSG for confirmation of tubal occlusion after microinsert sterilization. The efficacy of the microinsert system after confirmation of tubal occlusion is greater than 99%.

Microinserts are successfully placed bilaterally during more than 90% of procedures. Inability to visualize the tubal ostia is the most common cause of failed placement. Adherence to postoperative HSG is low; one study showed that only 12% of women returned after microinsert placement at a university clinic. A retrospective review of HSG results from more than 200 women after successful placement of microinserts revealed complete occlusion in 84% at 3 months postprocedure. Of women with tubal patency at 3 months, 94% had tubal occlusion at 6-month follow-up HSG. Therefore, repeating the HSG in 3 months is the best next step for the described patient.

The incidence of tubal perforation after microinsert placement is 1–3%. Nonocclusion of the tubes does not categorically indicate perforation. Intraoperative findings that increase the concern for perforation include failure of retraction of the black positioning marker on the delivery system and the visualization of the coil being "sucked up" into the tube. Tubal perforation also has been described after cases in which coil placement appeared to be uncomplicated.

Diagnostic laparoscopy should be considered in the event of suspected tubal perforation, and the implants should be removed in a timely fashion if perforation has occurred. Because perforation is not suspected, laparoscopy would not be indicated in this patient at this time.

Three-dimensional and two-dimensional ultrasonography have been proposed as methods to determine correct microinsert placement. In more than 600 women, 86% of microinserts were visualized in the correct location, prompting researchers to suggest that the use of ultrasonography could result in diminished need for HSG. European researchers have calculated that postoperative HSG would be required in 14% of women screened with three-dimensional ultrasonography and 27% of those screened with two-dimensional ultrasonography. Nevertheless, in the United States, ultrasonography is not approved by the U.S. Food and Drug Administration as a method to confirm postprocedure tubal occlusion after hysteroscopic sterilization.

The presence of tubal sterilization inserts is not a contraindication to MRI, and the nickel coils have a characteristic appearance on MRI. In the described patient, the location of the coils seems to be appropriate, so MRI evaluation is not necessary. Magnetic resonance imaging has not been evaluated as a method to assess tubal occlusion.

Gerritse MB, Veersema S, Timmermans A, Brolmann HA. Incorrect position of Essure microinserts 3 months after successful bilateral placement. Fertil Steril 2009;91:930.e1–5.

Kaneshiro B, Grimes DA, Lopez LM. Pain management for tubal sterilization by hysteroscopy. Cochrane Database of Systematic Reviews 2012, Issue 8. Art. No.: CD009251. DOI: 10.1002/14651858.CD009251.pub2.

Legendre G, Levaillant JM, Faivre E, Deffieux X, Gervaise A, Fernandez H. 3D ultrasound to assess the position of tubal sterilization microinserts. Hum Reprod 2011;26:2683–9.

Mercier RJ, Zerden ML. Intrauterine anesthesia for gynecologic procedures: a systematic review. Obstet Gynecol 2012;120:669–77.

Savage UK, Masters SJ, Smid MC, Hung YY, Jacobson GF. Hysteroscopic sterilization in a large group practice: experience and effectiveness. Obstet Gynecol 2009;114:1227–31.

Shavell VI, Abdallah ME, Diamond MP, Kmak DC, Berman JM. Post-Essure hysterosalpingography compliance in a clinic population. J Minim Invasive Gynecol 2008;15:431–4.

Thiel J, Suchet I, Tyson N, Price P. Outcomes in the ultrasound follow-up of the Essure micro-insert: complications and proper placement. J Obstet Gynaecol Can 2011;33:134–8.

Thoma V, Chua I, Garbin O, Hummel M, Wattiez A. Tubal perforation by ESSURE microinsert. J Minim Invasive Gynecol 2006;13:161–3.

127

Cytology screening in adolescents

A 17-year-old nulligravid adolescent girl comes to your office for her first gynecologic visit. She asks for sexually transmitted infection (STI) screening and a Pap test. She has been sexually active with one male partner for the past year and has been intermittently using condoms. She has not yet completed the human papillomavirus (HPV) vaccination series. Her medical history is significant for congenitally acquired human immunodeficiency virus (HIV) infection and a history of chlamydial infection from a previous partner. Her family history is significant for cervical dysplasia treated by cone biopsy in her mother. You counsel her that the reason cytologic screening is indicated for her is her

(A) incomplete HPV vaccination series
(B) history of chlamydia
(C) maternal history of cervical dysplasia
* (D) HIV-positive status
(E) unprotected sexual activity

Cervical cancer screening holds different risk–benefit considerations for women at different ages, as reflected in age-specific screening recommendations. In line with the guidelines from the American Society for Colposcopy and Cervical Pathology and the U.S. Preventive Services Task Force, the American College of Obstetricians and Gynecologists recommends that women younger than 21 years should not be screened for cervical cancer or HPV regardless of the age of sexual initiation or the presence of other behavior-related risk factors. This recommendation is based on the very low incidence of invasive cervical cancer in patients younger than 21 years and the lack of data that screening is effective at reducing the rate of cervical cancer in this age group. Only 0.1% of cases of cervical cancer occur before age 20 years, or approximately 1–2 cases per year per 1,000,000 females aged 15–19 years. Although the prevalence of HPV is high among sexually active adolescents, the immune system, particularly in young women, effectively clears the HPV infection in 1–2 years. Most cervical abnormalities that occur related to HPV infection in this age group resolve spontaneously and require no treatment.

Several vaccines are available to prevent infection with the HPV subtypes that cause most cases of cervical cancer; two of these vaccines also prevent the HPV subtypes that cause most cases of genital warts. The Advisory Committee on Immunization Practices of the Centers for Disease Control and Prevention (CDC) and the American College of Obstetricians and Gynecologists recommend administration of the vaccine to females aged 9–26 years. Although the vaccine will have optimal effect when given to girls before any exposure to HPV, girls and women can and should be offered the vaccine even after viral exposure. At the time of publication, the HPV vaccines available in the United States are administered in three shots over 6 months, although the vaccination series should be completed even if there is a delay between two of the doses. Failure to complete the HPV vaccination series is not an indication for cytologic screening in adolescents.

The CDC estimates that young people aged 15–24 years acquire one half of all new STIs, approximately 10 million infections annually, and that 25% of sexually active adolescent females have an STI, such as chlamydial infection or HPV. Adolescents are at a higher risk of STIs for a number of behavioral, biologic, and cultural reasons. The high incidence of STIs among adolescents also may be due to multiple barriers to accessing quality STI prevention services. A history of chlamydial infection does not change the recommendation to delay routine cervical cancer screening until age 21 years. Similarly, although teenage patients should be counseled about safer sex practices and condom use, a history of unprotected sex is not an indication for early cytologic screening.

A family history of cervical cancer is a risk factor for development of cervical cancer; it is unclear if this is because of an inherited impaired ability to clear an HPV infection or social factors that might be shared with family members. Overall, cervical dysplasia is more closely related to HPV infection than to family history. A history of dysplasia in the described patient's mother does not warrant early cytology screening.

Infection with HIV or other immunocompromising diseases is one of the only exceptions to the recommendation not to provide routine cervical cancer screening before age 21 years. In the case of this patient, cytologic screening is indicated because of her HIV-positive status.

Women infected with HIV are at increased risk of high-risk HPV infection and subsequent dysplasia. The incidence, prevalence, and persistence of HPV, including high-risk subtypes, are higher in the setting of HIV infection and increase with worsening immunosuppression (ie, decreasing CD4 cell count and increasing viral load). Because of their weakened immunity, girls and women who are infected with HIV should have cytology screening. Adolescents who have weakened immune systems from an organ transplant or from long-term steroid therapy should be screened twice in the first year after they become sexually active and annually thereafter. Additionally, HIV infection is not considered a contraindication to HPV vaccine administration, and the CDC recommendations for HPV vaccination of children and adolescents should be followed for populations with or without HIV.

Cervical cancer screening and prevention. Practice Bulletin No. 168. American College of Obstetricians and Gynecologists. Obstet Gynecol 2016;128:e1–20.

Gynecologic care for women with human immunodeficiency virus. Practice Bulletin No. 117. American College of Obstetricians and Gynecologists. Obstet Gynecol 2010;117:1492–509.

Moscicki AB, Ellenberg JH, Crowley-Nowick P, Darragh TM, Xu J, Fahrat S. Risk of high-grade squamous intraepithelial lesion in HIV-infected adolescents. J Infect Dis 2004;190:1413–21.

128

Screening for intimate partner violence

A 26-year-old woman, gravida 3, para 3, presents for the third time with a vague report of worsening headaches and body aches. On examination, you notice bruises on her breasts and inner thighs. Last year, she received a cytologic test result of low-grade squamous intraepithelial lesion and underwent fine-needle aspiration of a breast lesion found to be ductal carcinoma in situ (DCIS). She has no family history of breast or gynecologic malignancies and smokes a pack of cigarettes per day. The greatest threat to her immediate health can be determined today by screening for

(A) lung cancer
(B) breast cancer
* (C) intimate partner violence (IPV)
(D) substance abuse
(E) cervical cancer

Intimate partner violence is a major public health concern, with 1.3–5.3 million women experiencing IPV every year. The lifetime incidence of IPV is thought to range from 22% to 39%. Intimate partner violence spans a range of abusive behaviors, from psychologic aggression to physical and sexual violence and rape. The financial costs are high ($2–7 million annually), as are the effects on health, which can include injury, sexually transmitted infections, unintended pregnancies, psychologic distress, and death. Intimate partner violence during pregnancy—an especially high-risk time for abuse—can result in preterm birth and low birth weight. Chronic conditions associated with IPV include chronic pain, neurologic disorders, migraine headaches, anxiety disorders, depression, and substance abuse.

All patients should be screened for IPV without a partner in the room. The most immediately important screening for the described patient, who is otherwise healthy but has physical evidence concerning for physical abuse (bruising on breasts and inner thighs), is IPV screening. Screening for IPV is recommended by numerous professional organizations, including the American College of Obstetricians and Gynecologists (the College) and the American Medical Association. Intimate partner violence screening is an essential preventive health care service for adolescent girls and women because it is an important aspect of addressing women's safety and health concerns while also preventing future health problems. Numerous studies suggest that IPV screening tools can accurately identify women who are experiencing IPV. The harms of this screening are minimal, although obstetrician–gynecologists and other health care providers should be aware of the possibility of patient discomfort, loss of privacy, emotional distress, and even concerns about further abuse, which often increases when women are trying to leave abusive relationships. Safety plans are an important follow-up to the screening process. Although the described patient shows physical signs of abuse, many patients will have less overt signs such as chronic headaches, chronic pain, substance abuse, depression, or frequent visits with vague symptoms. These less objective findings should raise obstetrician–gynecologist and other health care provider awareness and allow for more targeted screening. Box 128-1 lists recommended screening questions.

Screening for IPV is the most important assessment this patient needs to undergo at this visit. However, there are other screening assessments from which she might benefit. As a smoker, she could benefit from tobacco use screening and cessation counseling, one of the most effective screening and preventive health actions. The "5 A's" model of Ask, Advise, Assess, Assist, and Arrange is an evidence-based approach to address smoking cessation. However, this is not an immediate threat to her health, so a referral or deferring counseling to a future visit would be appropriate. Although tobacco abuse is clearly associated with lung cancer, there are no good data to suggest a role for lung cancer screening in a young patient. The U.S. Preventive Services Task Force does recommend screening for lung cancer with low-dose

BOX 128-1

Sample Intimate Partner Violence Screening Questions

While providing privacy, screen for intimate partner violence during new patient visits, annual examinations, initial prenatal visits, each trimester of pregnancy, and the postpartum checkup.

Framing Statement

"We've started talking to all of our patients about safe and healthy relationships because it can have such a large impact on your health."*

Confidentiality

"Before we get started, I want you to know that everything here is confidential, meaning that I won't talk to anyone else about what is said unless you tell me that...(insert the laws in your state about what is necessary to disclose)."*

Sample Questions

"Has your current partner ever threatened you or made you feel afraid?"

(Threatened to hurt you or your children if you did or did not do something, controlled who you talked to or where you went, or gone into rages)†

"Has your partner ever hit, choked, or physically hurt you?"

("Hurt" includes being hit, slapped, kicked, bitten, pushed, or shoved.)†

For women of reproductive age:

"Has your partner ever forced you to do something sexually that you did not want to do, or refused your request to use condoms?"*

"Does your partner support your decision about when or if you want to become pregnant?"*

"Has your partner ever tampered with your birth control or tried to get you pregnant when you didn't want to be?"*

For women with disabilities:

"Has your partner prevented you from using a wheelchair, cane, respirator, or other assistive device?"‡

"Has your partner refused to help you with an important personal need such as taking your medicine, getting to the bathroom, getting out of bed, bathing, getting dressed, or getting food or drink, or threatened not to help you with these personal needs?"‡

*Family Violence Prevention Fund. Reproductive health and partner violence guidelines: an integrated response to intimate partner violence and reproductive coercion. San Francisco (CA): FVPF; 2010. Available at: http://www.futureswithoutviolence.org/userfiles/file/HealthCare/Repro_Guide.pdf. Retrieved October 12, 2011. Modified and reprinted with permission.

†Family Violence Prevention Fund. National consensus guidelines on identifying and responding to domestic violence victimization in health care settings. San Francisco (CA): FVPF; 2004. Available at: http://www.futureswithoutviolence.org/userfiles/file/Consensus.pdf. Retrieved October 12, 2011. Modified and reprinted with permission.

‡Center for Research on Women with Disabilities. Development of the abuse assessment screen-disability (AAS-D). In: Violence against women with physical disabilities: final report submitted to the Centers for Disease Control and Prevention. Houston (TX): Baylor College of Medicine; 2002. p. II-1–II-16. Available at http://www.bcm.edu/crowd/index.cfm?pmid=2137. Retrieved October 18, 2011. Modified and reprinted with permission.

Intimate partner violence. Committee Opinion No. 518. American College of Obstetricians and Gynecologists. Obstet Gynecol 2012;119:412–7.

computed tomography scan in patients aged 55–80 years with a significant smoking history (30 packs-per-year history).

Although recommendations regarding breast cancer screening vary between professional organizations, none suggest starting before age 40 years in a woman with no family history. Women older than 20 years should undergo clinical breast examinations every 1–3 years, per College recommendations. However, this patient was diagnosed with DCIS and should receive a referral to discuss treatment and surveillance options. Screening for breast cancer at this point is not the most appropriate next step, given her diagnosis. Although the DCIS diagnosis should not be ignored, it is not as immediate a threat to her health as ongoing violence in her relationship.

Substance abuse is a major public health concern. However, the U.S. Preventive Services Task Force has concluded that there is insufficient evidence to recommend widespread screening for substance abuse. The College does suggest annual screening for tobacco, alcohol, and other drug use, as well as screening during pregnancy. Cervical cancer has clear, although frequently changing, recommendations regarding screening. This 26-year-old patient had a diagnosis of low-grade squamous intraepithelial lesion, so she needs to undergo colposcopy. However, disease progression is slow, and this is not the most immediate threat to her health. The single most important screening she can undergo today is an assessment for IPV.

Committee on Preventive Services for Women, editor. Clinical preventive services for women: Closing the gaps. Washington, DC: Institute of Medicine; 2011. Available at: http://www.nap.edu/download.php?record_id=13181. Retrieved March 5, 2015.

Intimate partner violence. Committee Opinion No. 518. American College of Obstetricians and Gynecologists. Obstet Gynecol 2012; 119:412–7.

Nelson HD, Bougatsos C, Blazina I. Screening women for intimate partner violence: a systematic review to update the U.S. Preventive Services Task Force recommendation. Ann Intern Med 2012;156:796–808, W-279, W-280, W-281, W-282.

Tobacco use and women's health. Committee Opinion No. 503. American College of Obstetricians and Gynecologists. Obstet Gynecol 2011;118:746–50.

Well-woman recommendations. Available at: http://www.acog.org/About-ACOG/ACOG-Departments/Annual-Womens-Health-Care/Well-Woman-Recommendations. Retrieved March 12, 2015; June 16, 2016.

129

Diverticulitis

A 48-year-old obese woman, gravida 4, para 4, comes to your office with a 1-month history of lower abdominal pain. The pain is mostly crampy in nature and has been associated with intermittent constipation and soft stools. She reports occasional blood in her stools, which she attributes to her chronic hemorrhoids. She is up to date with all general health maintenance. Although her symptoms have not changed significantly over the past month, she is concerned because of a new-onset fever of 38.2°C (100.8°F) starting yesterday evening. On physical examination, she appears well, with the exception of a temperature of 38.0°C (100.4°F). Her abdomen is soft with mild tenderness to deep palpation in the left lower quadrant, which is confirmed on pelvic and rectal examinations. The next step in her evaluation should be

(A) colonoscopy
(B) flexible sigmoidoscopy
* (C) computed tomography (CT) scan
(D) pelvic ultrasonography
(E) diagnostic laparoscopy

Diverticular disease or diverticulosis describes the presence of uninflamed diverticula of the colon and is a common condition in Western and industrialized societies. In the United States, approximately 130,000 hospitalizations are attributed to diverticular disease annually. Prevalence rates of diverticulosis are similar in men and women, and the condition primarily occurs in the elderly. Approximately 80% of these patients are aged 50 years and older; however, this diagnosis needs to be considered in women younger than 50 years who present with fever, bowel symptoms, and localized abdominal pain. In contrast to diverticulosis, diverticulitis describes the inflammation of preexisting colonic diverticula and commonly is accompanied by gross or microscopic perforation.

Uncomplicated diverticulitis refers to the localized inflammation of colonic diverticula that occurs as a result of altered gut motility, increased luminal pressure, and a disordered colonic microenvironment. Approximately 90% of cases are confined to the sigmoid or descending colon. Complicated diverticulitis occurs when there is an abscess or phlegmon, fistula formation, stricture disease, bowel obstruction, or peritonitis. The clinical presentation of acute colonic diverticulitis varies depending on the extent of the disease process, and the diagnosis often is made using clinical signs and symptoms with supporting radiologic findings. The most commonly encountered clinical presentation includes obstipation and abdominal pain, which often is localized to the left lower quadrant, with low-grade fever and leukocytosis.

Computed tomography is recommended as the initial imaging study to evaluate acute diverticulitis. A CT scan enables identification of diverticular disease with a sensitivity of 93–97% and a specificity approaching 100%. Additionally, CT imaging enables the evaluation of other etiologies of abdominal pain that can mimic diverticulitis, such as inflammatory bowel disease, tuboovarian abscess, and appendicitis, and can characterize potential complications of diverticulitis, including perforation, abscess, fistula, obstruction, and bleeding. Thus, in addition to a thorough evaluation for all potential intra-abdominal processes, a CT scan can provide valuable information regarding the severity of disease and ultimately guide treatment planning for patients.

Colonoscopy and flexible sigmoidoscopy are useful diagnostic tools for evaluation of the colonic mucosa and readily can identify diverticular disease. However, patients with suspected acute diverticulitis are at an increased risk of further perforation or exacerbation of their disease with endoscopic evaluation in the acute setting. These studies are best deferred until 6 weeks after the acute flare, when inflammation has resolved; at this point, these studies are critical for the evaluation of underlying disease processes, such as cancer and inflammatory bowel disease. The primary role of lower endoscopy is to identify mucosal pathology, including benign and malignant neoplasia.

Pelvic ultrasonography is the preferred imaging modality for suspected obstetric or gynecologic disorders; however, its clinical utility is limited when gastrointestinal or urinary tract etiologies are suspected. The described patient has no signs or symptoms suggestive of an acute gynecologic process; thus, ultrasonography would not be the most appropriate next step in her evaluation.

Less than 10% of patients who require admission for acute diverticulitis will undergo acute surgical management. Indications for emergency operative intervention include uncontrolled sepsis, generalized peritonitis, uncontained visceral perforation, large undrainable abscess, and failure to respond to medical therapy. The ultimate determination of the need for surgical intervention will vary based on disease severity, the patient's age, and existing comorbidities. Surgical intervention, whether through an open or laparoscopic approach, would be premature at this time.

Based on the patient's fever, bowel symptoms, and left lower quadrant pain, acute diverticulitis is a likely source of her symptoms. A CT scan is the imaging test of choice because it would identify the presence of diverticulitis and exclude other potential intra-abdominal pathology.

Donaldson CK. Acute gynecologic disorders. Radiol Clin North Am 2015;53(6): 1293–307.

Jacobs DO. Clinical practice. Diverticulitis. N Engl J Med 2007;357:2057–66.

Morris AM, Regenbogen SE, Hardiman KM, Hendren S. Sigmoid diverticulitis: a systematic review. JAMA 2014;311:287–97.

Sartelli M, Moore FA, Ansaloni L, Di Saverio S, Coccolini F, Griffiths EA, et al. A proposal for a CT driven classification of left colon acute diverticulitis. World J Emerg Surg 2015;10:3. DOI: 10.1186/1749-7922-10-3.

130
Listeria in pregnancy

A 23-year-old woman, gravida 1, para 0, at 8 weeks of gestation comes to your office for her initial obstetric visit. She expresses concern about foods she should and should not eat during pregnancy. Particularly, she has heard that listeria is dangerous for pregnant women and wants to know the best way to avoid contracting a listeria infection. You recommend that she avoid the foods that have been implicated in past listeria outbreaks. In addition, you advise her that the best method of food handling and preparation of delicate produce to avoid listeria infection is to

(A) store foods in refrigerator
(B) clean all kitchen surfaces with bleach
(C) eat only organically grown products
* (D) rinse or wash all produce in free-running water

Listeria monocytogenes is a gram-positive bacteria that has been associated with invasive foodborne infections. Particularly at risk are pregnant women, newborns, and adults with weakened immune systems. For a woman with listeriosis, infections typically are self-limited, although the infection can be associated with a nonspecific influenza-like febrile illness. Infections of the fetus can occur transplacentally, particularly in the third trimester, and can lead to preterm labor, amnionitis, fetal loss, and early-onset neonatal sepsis. Neonatal infections possess a very high-case fatality rate (20–30%) and account for an estimated 500 deaths in the United States annually. Pregnant women are overly represented among all listeriosis cases. Latina women are at particularly high risk, possibly because of the practice of consuming fresh cheeses as a dietary supplement during pregnancy.

Counseling pregnant women on how to avoid exposure to listeria is important. Table 130-1 lists foods that are at high risk of containing listeria. Outbreaks have included processed ready-to-eat meats (hotdogs and deli meats) and dairy products made from unpasteurized milk (Mexican-style soft cheeses). Numerous cases have been associated with fresh produce (eg, melons, sprouts, strawberries, spinach, caramel apples) and ice cream that has been contaminated. Organic-growing practices do not necessarily decrease contamination. Listeria contamination may initiate anywhere in the food distribution chain, and an implicated source might be the soil or the manure used for fertilization.

Listeria can grow and spread even at refrigerated and freezing temperatures. Ready-to-eat foods (eg, hotdogs, deli meats, leftovers) should be reheated until steaming hot before consumption. Prepared food or leftovers should be consumed quickly or discarded because bacterial growth is not inhibited by refrigeration. Prevention or avoidance of cross-contamination is an important preventive measure, and all utensils and surfaces should be cleaned, particularly after cutting raw meat or unprepared foods. The U.S. Food and Drug Administration suggests a sanitizing solution of 1 tablespoon of chlorine bleach added to 1 gallon (3.8 L) of hot water. This solution can be used by flooding the surface to be sanitized and allowing it to stand for 10 minutes before allowing it to dry. Spills should be wiped up immediately and internal surfaces in the refrigerator should be regularly cleaned. Handwashing with warm soapy water for more than

20 seconds before and after handling food or the sanitization process is recommended. However, simply cleaning kitchen surfaces is insufficient to prevent listeria because the contamination is in the food. The best method of handling foods to minimize the risk of listeriosis is to make sure that produce is washed and scrubbed (eg, melons, cucumbers) before cutting because listeria can be introduced from the outside surfaces. Delicate produce should be rinsed with free-running water, which is the best method of food handling and preparation to avoid listeria infection.

Symptoms of listeriosis can occur days to a few weeks after consumption of contaminated food. The practitioner must maintain a high index of suspicion for listeriosis in regard to high-risk individuals who experience fever or muscle aches. Such patients may or may not have gastrointestinal symptoms. Although listeria can be cultured on blood agar, special techniques are needed to recover

Table 130-1. Common Foods: Select the Lower Risk Options

Type of Food	Higher Risk	Lower Risk
Meat and poultry	• Raw or undercooked meat or poultry	• Meat or poultry cooked to a safe minimum internal temperature†
Seafood	• Any raw or undercooked fish or shellfish, or food containing raw or undercooked seafood (eg, sashimi, found in some sushi or ceviche). Refrigerated smoked fish. • Partially cooked seafood, such as shrimp and crab	• Previously cooked seafood heated to 74°C (165°F) • Canned fish and seafood • Seafood cooked to 63°C (145°F)
Milk	• Unpasteurized (raw) milk	• Pasteurized milk
Eggs	Foods that contain raw/undercooked eggs, such as: • Homemade Caesar salad dressings* • Homemade raw cookie dough* • Homemade eggnog*	*At home:* • Use pasteurized eggs/egg products when preparing recipes that call for raw or undercooked eggs. *When eating out:* • Ask if pasteurized eggs were used.
Sprouts	• Raw sprouts (alfalfa, bean, or any other sprout)	• Cooked sprouts
Vegetables	• Unwashed fresh vegetables, including lettuce/salads	• Washed fresh vegetables, including salads • Cooked vegetables
Cheese	• Soft cheeses made from unpasteurized (raw) milk, such as: — Feta — Brie — Camembert — Blue-veined — Queso fresco	• Hard cheeses • Processed cheeses • Cream cheese • Mozzarella • Soft cheeses that are clearly labeled "made from pasteurized milk"
Hotdogs and deli meats	• Hotdogs, deli meats, and luncheon meats that have not been reheated‡	• Hotdogs, luncheon meats, and deli meats reheated to steaming hot or 74°C (165°F)‡
Pâtés	• Unpasteurized, refrigerated pâtés or meat spreads	• Canned or shelf-stable pâtés or meat spreads

*Tip: Most premade foods from grocery stores, such as Caesar dressing, premade cookie dough, or packaged eggnog, are made with pasteurized eggs.

†Tip: Use a food thermometer to check the internal temperature on the "Is It Done Yet?" chart in Food Safety for Pregnant Women (www.fda.gov/downloads/Food/ResourcesForYou/Consumers/SelectedHealthTopics/UCM312787.pdf) for specific safe minimum internal temperature.

‡Tip: Reheat hotdogs, deli meats, and luncheon meats before eating them because the bacteria *Listeria monocytogenes* grows at refrigerated temperatures (4.5°C [40°F] or below). Listeria may cause severe illness, hospitalization, or even death. Reheating these foods until they are steaming hot destroys these dangerous bacteria and makes these foods safe to eat.

U.S. Department of Agriculture, Food and Drug Administration. Food safety for pregnant women. Washington, DC; Silver Spring (MD): USDA; FDA; 2011. Available at: http://www.fda.gov/downloads/Food/FoodborneIllnessContaminants/UCM312787.pdf. Retrieved June 8, 2016.

from sites with mixed flora (eg, the vagina and rectum). The bacteria are morphologically similar to diphtheroids and streptococci and may be frequently mistaken for contaminants. If listeria infection is suspected, treatment with ampicillin is effective because listeria is uniformly sensitive to ampicillin.

The best prevention measure for listeria is fastidious attention to food preparation and avoidance of foods that have a high risk of contamination. The list of foods implicated in listeria outbreaks is growing. Safe food-handling practices should be discussed with pregnant patients, given that they are at high risk of serious infections. An important resource for patients about food safety during pregnancy may be found on the on the U.S. Food and Drug Administration website, available at www.fda.gov/downloads/Food/ResourcesForYou/Consumers/SelectedHealthTopics/UCM312787.pdf.

Jackson KA, Iwamoto M, Swerdlow D. Pregnancy-associated listeriosis. Epidemiol Infect 2010;138:1503–9.

Kourtis AP, Read JS, Jamieson DJ. Pregnancy and infection. N Engl J Med 2014;370:2211–8.

Lamont RF, Sobel J, Mazaki-Tovi S, Kusanovic JP, Vaisbuch E, Kim SK, et al. Listeriosis in human pregnancy: a systematic review. J Perinat Med 2011;39:227–36.

Management of pregnant women with presumptive exposure to Listeria monocytogenes. Committee Opinion No. 614. American College of Obstetricians and Gynecologists. Obstet Gynecol 2014;124:1241–4.

Silk BJ, Date KA, Jackson KA, Pouillot R, Holt KG, Graves LM, et al. Invasive listeriosis in the Foodborne Diseases Active Surveillance Network (FoodNet), 2004–2009: further targeted prevention needed for higher-risk groups. Clin Infect Dis 2012;54 Suppl 5:S396–404.

U.S. Department of Agriculture, Food and Drug Administration. Food safety for pregnant women. Washington, DC; Silver Spring (MD): USDA; FDA; 2011. Available at: http://www.fda.gov/downloads/Food/FoodborneIllnessContaminants/UCM312787.pdf. Retrieved June 18, 2016.

131
Nonspecific vaginitis

A 6-year-old girl is brought to your office by her mother because of a 7-day history of vaginal irritation and pruritus. She has no significant medical history and has not recently been ill or taken antibiotics. Her mother noticed that the girl's perineum was erythematous. She has been putting lotion on the affected area, which seems to provide temporary relief. However, her daughter is still very uncomfortable, and her symptoms seem to be worsening. Today, the girl's pulse is 105 beats per minute and her temperature is 36.7°C (98.1°F). You explain to the girl why examination of this area is necessary and how the examination will be performed. The girl is placed in her mother's lap to perform the examination. Physical findings include an erythematous vulva and a thin, clear nonodorous vaginal discharge. The most likely diagnosis is

(A) foreign body
(B) pinworm infection
* (C) nonspecific vaginitis
(D) *Candida* infection

Vulvovaginitis is inflammation of the vulvar and vaginal tissues. It is one of the most common reasons for visits to obstetrician–gynecologists. Common symptoms include pruritus, burning, irritation, and abnormal discharge. Because of differences in estrogen status of the vagina, causes of vulvovaginitis in girls are different than those in adult women. In premenarchal girls, the most likely cause is nonspecific vaginitis. In adults, however, the cause typically is specific vaginitis, namely bacterial vaginosis, candidiasis, or trichomoniasis. In contrast to premenarchal vaginitis, these three etiologies are responsible for 90% of cases of adult vaginitis.

In prepubertal girls, vulvovaginitis is the most common gynecologic concern. Typical symptoms are vaginal discharge, vulvar soreness, and irritation. Although not serious, such discharge may cause great anxiety to the girl and her parents because they may think it indicates serious pathology, a sign of abuse, or a threat to future fertility. Additionally, vulvovaginitis may disrupt school performance. In childhood, infection usually begins in the vulva and secondarily spreads to the vagina. Young girls are very susceptible to vulvovaginitis for several reasons. Vaginal epithelium in young girls is thin, and the pH of the vagina is elevated. This creates a favorable environment for bacterial growth. Anatomically, absence of pubic hair and labial fat pads put girls at risk because they act as anatomical barriers. Also, children often have poor hygiene after urination and defecation, which can lead to contamination of the vulva. Inadequate hand washing may add to this contamination and irritation.

Obtaining a history from the parent and the child is important to best ascertain the etiology of vaginitis. Information from the history should include duration of symptoms, presence of discharge, history of trauma or foreign body insertion, and overall hygiene habits. It is very important for the clinician to ask about the potential for abuse as well as whether the girl has experienced any bleeding. Either of those situations would warrant a more comprehensive evaluation. Classically, nonspecific vaginitis symptoms wax and wane, depending on the patient's hygiene and exposures, which only adds to caregivers' frustration.

When examining a child, it is important that the obstetrician–gynecologist or other health care provider explains to the child why the examination is necessary and how it will be performed. The parents should be reassured that the examination will be painless and nothing will be done to change or distort the girl's genital anatomy, such as altering the hymen. Examining a girl while she is sitting in her parent's lap may lead to better compliance during the examination. It is important to examine the perineum to assess hygiene and to make sure there are no underlying skin abnormalities, such as lichen sclerosus. With the labia spread laterally and with gentle downward traction, the lower aspect of the vagina and hymen can be visualized. If there is a significant vaginal discharge, testing for chlamydia and gonorrhea, performing a wet mount, or both, is appropriate.

Nonspecific vaginitis accounts for 75% of all cases of pediatric vulvovaginitis. It also has been referred to as irritant dermatitis. The described patient has typical symptoms of nonspecific vaginitis, including a scanty, nonpurulent discharge and vulvar irritation. Treatment of nonspecific vaginitis includes improving hygiene by educating the girl on proper hand washing and wiping from front to back after bowel movements. Wearing loose cotton underpants and avoiding tight-fitting clothing is recommended. Constipation should be treated if present. If the inflammation is due to a specific irritant, avoidance of the irritant, which may include bubble baths, is crucial. However, patients should be instructed to soak in clean, warm bath water at least daily when symptomatic. Applications of an inert barrier such as petroleum jelly to protect skin may be beneficial. If the symptoms persist after these interventions, assessment of the entire vagina by means of vaginoscopy may be indicated.

A vaginal foreign body usually presents with recurrent symptoms that are resistant to previous treatment recommendations. A malodorous, purulent discharge that may be blood-tinged is typical. Toilet paper unintentionally placed in the vagina is the most common foreign body discovered. Office vaginal lavage or vaginoscopy may be necessary to diagnose a foreign body. Because the described patient did not have abnormal discharge as a symptom, a foreign body as a cause for her symptoms is less likely.

Pinworm infection (*Enterobius vermicularis*) is a common cause of vulvar pruritus in children. Symptoms include perianal pruritus and nocturnal symptoms, because this is the time when mature pinworms lay eggs in this area. Diagnosis involves either inspecting the anal area at night or using adhesive tape to look for microscopic eggs.

Candidal vulvovaginitis is common in the adolescent and adult years. It is uncommon in children after they are out of diapers. In prepubescent girls, this infection occurs with diabetes mellitus, other immunocompromised states, or, very rarely, after antibiotic use. Physical findings include erythematous vulva, satellite lesions, and an adherent white discharge. Diagnosis is confirmed by demonstration of pseudohyphae on a 10% potassium hydroxide wet mount preparation.

Emans SJ. Office evaluation of the child and adolescent. In: Emans SJ, Laufer MR, editors. Goldstein's pediatric & adolescent gynecology. 6th ed. Philadelphia (PA): Wolters Kluwer Lippincott Williams & Wilkins; 2012. p. 1–20.

Garden AS. Vulvovaginitis and other common childhood gynaecological conditions. Arch Dis Child Educ Pract Ed 2011;96:73–8.

Kokotos F. Vulvovaginitis. Pediatr Rev 2006;27:116–7.

Vaginitis. ACOG Practice Bulletin No. 72. American College of Obstetricians and Gynecologists. Obstet Gynecol 2006;107:1195–206.

Van Eyk N, Allen L, Giesbrecht E, Jamieson MA, Kives S, Morris M, et al. Pediatric vulvovaginal disorders: a diagnostic approach and review of the literature. J Obstet Gynaecol can 2009;31:850–62.

132

Requirements of the American Institute of Ultrasound in Medicine

Your office will soon begin performing fetal surveys on low-risk obstetric patients. In order to meet the accreditation requirements of the American Institute of Ultrasound in Medicine (AIUM), each obstetrician in your practice who has completed residency or fellowship longer than 3 years ago must demonstrate that, in the past 36 months, he or she has attained at least 30 American Medical Association (AMA) Physician's Recognition Award (PRA) Category 1 Credits dedicated to diagnostic obstetric ultrasonography and

(A) personally performed 100 diagnostic obstetric ultrasonographic examinations
* (B) supervised, interpreted, and reported at least 300 diagnostic obstetric ultrasonographic examinations
(C) worked with at least one full-time or two part-time qualified Registered Diagnostic Medical Sonographer(s)
(D) passed the written competency examination developed by AIUM
(E) submitted at least five sample images of diagnostic obstetric ultrasonographic examinations

The AIUM has specified guidelines for physicians who are responsible for interpreting ultrasonographic examinations. Physicians not only must provide evidence of training and competence needed for interpretation of diagnostic ultrasonography, but they should maintain their training. Per AIUM, physicians performing diagnostic obstetric ultrasonography must have completed an approved residency, fellowship, or postgraduate training program in which they were involved with the performance, evaluation and interpretation, and reporting of at least 300 obstetric ultrasonographic examinations under the supervision of a qualified physician. Physicians who completed such training more than 3 years ago must demonstrate that, in the past 36 months, they have attained at least 30 AMA PRA Category 1 Credits dedicated to diagnostic obstetric ultrasonography and supervision–performance, interpretation, and reporting of at least 300 diagnostic obstetric ultrasonographic examinations.

For physicians who did not receive the required training in diagnostic obstetric ultrasonography, AIUM has stipulated that they still may interpret scans if they can document appropriate clinical experience as evidenced by, in the past 36 months, attainment of at least 50 AMA PRA Category 1 Credits dedicated to diagnostic obstetric ultrasonography and supervision, interpretation, and reporting of at least 300 diagnostic obstetric ultrasonographic examinations under the supervision of a qualified physician.

Part of the reason for these stringent criteria for those who continue to interpret diagnostic obstetric ultrasonographic examinations is that ultrasonographic training has not been consistently adequate. The Council on Resident Education in Obstetrics and Gynecology conducted a survey in 2000–2003 to assess the quality of ultrasonographic training from the perspective of the program directors and the residents in training. In fact, many directors reported that there were few formal requirements for ultrasonographic training and evaluation. Also, despite the perceived importance of hands-on training, most residents reported that their program did not require them to perform or interpret diagnostic scans.

The obstetricians in the practice will need at least 30 AMA PRA Category 1 Credits dedicated to diagnostic ultrasonography in the past 3 years. The number of ultrasonographers in a physician's practice does not affect AIUM accreditation. There is no written competency examination for interpretation of ultrasonographic examinations. Submission of images is not required for AIUM certification.

American Institute of Ultrasound in Medicine. Training guidelines for physicians who evaluate and interpret diagnostic obstetric ultrasound examinations. AIUM official statements 59. Laurel (MD): AIUM; 2015. Available at: http://www.aium.org/officialStatements/59. Retrieved June 15, 2016.

Lee W, Hodges AN, Williams S, Vettraino IM, McNie B. Fetal ultrasound training for obstetrics and gynecology residents. Obstet Gynecol 2004;103:333–8.

133–136

Cervical cytology screening

Match the patient (133–136) with the preferred test (A–E).

(A) Cervical cytology now
(B) Cervical cytology and human papillomavirus (HPV) cotesting now
(C) HPV testing now
(D) Cervical cytology and HPV cotesting in 3 years
(E) Screening for cervical cancer not indicated

133. E. A 66-year-old healthy woman with lifetime normal cervical cancer screening

134. B. A 65-year-old woman with mild cervical dysplasia (ie, cervical intraepithelial neoplasia [CIN] 1) on biopsy 1 year ago

135. C. A 65-year-old woman has had lifetime negative cervical cancer screening. Cervical cytology 1 month ago was negative for dysplasia or malignancy but showed insufficient endocervical cells.

136. A. A 65-year-old woman had primary cervical HPV screening 1 month ago. The screening test result was positive for high-risk HPV and reflex negative for HPV subtypes 16 and 18.

Screening for cervical cancer is not recommended in women older than 65 years who have a history of adequate screening. *Adequate screening* is defined as two consecutive negative HPV tests or three consecutive negative Pap tests within 10 years of screening cessation. One of the negative tests must have been performed within 5 years of cessation. Therefore, Patient 133 does not require screening. Women older than 65 years who have never been screened should undergo screening for cervical cancer. Resumption of screening after age 65 years is not recommended, even in women with new partners, given that a new HPV infection is unlikely to lead to cancer in the patient's lifetime. Similar to those in younger women, most new HPV infections will clear spontaneously in women older than 65 years. Women with human immunodeficiency virus (HIV) require more frequent screening. Guidelines that recommend against continued screening for women older than 65 years who meet criteria cite an increased risk of harm from continued screening. Modeling data have shown that screening after age 65 years leads to significant increases in colposcopies as a result of false-positive screening test results and to a slight gain in life expectancy.

Initial follow-up for women older than 65 years with mild cervical dysplasia preceded by lesser abnormalities, such as low-grade squamous intraepithelial lesion, atypical squamous cells of undetermined significance, or positive test results for HPV subtypes 16 or 18, does not differ from that for women younger than 65 years. The recommended screening for Patient 134 is cotesting 1 year after her diagnosis of CIN 1. Women with a history of CIN 2, CIN 3, or adenocarcinoma in situ should continue screening for 20 years after treatment, even if this requires screening after age 65 years. Surveillance guidelines after biopsy-proven or treated cervical dysplasia for women older than 65 years are the same as those for women aged 30–64 years.

Guidelines for management of women with cytology that is negative for dysplasia but with insufficient or absent endocervical cells or transformation zone, as with Patient 135, recommend HPV testing now (preferred) or repeat cytology in 3 years. This should be done even if the cytology will be performed after age 65 years.

The American Society for Colposcopy and Cervical Pathology (ASCCP) supports primary HPV screening as an acceptable alternative to cytology-based screening schemes for women older than 25 years because HPV-based screening has the same or improved efficacy for the detection of high-grade dysplasia compared with cytology alone. Studies have shown decreased incidence of cervical cancer and high-grade lesions after 3–6 years of follow-up in women initially screened with HPV compared with women screened using cytology alone. Patients with positive HPV test results, such as Patient 136, should undergo reflex genotyping to triage women to colposcopy (positive for HPV 16 or 18) or immediate cervical cytology.

The ASCCP management guidelines for cervical cancer screening are updated on a regular basis and can be found on the ASCCP website (www.asccp.org/). A mobile app is also available to download on this website.

Huh WK, Ault KA, Chelmow D, Davey DD, Goulart RA, Garcia FA, et al. Use of primary high-risk human papillomavirus testing for cervical cancer screening: interim clinical guidance. Gynecol Oncol 2015;136:178–82.

Kulasingam SL, Havrilesky L, Ghebre R, Myers ER. Screening for cervical cancer: A decision analysis for the U.S. Preventive Services Task Force. AHRQ publications no. 11-05157-EF-1. Rockville (MD): Agency for Healthcare Research and Quality; 2011. Retrieved June 17, 2016.

Saslow D, Solomon D, Lawson HW, Killackey M, Kulasingam SL, Cain JM, et al. American Cancer Society, American Society for Colposcopy and Cervical Pathology, and American Society for Clinical Pathology screening guidelines for the prevention and early detection of cervical cancer. J Low Genit Tract Dis 2012;16:175–204.

Sawaya GF, Grady D, Kerlikowske K, Valleur JL, Barnabei VM, Bass K, et al. The positive predictive value of cervical smears in previously screened postmenopausal women: the Heart and Estrogen/progestin Replacement Study (HERS). Ann Intern Med 2000;133:942–50.

Services Task Force recommendation statement. U.S. Preventive Services Task Force [published erratum appears in Ann Intern Med 2013;158:852]. Ann Intern Med 2012;156:880,91, W312.

137–141

Industry support

For each physician–industry relationship scenario (137–141), consider whether each is required or exempt from reporting to the Centers for Medicare and Medicaid Services (CMS) under the Physician Payments Sunshine Act (A or B).

(A) Required
(B) Exempt

137. A. A physician's spouse owns stock in a group purchasing organization that negotiates contracts between device manufacturers and hospitals.

138. B. A pharmaceutical company donates samples of oral contraceptives to a private physician's office to dispense to patients.

139. B. A manufacturing company donates a colposcope for use in providing charity care.

140. B. A pharmaceutical company provides buffet meals and coffee to be available to all participants at the Annual Clinical and Scientific Meeting of the American College of Obstetricians and Gynecologists.

141. B. A pharmaceutical company pays speaking fees and reimburses travel for a nurse practitioner to speak at a continuing medical education event.

Financial relationships between physicians and industry have long been a subject for ethical debate. Collaboration can facilitate development of new products that may improve care. However, conflict of interest can develop between a physician's financial interest and the goals of research, education, or patient care. Pharmaceutical and device manufacturers devote significant amounts of their budgets to marketing, and a 2009 national survey found that nearly 84% of physicians had some financial relationship with industry. It has been demonstrated that even nominal gifts and subtle marketing messages can influence physician prescribing practices, and physicians often are unaware of this influence. The growing awareness that physician–industry relationships can bias physician decision making has led to the development of conflict-of-interest policies by professional bodies, medical journals, and academic institutions, as well as state and national laws requiring the disclosure of certain financial interests. However, these policies and reporting systems have been inconsistent and fragmented. The Medicare Payment Advisory Commission and the Institute of Medicine have called for greater transparency and the establishment of a standardized, nationwide, mandatory public reporting program. In response to these concerns, the Physician Payments Sunshine Act was incorporated into the Affordable Care Act (ACA) of 2010.

The Physician Payments Sunshine Act, section 6002 of the ACA, requires that manufacturers and group purchasing organizations report to CMS on three types of payments or "transfers of value" to physicians and teaching hospitals. The first covers general payments or transfers of value, such as meals, travel reimbursement, and consulting fees. The second covers ownership and investment interests held by physicians and their immediate family members. The third covers research, including payments for participation in preclinical research, clinical trials, or other product development activities. These payments or transfers of value are further classified into 15 categories, as listed in Box 137–141-1. The federal program that collects this information and makes it publicly available is called the National Physician Payment Transparency Program, or Open Payments. The burden of reporting is on the manufacturer or group purchasing organizations. After data are reported, they are collated and posted. Then physicians, teaching hospitals, group purchasing organizations, and manufacturers have 45 days to review the data and an additional 15 days to dispute and correct the data. After that point, if a dispute has not been resolved, the data will be published by CMS with a notation that the data are under dispute. Penalties of $1,000–$10,000 per unreported payment may be applied to manufacturers and group purchasing organizations that fail to report. Larger penalties of up to $1 million may be applied in cases of deliberate failures to report. Although payment for research must be reported, there is a provision allowing for a delay in reporting of payments made in support of products that are under development. Public disclosure of such payments can be delayed for 4 years or until U.S. Food and Drug Administration approval, whichever comes first.

BOX 137–141-1

Categories of Reportable Payments Under the Physician Payments Sunshine Act

- Consulting fees
- Compensation for services other than consulting (such as speaker fees)
- Honoraria
- Gifts
- Entertainment
- Food and beverage
- Travel and lodging
- Education
- Research
- Charitable contributions
- Royalty or license
- Current or prospective ownership or investment interest
- Compensation for serving as faculty or speaker for continuing medical education
- Grants
- Space rental or facility fees (teaching hospital only)

Centers for Medicaid and Medicare Services. Open Payments (Physician Payments Sunshine Act). Fact sheet for physicians. Baltimore (MD): CMS; 2015. Available at: https://www.cms.gov/regulations-and-guidance/legislation/national-physician-payment-transparency-program/downloads/physician-fact-sheet.pdf. Retrieved June 13, 2016.

The Physician Payments Sunshine Act requires that manufacturers and group purchasing organizations report on interests held by physicians and their immediate family members. The stock ownership by a physician's spouse in Scenario 137, therefore, must be reported.

Certain transactions and transfers are exempt from disclosure, such as payments under $10 (as long as they do not total over $100 annually), educational materials intended solely for patients, or product samples. A list of financial relationships exempt from reporting is shown in Box 137–141-2. Pharmaceutical samples donated to

BOX 137–141-2

Exemptions to the Physician Payments Sunshine Act

- Certified and accredited continuing medical education
- Buffet meals, snacks, soft drinks, or coffee generally available to all participants of a large-scale conference or similar large-scale event
- Product samples intended for patient use, not sale
- Educational materials intended for patient use
- Loan of a medical device for a short-term trial not to exceed 90 days
- Items or services provided under a contractual warranty
- A transfer of anything of value to a physician when the physician is a patient and not acting in his or her professional capacity as a physician
- Discounts and rebates
- In-kind items used in provision of charity care
- Dividend or other profit distribution from or ownership or investment in a publicly traded security and mutual fund
- Payments for provision of health care to employees under a self-insured plan offered by an applicable manufacturer
- Transfer of anything of value to a physician who is a licensed nonmedical professional for the nonmedical professional services of such licensed nonmedical professional (such as obtaining legal advice from a physician who is licensed to practice law)
- A transfer of value that is related to the services of the physician with respect to a civil or criminal action or an administrative proceeding in the case of a physician who is a covered recipient
- A transfer of anything of value less than $10, unless the aggregate amount exceeds $100 during the calendar year

Adapted from Centers for Medicaid and Medicare Services. Open Payments (Physician Payments Sunshine Act). Fact sheet for physicians. Baltimore (MD): CMS; 2015. Available at: https://www.cms.gov/regulations-and-guidance/legislation/national-physician-payment-transparency-program/downloads/physician-fact-sheet.pdf. Retrieved June 13, 2016.

a physician's office to be dispensed to patients, as in Scenario 138, do not need to be reported under the Physician Payments Sunshine Act (notably, according to a separate provision of the ACA, manufacturers must report to the U.S. Food and Drug Administration the type and quantity of medicines requested from and distributed to physicians as samples). Donations of in-kind items for the provision of charity care, such as the donation of the colposcope in Scenario 139, are exempt from reporting. Also exempt are buffet meals, snacks, soft drinks, or coffee generally available to all participants of large-scale conferences, such as the Annual Clinical and Scientific Meeting of the American College of Obstetricians and Gynecologists, described in Scenario 140.

For the purpose of reporting requirements, a *physician* is defined by CMS as a professional who is legally authorized to practice medicine (Box 137–141-3). The Physician Payments Sunshine Act excludes certain categories of health care providers, such as physician assistants, nurse practitioners, and medical residents. Therefore, the payment of speaking fees and reimbursement to a nurse practitioner, as in Scenario 141, does not need to be reported.

BOX 137–141-3

Covered Recipients Under the Physician Payments Sunshine Act

- Doctor of Medicine
- Doctor of Osteopathic Medicine
- Doctor of Dental Medicine
- Doctor of Dental Surgery
- Doctor of Podiatric Medicine
- Doctor of Optometry
- Doctor of Chiropractic Medicine

Centers for Medicaid and Medicare Services. Open Payments (Physician Payments Sunshine Act). Fact sheet for physicians. Baltimore (MD): CMS; 2015. Available at: https://www.cms.gov/regulations-and-guidance/legislation/national-physician-payment-transparency-program/downloads/physician-fact-sheet.pdf. Retrieved June 13, 2016.

American Medical Association. Sunshine act FAQs. Chicago (IL): AMA; 2016. Available at: http://www.ama-assn.org/ama/pub/advocacy/topics/sunshine-act-and-physician-financial-transparency-reports/sunshine-act-faqs.page. Retrieved June 13, 2016.

Centers for Medicaid and Medicare Services. Open Payments (Physician Payments Sunshine Act). Fact sheet for physicians. Baltimore (MD): CMS; 2015. Available at: https://www.cms.gov/regulations-and-guidance/legislation/national-physician-payment-transparency-program/downloads/physician-fact-sheet.pdf. Retrieved June 13, 2016.

Professional relationships with industry. Committee Opinion No. 541. American College of Obstetricians and Gynecologists. Obstet Gynecol 2012;120:1243–9.

Richardson E. Health policy brief: the physician payments sunshine act. Health affairs. Bethesda (MD): Health Affairs; 2014. p. 1–6. Available at: http://healthaffairs.org/healthpolicybriefs/brief_pdfs/healthpolicybrief_127.pdf. Retrieved June 13, 2016.

142–146

Colon cancer screening recommendations

For each patient (142–146), select the most appropriate cancer screening (A–C).

(A) Colonoscopy now
(B) Colonoscopy beginning at age 50 years
(C) Colonoscopy not recommended

142. B. A 47-year-old Asian woman with no personal or family history of malignancy comes to your office for a routine well-woman examination. She has undergone mammography and routine Pap tests that have all been normal to date.

143. A. A 25-year-old white woman with a known diagnosis of Lynch syndrome visits your office for a routine well-woman examination. The earliest age of cancer diagnosis in her family is age 35 years. She has not yet undergone endometrial or colorectal cancer screening but has had no symptoms.

144. A. A 46-year-old African American woman with no personal or family history of malignancy comes to your office for an annual well-woman examination. She has undergone mammography and routine Pap tests that have all been normal to date.

145. C. A 78-year-old African American woman with no personal or family history of malignancy comes to your office for a well-woman examination. She is up to date with all of her general health maintenance. Her last colonoscopy was 10 years ago and the result was normal. She denies any gastrointestinal symptoms.

146. A. A 40-year-old white woman with a personal history of Crohn disease diagnosed at age 30 years comes to your office for her annual well-woman examination. Her first colonoscopy was performed at the time of her diagnosis of inflammatory bowel disease. Her Crohn disease is under good control.

Colorectal cancer is the third leading cause of cancer-related deaths in women, with approximately 24,000 deaths annually in the United States. In 2015, an estimated 93,090 new cases of colon cancer and 39,601 new cases of rectal cancer occurred in the United States. Risk factors for colorectal cancer include a personal history of inflammatory bowel disease; a personal or family history of colorectal cancer or polyps; genetic predisposition; and lifestyle factors, including alcohol consumption, poor dietary habits, obesity, tobacco use, and sedentary lifestyle. The goal of colorectal cancer screening is to reduce mortality through early detection and cancer prevention. Screening for colorectal cancer is a well-accepted modality to promote early detection, removal of adenomatous polyps, and reduction of mortality by detection of early disease. However, despite consensus among many health care organizations regarding the importance of screening modalities, only 65% of respondents among U.S. women aged 50–75 years report screening with either colonoscopy or sigmoidoscopy in the past 10 years or fecal occult blood testing in the past year.

The most complete and effective screening modality for colorectal cancer is colonoscopy performed at 10-year intervals (if results are normal). Routine colorectal cancer screening for an average-risk woman should begin at age 50 years. Colonoscopy provides a thorough evaluation of the colon and rectum in a single setting and enables biopsy or removal of colonic polyps. Screening with polyp removal using colonoscopy results in an 83% reduction in mortality from colon cancer. Downsides of colonoscopy include costs, risk of serious complications, dietary and bowel preparation, and need for a chaperone after the procedure. For women at increased risk of colorectal cancer, screening with colonoscopy should be initiated at age 40 years or at 10 years younger than the age at which the youngest affected relative was diagnosed with colorectal cancer.

Patient 142 should have routine colorectal cancer screening. Her Asian race does not put her at higher risk. She is of average risk and has no personal or family history of colorectal cancer.

Patient 143 has a diagnosis of Lynch syndrome. Women known to have Lynch syndrome should have colonoscopy every 1–2 years beginning at age 20–25 years or 2–5 years before the earliest cancer diagnosis in the family, whichever is earlier. This screening should be performed regardless of the presence or absence of symptoms.

African American women have been shown to exhibit a higher incidence of colorectal cancer as well as decreased survival compared with their white counterparts. Patient 144 has no personal or family history of colorectal cancer; however, given her race, she warrants earlier screening. Current recommendations suggest that screening by colonoscopy should begin in this high-risk group at age 45 years.

Patient 145 falls into a high-risk group even though she has had no personal or family history of colorectal cancer and is symptom free. In general, routine colorectal cancer screening should be discontinued at age 75 years, so a colonoscopy would not be indicated in this patient.

Patient 146 is at an increased risk of developing colorectal cancer because of her personal history of inflammatory bowel disease. According to the National Comprehensive Cancer Network Panel, surveillance colonoscopy should be initiated 8–9 years after the onset of symptoms in individuals with a personal history of inflammatory bowel disease and performed every 1–2 years thereafter. Thus, Patient 146 should receive a screening colonoscopy now, despite the absence of symptoms.

A variety of additional screening tests exist, each with their own advantages and limitations. However, abnormalities noted on other screening modalities require prompt referral for diagnostic colonoscopy. Flexible sigmoidoscopy can be performed at 5-year intervals and results in a 60–80% reduction in mortality from left-sided colonic lesions. Compared with colonoscopy, flexible sigmoidoscopy is technically easier to perform, requires less preparation, has fewer complications, and can be performed without sedation. However, a notable limitation is its inability to visualize the distal colon; as a result, it will miss a significant number of right-sided lesions. Right-sided lesions presently account for 65% of advanced colorectal neoplasia in women.

Digital rectal examination and stool guaiac testing result in a 15–33% reduction in mortality from colon cancer. However, guaiac-based stool testing has several limitations, including false-negative rates with cases of colorectal cancer that have minimal or only intermittent bleeding, as well as false-positive results due to upper gastrointestinal bleeding or reaction with nonhuman products present in food. Therefore, in-office single-stool guaiac fecal occult blood testing for colorectal cancer screening is not an acceptable stool test and is not recommended. If guaiac fecal occult blood testing is performed, it is recommended that samples should be obtained on three separate occasions while adhering to a specific diet in order to obtain the most accurate results. High-sensitivity guaiac testing and fecal immunochemical testing with high sensitivity for cancer are noninvasive tests that can be performed annually; fecal immunochemical testing results in a 74% reduction in colorectal cancer mortality.

Newer technologies include computed tomography colonography (ie, virtual colonoscopy) and fecal DNA testing. One-time testing with computed tomography colonography is ineffective, and negative tests should be repeated annually. High-sensitivity guaiac testing has replaced older conventional guaiac-based stool testing and requires two samples from each of three consecutive bowel movements. Both studies must be performed annually to be effective, and all positive results require further diagnostic evaluation. Because of these limitations, a combination of annual high-sensitivity guaiac fecal occult blood testing or fecal immunochemical testing in conjunction with flexible sigmoidoscopy every 5 years probably is superior to either method alone. Fecal DNA testing techniques currently are evolving and have shown promising early results in enabling the detection of genetic mutations related to colorectal cancer. Current evidence suggests increased sensitivity over guaiac fecal occult blood testing in detecting precancerous and cancerous lesions; however, this test currently is not recommended for routine screening.

Colorectal cancer screening strategies. Committee Opinion No. 609. American College of Obstetricians and Gynecologists. Obstet Gynecol 2014;124:849–55.

Levin TR, Corley DA. Colorectal-cancer screening—coming of age. N Engl J Med 2013;369:1164–6.

National Comprehensive Cancer Network. Colon cancer. NCCN Clinical Practice Guidelines in Oncology, version 2.2016 [after login]. Ft. Washington (PA): NCCN; 2016. Available at: https://www.nccn.org/professionals/physician_gls/pdf/colon.pdf. Retrieved June 20, 2016.

Paquette IM, Ying J, Shah SA, Abbott DE, Ho S. African Americans should be screening at an earlier age for colorectal cancer. Gastrointest Endosc 2015;82:878–83.

Theodore R, Levin R, Corley DA. Colorectal cancer screening—coming of age. N Engl J Med 2013;1164–6.

Vrees RA. Colon cancer screening: a clinical update for the obstetrician/gynecologist. Postgraduate Obstetrics and Gynecology 2015;35(19): 1–6.

147–150

Pneumococcus vaccination in adults

For each patient (147–150), select the indicated vaccine or vaccines (A–E).

(A) 13-valent pneumococcal conjugate vaccine (PCV13)
(B) 23-valent pneumococcal polysaccharide vaccine (PPSV23)
(C) PCV13 now and PPSV23 in 6–12 months
(D) PPSV23 followed by PCV13 in 12 months
(E) Pneumococcal vaccination is not indicated

147. C. A 65-year-old woman with diabetes mellitus comes to your office for her annual well-woman examination. She asks you whether she should receive PCV13, which she saw advertised in a magazine. You review her vaccination history and see that she received PPSV23 at age 60 years because of her diabetes.

148. B. A 24-year-old women with sickle cell disease comes to your office for a new obstetric visit at 12 weeks of gestation. You review her immunization history and see that she previously received PCV13 at age 19 years and has received no other immunizations since then.

149. A. A 68-year-old woman comes to your clinic for her annual well-woman examination. Your records indicate that she received PPSV23 at age 65 years.

150. B. A 27-year-old woman visits your office for prepregnancy counseling. She has a history of severe asthma requiring daily maintenance therapy. She has no prior history of pneumococcal vaccination.

Pneumococcal disease is responsible for more mortality in the United States each year than all other vaccine-preventable diseases combined. In spite of appropriate therapy, pneumococcal bacteremia has a mortality rate of approximately 15% among adults and up to 60% in the elderly. Immunization with PPSV23 has been a proven strategy for more than a decade to prevent the serious illnesses caused by *Streptococcus pneumoniae* (pneumococcus, which includes pneumonia, meningitis, and bacteremia in adults 65 years and older or earlier in individuals with medical conditions that predispose them to pneumococcal infection). In August 2014, the Advisory Committee on Immunization Practices (ACIP) also recommended routine vaccination with PCV13 for adults 65 years and older. This recommendation was based on a randomized placebo-controlled trial of 85,000 adults 65 years and older that demonstrated enhanced protection with the addition of PCV13 in individuals who had already received age-directed PPSV23.

Although there are more than 90 serotypes of pneumococcus, 20–25% of cases of invasive pneumococcal disease and 10% of community-acquired cases of pneumonia are caused by pneumococcal isolates covered by PCV13. Twelve serotypes of pneumococcus are common to PCV13 and PPSV23. However, 38% of cases of invasive pneumococcal disease in adults are caused by serotypes of pneumococcus unique to PPSV23. Another study that evaluated the immune response of both vaccines showed that adults who received PCV13 as the initial vaccine followed by a dose of PPSV23 had significantly higher antibody responses than adults who received PPSV23 followed by PCV13. These data have led to the recommendation from ACIP that PCV13 and PPSV23 should be administered routinely in series to all adults 65 years and older. Figure 147–150-1 shows the recommended sequential administration intervals for PCV13 and PPSV23.

Currently, PCV13 is recommended for adults 19 years and older who have immunocompromising conditions, functional or anatomic asplenia, cerebrospinal fluid leak, or cochlear implants. The PCV13 vaccine is contraindicated in individuals known to have a severe allergic reaction to any component of PCV13, PCV7, or any diphtheria toxoid-containing vaccine. Medical conditions and other indications for PCV13, PPSV23, or both, are listed in Table 147–150-1.

Patient 147 received PPSV23 at age 60 years because diabetes mellitus is a risk factor for pneumococcal disease. Now, at age 65 years, she qualifies for the age-directed vaccination with PCV13. However, she also is due for her repeat vaccination with PPSV23 because 5 years have lapsed since she received her last dose. She

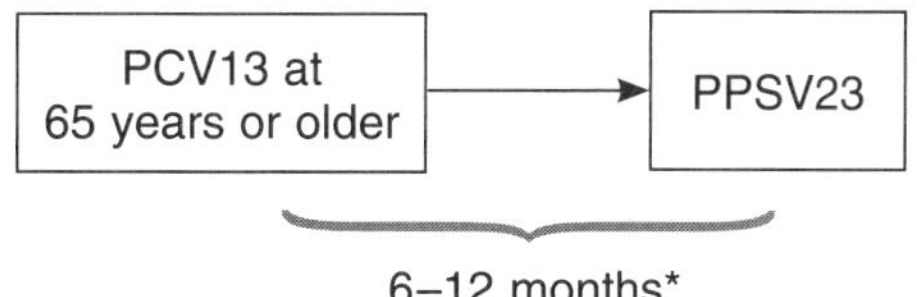

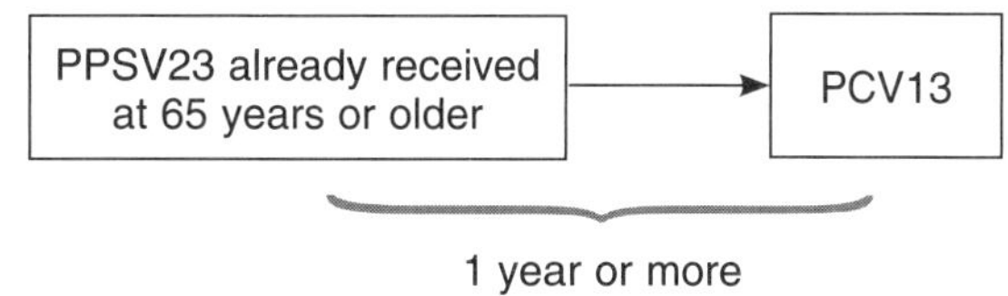

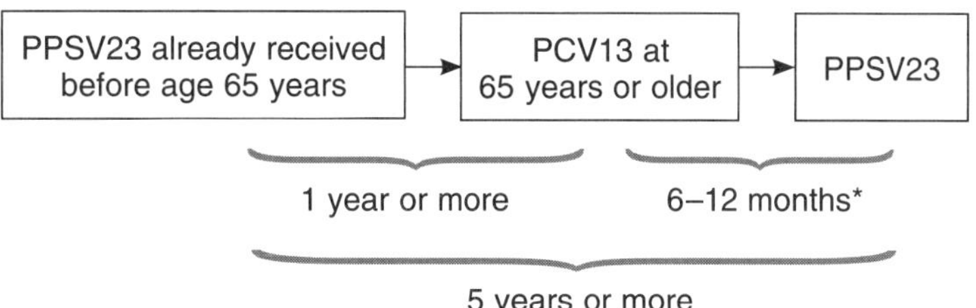

FIGURE 147–150-1. Sequential administration and recommended intervals for PCV13 and PPSV23 for adults aged 65 years and older – Advisory Committee on Immunization Practices, United States. Abbreviations: PCV13, 13-valent pneumococcal conjugate vaccine; PPSV23, 23-valent pneumococcal polysaccharide vaccine. *Minimum interval between sequential administration of PCV13 and PPSV23 is 8 weeks; PPSV23 can be given later than 6–12 months after PCV13 if this window is missed. (Tomczyk S, Bennett NM, Stoecker C, Gierke R, Moore MR, Whitney CG, et al. Use of 13-valent pneumococcal conjugate vaccine and 23-valent pneumococcal polysaccharide vaccine among adults aged >/=65 years: recommendations of the Advisory Committee on Immunization Practices [ACIP]. Centers for Disease Control and Prevention. MMWR Morb Mortal Wkly Rep 2014;63:822–5.)

should receive PCV13 now and return to the clinic in 6–12 months for a second PPSV23 vaccination. The recommended sequencing interval for PPSV23 after PCV13 is 6–12 months.

Patient 148 appropriately received PCV13 at age 19 years because she has sickle cell disease. As shown in Table 147–150-1, she also should be vaccinated with PPSV23. Because more than 6–12 months have elapsed since she received PCV13, she should receive PPSV23 now. Pregnancy is not a contraindication to pneumococcal vaccination because it is not a live bacterium. Adults aged 19–64 years with sickle cell disease or other chronic medical conditions also should receive a second booster dose of PPSV23 at 5 years after the first dose. No additional boosters would be required until the age-directed dose at age 65 years.

Patient 149 received her age-appropriate vaccination with PPSV23 at age 65 years, according to the ACIP guidelines before 2014. Current recommendations also call for vaccination with PCV13 starting at age 65 years. Given that it has been more than 12 months since she received PPSV23, she can be given PCV13 at this visit. Even though the preferred order is PCV13 first followed by PPSV23, it is not recommended to administer another PPSV23 in the future. Adults who receive PPSV23 at or after age 65 years need no further booster doses of PPSV23 even if they have chronic underlying diseases.

Patient 150 is age 27 years; PPSV23 is indicated because of her history of chronic lung disease. She does not require vaccination with PCV13, as noted in Table 147–150-1.

It is important to check regularly for updated recommendations in adult immunization guidelines. As additional studies become available, ACIP adjusts recommendations based on the Grading of Recommendations, Assessment, Development, and Evaluation framework. More information is available on the ACIP website at www.cdc.gov/vaccines/acip/.

TABLE 147–150-1. Medical Conditions or Other Indications for Administration of PCV13, and Indications for PPSV23 Administration and Revaccination for Adults 19 Years or Older

		PCV13	PPSV23*	
Risk Group	Underlying Medical Condition	Recommended	Recommended	Revaccination at 5 years after first dose
Immunocompetent individuals	Chronic heart disease†		✓	
	Chronic lung disease‡		✓	
	Diabetes mellitus		✓	
	CSF leaks	✓	✓	
	Cochlear implants	✓	✓	
	Alcoholism		✓	
	Chronic liver disease		✓	
	Cigarette smoking		✓	
Individuals with functional or anatomic asplenia	Sickle cell disease/other hemoglobinopathies	✓	✓	✓
	Congenital or acquired asplenia	✓	✓	✓
Immunocompromised individuals	Congenital or acquired immunodeficiencies§	✓	✓	✓
	HIV infection	✓	✓	✓
	Chronic renal failure	✓	✓	✓
	Nephrotic syndrome	✓	✓	✓
	Leukemia	✓	✓	✓
	Lymphoma	✓	✓	✓
	Hodgkin disease	✓	✓	✓
	Generalized malignancy	✓	✓	✓
	Iatrogenic immunosuppression‖	✓	✓	✓
	Solid organ transplant	✓	✓	✓
	Multiple myeloma	✓	✓	✓

Abbreviations: CSF, cerebrospinal fluid; HIV, human immunodeficiency virus; PCV13, 13-valent pneumococcal conjugate vaccine; PPSV23, 23-valent pneumococcal polysaccharide vaccine.

*All adults 65 years or older should receive a dose of PPSV23, regardless of previous history of vaccination with pneumococcal vaccine.

†Including congestive heart failure and cardiomyopathies

‡Including chronic obstructive pulmonary disease, emphysema, and asthma

§Includes B- (humoral) or T-lymphocyte deficiency, complement deficiencies (particularly C1, C2, C3, and C4 deficiencies), and phagocytic disorders (excluding chronic granulomatous disease)

‖Diseases requiring treatment with immunosuppressive drugs, including long-term systemic corticosteroids and radiation therapy

Centers for Disease Control and Prevention. PCV13 (pneumococcal conjugate) vaccine: Recommendations, scenarios and Q&As for healthcare professionals about PCV13 for adults. Atlanta (GA): CDC; 2015. Available at http://www.cdc.gov/vaccines/vpd-vac/pneumo/vac-pcv13-adults.htm. Retrieved June 17, 2016.

Advisory Committee on Immunization Practices (ACIP). Available at http://www.cdc.gov/vaccines/acip/. Retrieved June 17, 2016.

Centers for Disease Control and Prevention. PCV13 (pneumococcal conjugate) vaccine: Recommendations, scenarios and Q&As for healthcare professionals about PCV13 for adults. Atlanta (GA): CDC; 2015. Available at http://www.cdc.gov/vaccines/vpd-vac/pneumo/vac-pcv13-adults.htm. Retrieved June 17, 2016.

Centers for Disease Control and Prevention (CDC), Advisory Committee on Immunization Practices. Updated recommendations for prevention of invasive pneumococcal disease among adults using the 23-valent pneumococcal polysaccharide vaccine (PPSV23). Centers for Disease Control and Prevention, Advisory Committee on Immunization Practices. MMWR Morb Mortal Wkly Rep 2010;59:1102–6.

Licensure of 13-valent pneumococcal conjugate vaccine for adults aged 50 years and older. Centers for Disease Control and Prevention. MMWR Morb Mortal Wkly Rep 2012;61:394–5.

Tomczyk S, Bennett NM, Stoecker C, Gierke R, Moore MR, Whitney CG, et al. Use of 13-valent pneumococcal conjugate vaccine and 23-valent pneumococcal polysaccharide vaccine among adults aged >/=65 years: recommendations of the Advisory Committee on Immunization Practices (ACIP). Centers for Disease Control and Prevention. MMWR Morb Mortal Wkly Rep 2014;63:822–5.

151–154

Prevention strategies

Select the most appropriate category of prevention strategy (A–C) for each patient (151–154).

(A) Primary prevention
(B) Secondary prevention
(C) Tertiary prevention

151. A. A 14-year-old patient presents for a school sports physical examination. She is not yet sexually active and has no acute concerns. After performing her examination and age-appropriate counseling, you recommend she start the human papillomavirus (HPV) vaccine series.

152. B. You call a 36-year-old patient to review results from the colposcopy you performed last week. The colposcopy was adequate, and one of the biopsies revealed cervical intraepithelial neoplasia grade 2/3. You recommend that she undergo a loop electrosurgical excision procedure (LEEP).

153. B. A 34-year-old patient, gravida 1, para 1, presents for her annual examination. Last year, her Pap test was normal; HPV testing was positive, but negative for high-risk subtypes 16 and 18. Today you perform a Pap test and HPV tests.

154. C. A 92-year-old patient is brought to your office by her daughter because of vaginal bleeding. On speculum examination, a necrotic, ulcerated lesion obliterates most of her cervix. Although you do not yet have a tissue diagnosis, you want to prepare her and her family for the likely diagnosis of cervical cancer and possible management options, such as palliative radiation and hospice care.

Disease prevention is an important goal of office obstetrics and gynecology practice. Prevention entails a wide range of interventions that reduce the risk of threats to personal or population-level health. These interventions are categorized as primary, secondary, or tertiary preventions, depending on when within a disease pathway they are used.

Primary prevention refers to preventing a disease process before it occurs through prevention of exposures that may cause the disease. This prevention includes changing unsafe behaviors that may result in exposure, disease, or injury or improving resistance to disease or injury in the case of an exposure. An often described example of primary prevention is vaccination, but public health measures such as folic acid supplementation of foods or bicycle helmet regulations are other common examples. Primary prevention offers the potential for the largest effect because it begins before any disease process or exposure has started and often can be implemented at a population level.

Patient 151 has yet to be exposed to HPV, so the HPV vaccination should improve her resistance if the exposure occurs. There are three HPV vaccines currently approved for use in the United States, all with varying degrees of virus coverage: bivalent, quadrivalent, and 9-valent. The Centers for Disease Control and Prevention recommends vaccination of nonpregnant women aged 11–26 years with the 9-valent vaccine, which protects against HPV types 6, 11, 16, 18, 31, 33, 45, 52, and 58; these are the virus types responsible for most cases of cervical cancer and anogenital warts. If a patient has initiated an unknown vaccine type, it is appropriate to continue the series with any available vaccine with a goal of transitioning to the 9-valent product. Human papillomavirus vaccines have the potential to significantly decrease the burden of cervical cancer in the United States and around the world if adopted widely.

Secondary prevention decreases the effect of a disease or injury that has already occurred. This prevention is accomplished mainly by early detection and prompt treatment to halt or slow disease progression. The most common forms of secondary prevention in gynecology are cervical cancer screening and mammography.

Patient 152 will benefit from secondary prevention by undergoing LEEP. Performing LEEP can serve diagnostic and therapeutic purposes and is intended to decrease her risk of progression to cancer. Although LEEP is a surgical procedure, in this case it would be considered a form of secondary prevention because it is addressing a precancerous lesion.

Patient 153 also will benefit from secondary prevention through a Pap test and HPV testing. She has already been exposed to HPV, so preventive interventions are aimed at minimizing its effect. The progression of HPV infection and the associated changes within the cervical epithelium are well established. Thus, ongoing screening can detect changes before progression to cancer and offer an early window for treatment (as seen in Patient 152).

Tertiary prevention refers to interventions that reduce or eliminate long-term impairments or disabilities, minimize suffering, and promote lifestyle adjustments for chronic conditions. The overall goal of tertiary prevention is to reduce complications and suffering by treating disease.

Tertiary prevention of cervical cancer includes the diagnosis of cancer and treatment of confirmed cases with surgery, radiation, and sometimes chemotherapy. Palliative care is offered when the disease state is incurable or the patient cannot tolerate or declines more aggressive measures. If Patient 154 is confirmed to have cervical cancer, a conversation regarding goals of care and assessment of other comorbidities will guide what tertiary prevention strategies would be offered to maximize her comfort and minimize the effect of the disease on her life.

Cervical cancer screening and prevention. Practice Bulletin No. 157. American College of Obstetricians and Gynecologists. Obstet Gynecol 2016;127:e1–20.

Petrosky E, Bocchini JA Jr, Hariri S, Chesson H, Curtis CR, Saraiya M, et al. Use of 9-valent human papillomavirus (HPV) vaccine: updated HPV vaccination recommendations of the advisory committee on immunization practices. Centers for Disease Control and Prevention. MMWR Morb Mortal Wkly Rep 2015;64:300–4.

155–157

Evaluation of asthma in a pregnant patient

For each patient with asthma (155–157), choose the most appropriate intervention to manage her symptoms and reduce the risk of complications during pregnancy (A–D).

(A) Theophylline
(B) Low-dose daily inhaled corticosteroid
(C) High-dose inhaled corticosteroid and a long-acting inhaled β-agonist
(D) 2–4 puffs of a short-acting β-agonist as needed

155. D. A 25-year-old woman, gravida 3, para 2, at 24 weeks of gestation has asthma symptoms once a week. Her peak expiratory flow is 90% of her personal best, and she states that her asthma does not interfere with daily activity.

156. B. A 40-year-old woman, gravida 10, para 9, at 36 weeks of gestation states that she requires her albuterol inhaler four times per week. Her peak expiratory flow is 90% of her personal best. She reports some mild interference with daily activities.

157. C. A 35-year-old primigravid woman at 12 weeks of gestation has frequent asthma exacerbations. Her peak expiratory flow is 50% of her personal best, and she reports that her asthma wakes her up four to seven times per week.

Asthma complicates 4–8% of pregnancies. Asthmatic symptoms typically worsen for 30% of women and improve for 23% of women during pregnancy. Those with well-controlled asthma can have excellent obstetric outcomes. However, poorly controlled or severe asthma may be associated with an increased risk of preterm birth, preeclampsia, growth restriction, and maternal morbidity and mortality. As stated by the National Asthma Education and Prevention Program, "it is safer for pregnant women with asthma to be treated with asthma medications than it is for them to have asthma symptoms and exacerbations."

The optimal management of asthma and prevention of acute asthmatic exacerbations is essential to maternal and fetal well-being because prevention of hypoxic episodes in the mother will help to maintain adequate oxygenation for the fetus. Asthma management includes monitoring of lung function with pulmonary function testing, avoidance of triggers (such as tobacco smoke, mold, dust mite exposure, animal dander, and cockroaches), and a step-care approach to pharmacologic therapy based on the severity of the patient's asthma. Asthma generally is managed the same way in pregnant women as in nonpregnant women because typical asthma medications are considered safe during pregnancy. If asthma is well controlled with medications before pregnancy, it is recommended to continue the same medication regimen during pregnancy. A patient should seek medical care immediately if an asthma flare does not respond to therapy.

The National Asthma Education and Prevention Program Asthma and Pregnancy Working Group defined categories of asthma according to objective pulmonary function testing and occurrence of daytime and nighttime symptoms (Table 155–157-1). Most exacerbations occur between 24 weeks and 36 weeks of gestation. Baseline peak flow measurement should be obtained with the patient in the upright standing position. The patient should take a deep breath, hold it, and then place the peak flow mouthpiece between her teeth. She should then blow out hard and fast in a single blow. She should repeat this process three times. The highest number is considered her personal best peak flow.

Asthma therapy usually is divided into rescue therapy (typically a short-acting β-agonist such as albuterol) to provide immediate relief of asthma exacerbations and maintenance medications (typically inhaled corticosteroids) that provide long-term control and prevention of asthma exacerbations for those with persistent asthma. Patients with intermittent asthma require only an inhaled short-acting β-agonist as needed, whereas patients with persistent asthma need additional treatment, which follows a step therapy (Box 155–157-1). If patients who previously were considered to have intermittent asthma are routinely requiring short-acting β-agonist use more than twice weekly, the addition of an inhaled steroid (eg, budesonide or fluticasone) to the asthma management plan is recommended. If the inhaled steroid does not improve asthma exacerbations and patients require

TABLE 155–157-1. Classification of Asthma Severity and Control in Pregnant Patients

Asthma Severity* (Control†)	Symptom Frequency	Nighttime Awakening	Interference With Normal Activity	FEV_1 or Peak Flow (Predicted Percentage of Personal Best)
Intermittent (well controlled)	2 days per week or less	Twice per month or less	None	More than 80%
Mild persistent (not well controlled)	More than 2 days per week, but not daily	More than twice per month	Minor limitation	More than 80%
Moderate persistent (not well controlled)	Daily symptoms	More than once per week	Some limitation	60–80%
Severe persistent (very poorly controlled)	Throughout the day	Four times per week or more	Extremely limited	Less than 60%

Abbreviation: FEV1, forced expiratory volume in the first second of expiration

*Assess severity for patients who are not taking long-term-control medications.

†Assess control in patients taking long-term-control medications to determine whether step-up therapy, step-down therapy, or no change in therapy is indicated.

Asthma in pregnancy. ACOG Practice Bulletin No. 90. American College of Obstetricians and Gynecologists. Obstet Gynecol 2008;111:457–64.

daily rescue inhaler use, then a combined inhaled steroid/long-acting β-agonist should be prescribed instead. In general, appropriate classification of asthma severity (Table 155–157-1) is recommended in order to optimize treatment (Box 155–157-1).

Patient 155 has intermittent asthma that is well controlled; she has symptoms fewer than 2 days a week, peak flow greater than 80%, and no interference with daily activities. Therefore, she does not need to escalate therapy and can be managed with a short-acting β-agonist (such as albuterol) as needed. Patient 156 has mild persistent asthma that is not well controlled, as is evidenced by her symptom frequency greater than 2 days and less than 7 days per week, her peak flow of 90%, and minor limitations of daily activities. She would be best managed with a low-dose inhaled corticosteroid. Patient 157 has severe persistent asthma that is very poorly controlled, as evidenced by her peak flow less than 60% and her four to seven nighttime awakenings per week. She should be managed with a high-dose inhaled corticosteroid and a long-acting β-agonist (such as salmeterol). An oral corticosteroid may need to be added to her regimen. Consultation with maternal–fetal medicine or pulmonology specialists is recommended.

The published literature is contradictory with regard to the use of stress-dose steroids during labor for patients who have recently required oral steroids; however, most patients will not require this treatment. They should continue their usual dose of steroids throughout labor or perioperatively. Exceptions are patients with primary renal failure or pituitary axis disorders. If required, stress-dose steroids are safe to use during labor and delivery if the patient has required substantial systemic corticosteroid treatment before delivery. It also is important to note that certain medications commonly used in obstetrics can worsen asthma. These include prostaglandin $F_{2\alpha}$, ergonovine, and indomethacin (in patients who are aspirin allergic).

BOX 155–157-1

Step Therapy Medical Management of Asthma During Pregnancy

Intermittent Asthma

No daily medications, albuterol as needed

Mild Persistent Asthma

Preferred—Low-dose inhaled corticosteroid

Alternative—Cromolyn, leukotriene receptor antagonist, or theophylline (serum level 5–12 micrograms/mL)

Moderate Persistent Asthma

Preferred—Low-dose inhaled corticosteroid and salmeterol or medium-dose inhaled corticosteroid or (if needed) medium-dose inhaled corticosteroid and salmeterol

Alternative—Low-dose or (if needed) medium-dose inhaled corticosteroid and either leukotriene receptor antagonist or theophylline (serum level 5–12 micrograms/mL)

Severe Persistent Asthma

Preferred—High-dose inhaled corticosteroid and salmeterol and (if needed) oral corticosteroid

Alternative—High-dose inhaled corticosteroid and theophylline (serum level 5–12 micrograms/mL) and oral corticosteroid if needed

Modified from Asthma in pregnancy. ACOG Practice Bulletin No. 90. American College of Obstetricians and Gynecologists. Obstet Gynecol 2008;111:457–64.

Asthma in pregnancy. ACOG Practice Bulletin No. 90. American College of Obstetricians and Gynecologists. Obstet Gynecol 2008; 111:457–64.

Expert Panel Report 3 (EPR-3): Guidelines for the Diagnosis and Management of Asthma—Summary Report 2007. National Asthma Education and Prevention Program [published erratum appears in J Allergy Clin Immunol 2008;121:1330]. J Allergy Clin Immunol 2007;120:S94–138.

Schatz M, Dombrowski MP, Wise R, Thom EA, Landon M, Mabie W, et al. Asthma morbidity during pregnancy can be predicted by severity classification. J Allergy Clin Immunol 2003;112:283–8.

158–161
Health maintenance choices

For each patient (158–161), select the interval (A–E) when her next screening or vaccination should be performed.

(A) 1 year
(B) 3 years
(C) 5 years
(D) 10 years
(E) never

158. D. A 50-year-old white woman with no family history of colorectal cancer has normal screening colonoscopy.

159. B. A 23-year-old woman has normal cervical cytology.

160. A. A 31-year-old woman, gravida 1, receives the influenza vaccine at 23 weeks of gestation.

161. A. A 33-year-old woman undergoes depression screening during her annual well-woman examination. She has no personal history of psychiatric disorders.

A health maintenance examination is an opportunity for obstetrician–gynecologists and other health care providers to promote a healthy lifestyle and discuss disease prevention. Although there is no uniform consensus on the frequency of this examination, the American College of Obstetricians and Gynecologists (the College) recommends an annual visit. During the annual examination, screening tests and vaccine strategies should be reviewed in order to promote health and provide preventive care. Additionally, a thorough history should be taken, including medical, social, and family history. A comprehensive review of systems will help elicit other risk factors that should be addressed. Vital signs to be obtained include weight, height, blood pressure, and body mass index (calculated as weight in kilograms divided by height in meters squared [kg/m^2]). A general physical examination should be performed, which will help detect abnormalities. Clinical breast and pelvic examinations should be performed for all patients aged 21 years or older.

Because Patient 158 has no risk factors, she appropriately began screening for colorectal cancer at age 50 years. The College recommends colonoscopy as the preferred screening test for women 50 years and older. African American women should begin colorectal cancer screening at age 45 years. The U.S. Preventive Services Task Force (USPSTF) recommends screening for colorectal cancer using fecal occult blood testing, sigmoidoscopy, or colonoscopy in adults beginning at age 50 years and continuing until age 75 years. In the absence of pathology, follow-up colonoscopy every 10 years is the most effective screening regimen, as recommended by the College and USPSTF. Recent guidelines published by the U.S. Multi-Society Task Force on Colorectal Cancer provide a regimen for surveillance of adenomas discovered at screening colonoscopy. If a low-risk adenoma (tubular adenoma less than 10 mm) is discovered on screening colonoscopy, the first surveillance colonoscopy should be performed in 5–10 years. If an advanced adenoma (10 mm or more), high-grade dysplasia, or villous histology is noted on screening colonoscopy, the patient should undergo her first surveillance colonoscopy in 3 years.

The American Cancer Society, American Society for Colposcopy and Cervical Pathology, American Society for Clinical Pathology, and the College update their guidelines on a regular basis for cervical cancer screening. Cervical cancer screening should begin at age 21 years. Women aged 21–29 years should undergo cervical cytology alone every 3 years. For women aged 30–65 years, cotesting with cytology and human papillomavirus testing every 5 years is recommended. Cervical cancer screening is no longer indicated for women older than 65 years. Because Patient 159 is age 23 years and has normal cytology results, cervical cytology should be repeated every 3 years. Completion of the human papillomavirus vaccine series has no effect on recommendations regarding cervical cancer screening.

The Centers for Disease Control and Prevention recommends annual influenza vaccination for everyone 6 months and older. Vaccination to prevent influenza is particularly important for women who are or will be pregnant during the influenza season. Because Patient 160 just received the influenza vaccine during her pregnancy, she should receive the next vaccination in 1 year.

The USPSTF recommends routine screening for depression in clinical practices that have systems in place to ensure accurate diagnosis, effective treatment, and follow-up. Depression that is diagnosed is treated effectively in approximately 85% of cases. The following two questions may be as effective as using longer screening measures: 1) "Over the past two weeks, have you ever felt down, depressed, or hopeless?" and 2) "Have you felt little interest or pleasure in doing things?" Patient 161 underwent depression screening at her annual examination, so the next screening should occur in 1 year.

American College of Obstetricians and Gynecologists. Guidelines for women's health care: a resource manual. 4th edition. Washington, DC: American College of Obstetricians and Gynecologists; 2014.

Cervical cancer screening and prevention. Practice Bulletin No. 157. American College of Obstetricians and Gynecologists. Obstet Gynecol 2016;127:e1–20.

Colorectal cancer screening strategies. Committee Opinion No. 609. American College of Obstetricians and Gynecologists. Obstet Gynecol 2014;124:849–55.

Grohskopf LA, Olsen SJ, Sokolow LZ, Bresee JS, Cox NJ, Broder KR, et al. Prevention and control of seasonal influenza with vaccines: recommendations of the Advisory Committee on Immunization Practices (ACIP) — United States, 2014-15 influenza season. Centers for Disease Control and Prevention. MMWR Morb Mortal Wkly Rep 2014;63:691–7.

Lieberman DA, Rex DK, Winawer SJ, Giardiello FM, Johnson DA, Levin TR. Guidelines for colonoscopy surveillance after screening and polypectomy: a consensus update by the US Multi-Society Task Force on Colorectal Cancer. United States Multi-Society Task Force on Colorectal Cancer. Gastroenterology 2012;143:844–57.

O'Connor E, Rossom RC, Henninger M, Groom HC, Burda BU. Primary care screening for and treatment of depression in pregnant and postpartum women: evidence report and systematic review for the US Preventive Services Task Force. JAMA 2016;315:388–406. DOI:10.1001/jama.2015.18948.

Siu AL, Bibbins-Domingo K, Grossman DC, Baumann LC, Davidson KW, Ebell M, et al. Screening for depression in adults: U.S. Preventive Services Task Force recommendation statement. U.S. Preventive Services Task Force. JAMA 2016;315:380–7.

Workowski KA, Bolan GA. Sexually transmitted diseases treatment guidelines, 2015. Centers for Disease Control and Prevention [published erratum appears in MMWR Recomm Rep 2015;64:924]. MMWR Recomm Rep 2015;64:1–137.

162–166

Diagnosis of skin conditions

For each patient (162–166), select the most likely diagnosis (A–E).

(A) Contact dermatitis
(B) Lichen planus
(C) Tinea cruris
(D) Lichen simplex chronicus
(E) Lichen sclerosus

162. B. A 48-year-old woman has a 1-year history of intense vulvar itching, burning, and generalized soreness with associated yellow discharge. She has not been able to have intercourse for the past 6 months because of dyspareunia. She also mentions intermittent sores at the bottom of her gumline (Fig. 162–166-1; see color plate).

163. A. A 25-year-old woman has erythema, edema, and fissures on the vulva that, over the past several days, have evolved into erosions. She reports pruritus as well as pain and intense burning (Fig. 162–166-2; see color plate).

164. E. A 62-year-old woman reports a 6-month history of vulvar itching. She was recently treated for recurrent vulvovaginal candidiasis with some improvement in her symptoms, which was short lived. On examination, you note ivory white and shiny tissue throughout her labia minora with areas of confluent white patches (Fig. 162–166-3; see color plate).

165. D. A 21-year-old woman is referred to you by her primary care physician because of recurrent yeast infections. For the past 8 months, she has suffered from intense vulvar and perianal pruritus, and her symptoms are affecting her ability to sleep at night. She reports that she cannot stop scratching. On examination, you note that the labia minora are erythematous and swollen and that the labia majora appear pale and leathery with multiple areas of excoriations noted (Fig. 162–166-4; see color plate).

166. C. A 45-year-old woman has a pruritic rash that started on the left labium majus approximately 10 days ago and has spread to include the inner thigh and pubic area. On physical examination, you see a pale red skin eruption with sharply defined margins involving the entire left side of the vulva, intercrural fold, inner thigh, buttocks, and groin, extending onto the mons pubis. The leading edges are more intensely erythematous and demonstrate scaling (Fig. 162–166-5; see color plate).

Vulvovaginal concerns are responsible for more than 10 million office visits in the United States annually and are among the most common problems encountered by family practitioners, gynecologists, and dermatologists. Vulvovaginal disorders are common, often chronic conditions that typically present with either pruritus or pain and can significantly disrupt a woman's quality of life, particularly with respect to her general sense of well-being and sexual functioning. These symptoms can occur in the presence of obvious skin changes or with little-to-no visible evidence of dermatologic disease. *Vulvodynia* is defined as the constellation of burning, stinging rawness, or soreness; can occur with or without concurrent pruritus; and can be further classified based on whether symptoms are generalized or localized and provoked or spontaneous.

Patient 162 has lichen planus, an inflammatory autoimmune disorder that affects skin and mucous membranes. The etiology remains largely unknown but is thought to be T-cell mediated. Characteristic skin lesions are intensely pruritic, violaceous papules and plaques that often result in erosion and ulceration of the vulvar tissue. Approximately 70% of patients have involvement of the vagina, which can lead to friable mucosa and significant yellow discharge. Dyspareunia and postcoital bleeding are common symptoms when vaginal stenosis and synechiae develop from untreated cases. Wickham striae are the fine, white, lacey reticulated pattern often seen on the buccal mucosa. The most commonly affected areas include the skin of the wrists, forearms, shins, ankles, lower back, oral cavity, genital mucous membranes, scalp, and nails. Despite the severe pruritus that accompanies this disorder, excoriations are rarely present. Spontaneous remission of vulvovaginal lichen planus is quite poor, and this disorder is chronic, is often progressive and recurring, and requires long-term maintenance. As such, lifestyle modifications remain a cornerstone of therapy. In addition to strict vulvar hygiene, super potent topical steroids or, on occasion, systemic corticosteroids offer the best chance for symptom relief (Table 162–166-1). Additional treatment options for more refractory cases include topical and local cyclosporine, topical tacrolimus, hydroxychloroquine, oral retinoids, methotrexate, azathioprine, and cyclophosphamide (Box 162–166-1). Only one third of patients will experience resolution of symptoms and recurrence is almost certain. Furthermore, with lichen planus, the risk of progression to vulvar cancer is approximately 3–6%.

Patient 163 has contact dermatitis, one of the most frequently encountered vulvovaginal conditions seen in ambulatory settings. It is a condition that predominantly affects the vulva and can present in a variety of patterns, including acute, subacute, and chronic forms. Contact dermatitis often is avoidable and can be induced by a specific irritant or allergy. However, vulvar dermatitis is more commonly caused by exposure to a chemical or physical irritant than by a cell-mediated allergic response. Seemingly benign behaviors such as bathing in a tub or use of sanitary napkins or incontinence pads, feminine hygiene products, topical medications, and condoms can result in contact dermatitis. Physical examination findings range from mild erythema and edema to scaling, marked erythema, fissures, ulcers, and erosions in more severe cases. The evaluation of contact dermatitis always should exclude vulvovaginal candidiasis. Primary prevention with good vulvar hygiene and avoidance of potential irritants is key to the management of contact dermatitis.

Patient 164 has lichen sclerosus, a chronic, progressive inflammatory skin disease that often affects the genital area. Vulvar pruritus is the most common symptom and ranges from mild and intermittent to intense, constant, and intractable. Additional prominent symptoms include vulvar burning and dyspareunia. However, almost one third of women who have this condition are asymptomatic. Although the exact pathogenesis remains unknown, lichen sclerosus is thought to be autoimmune in origin, with a familial predisposition. Additional potential etiologies include infectious or environmental factors. There is a bimodal distribution, with peak incidence during the prepubertal or postmenopausal years. Lichen sclerosus leads to characteristic changes in the color and architecture of the vulva. Notably, the skin exhibits hypopigmented, ivory white patches or plaques that may coalesce to form a figure eight or hourglass appearance around the vulva and anus in conjunction with a

TABLE 162–166-1. Common Topical Steroid Formulations

Class	Name	Common Uses
Class I (super potency)	Clobetasol propionate (0.05% cream, ointment)*	Lichen sclerosus
	Halobetasol propionate (0.05% cream, ointment)	Lichen planus
Class II (high potency)	Fluocinonide (0.05%)	Psoriasis, lichen simplex chronicus
Class III	Betamethasone valerate (0.1% ointment)	Lichen simplex chronicus, maintenance of lichen sclerosus
Class IV (medium potency)	Triamcinolone (0.1% cream), hydrocortisone valerate (0.2% ointment)	Eczema, mild irritation, maintenance of lichen sclerosus
Class V	Hydrocortisone butyrate (0.1% cream), betamethasone valerate (0.1% cream), hydrocortisone valerate (0.2% cream)	Eczema, mild irritation
Class VI (low potency)	Fluocinolone acetonide (0.01%), desonide (0.05%)	Mild irritation
Class VII (mild)	Hydrocortisone (1.0%, 2.5%)	Mild eczema, maintenance

*Creams tend to work better in the vagina because of better absorption. Ointments work well on the vulva because they are less irritating than creams, solutions, jellies, or lotions and provide a soothing barrier.

Boardman LA, Kennedy CM. Vulvar disorders. Clin Update Womens Health Care 2009;VIII(2):1–117.

BOX 162–166-1

Topical Antifungals

Allylamines—Inhibit squalene epoxidase, reducing cell membrane ergosterol synthesis
- Naftifine
- Terbinafine

Hydroxypyrimidine—Chelates polyvalent cations and inhibits cell membrane transfer
- Ciclopirox

Benzylamines—Inhibit squalene epoxidase, reducing cell membrane ergosterol synthesis
- Butenafine

Thiocarbamate—Inhibit squalene epoxidase, reducing cell membrane ergosterol synthesis
- Tolnaftate

Azoles—Reduce cell membrane ergosterol synthesis, increase membrane permeability
- Clotrimazole
- Ketoconazole
- Miconazole
- Oxiconazole
- Sertaconazole
- Sulconazole
- Luliconazole
- Econazole
- Efinaconazole

Polyene—Bind cell membrane sterols, increasing permeability
- Nystatin

waxy texture of wrinkling of the epidermis commonly described as "cigarette paper." The most commonly affected area is the medial labia majora, followed by the interlabial creases, labia minora, clitoris, clitoral hood, and posterior fourchette. The vaginal mucosa typically is spared in lichen sclerosus, but approximately 30–60% of women will have perianal involvement. Approximately 2–5% of patients who have lichen sclerosus will have coexisting squamous cell carcinoma, so diagnosis should be confirmed by biopsy. Given the chronic nature of this disease, treatment options focus primarily on symptom management rather than cure, with super potent topical corticosteroids as a mainstay of therapy.

Patient 165 has lichen simplex chronicus, which is a chronic eczematous disease that results from a chronic itch–scratch cycle. Although the exact incidence is unknown, lichen simplex chronicus accounts for 10–35% of women seen in specialty vulvar clinics. It typically presents in mid-to-late adult life but also can occur in childhood. This vulvar disorder often occurs in response to an inciting process that could be environmental (eg, tight clothing, feminine products) or dermatologic (eg, candidiasis, lichen sclerosus). Atopic dermatitis (ie, eczema) also can trigger lichen simplex chronicus, and many affected women will have a personal or family history of atopy. Symptoms typically include intractable vulvar pruritus that is often worst at night and leads to unconscious scratching that can result in bleeding. With long-standing disease, the skin undergoes lichenification with thick, leathery hyperpigmented areas. Excoriations from chronic scratching are also common. Yeast and bacterial infections should be ruled out because they may be the underlying cause or inciting event for lichen simplex chronicus. The primary goal of therapy is to stop the itch–scratch cycle by removing any irritants, treating underlying disease or infections, and allowing the vulvar skin to heal.

Patient 166 has tinea cruris, which is a fungal infection of the keratinized skin caused by one of the dermatophytes: *Trichophyton, Microsporum*, or *Epidermophyton*. It is commonly misdiagnosed as a *Candida* (ie, yeast infection) and also can be confused with contact dermatitis (ie, eczema). It presents as an intensely pruritic, pale red rash with sharply demarcated and scaly borders. It spreads in an advancing, annular pattern from the labia majora to the intercrural folds, inner and upper thigh, inguinal region, buttocks, and the mons pubis. Occasionally, it can start at multiple sites and become large and contiguous. A 10% potassium hydroxide preparation can confirm segmented and branching hyphae, which excludes eczema in the differential diagnosis. The sample should be taken by using a scalpel blade to scrape scale from the leading edge of the rash onto a glass microscope slide, applying several drops of 10% potassium hydroxide, covering with a cover slip, and heating the slide with a match or alcohol lamp for 3–4 seconds. Slight compression of the cover slip will aid in separating the squamous cells and hyphae. A culture can be used to confirm but requires special media.

Boardman LA, Kennedy CM. Vulvar disorders. Clin Update Womens Health Care 2009;VIII(2):1–117.

Diagnosis and management of vulvar skin disorders. ACOG Practice Bulletin No. 93. 2008;111:1243–53.

Hoang MP, Reuter J, Papalas MA, Edwards L, Selim MA. Vulvar inflammatory dermatoses: an update and review [published erratum appears in Am J Dermatopathol 2015;37:347]. Am J Dermatopathol 2014;36:689–704.

Prabhu A, Gardella C. Common vaginal and vulvar disorders. Med Clin N Am 2015;99:553–74.

Schlosser B, Mirowski G. Lichen sclerosus and lichen planus in women and girls. Clin Obstet Gynecol 2015;58:125–42.

Thorstensen KA, Birenbaum DL. Recognition and management of vulvar dermatologic conditions: lichen sclerosus, lichen planus, and lichen simplex chronicus. J Midwifery Womens Health 2012;57:260–75.

167–169

Gestational diabetes mellitus

The prevalence of gestational diabetes mellitus (GDM) in your practice is approximately 5%. Patients currently undergo the traditional 1-hour glucose challenge test (GCT) with a 50-g glucose load in the nonfasting state at 24–28 weeks of gestation. Patients with serum glucose values greater than your currently established 140 mg/dL cutoff then undergo the diagnostic 3-hour glucose tolerance test (GTT). You are considering decreasing the cutoff from 140 mg/dL to 130 mg/dL. For each parameter (167–169), choose how this change would affect the screening performance (A–C).

(A) Increases
(B) Decreases
(C) Unaffected

167. B. Specificity

168. B. Positive predictive value

169. A. Sensitivity

Gestational diabetes mellitus is defined as hyperglycemia that is first diagnosed during pregnancy. Although pregestational diabetes complicates up to 2% of pregnancies, the prevalence of GDM is directly proportional to that of type 2 diabetes in a given population.

All pregnant women should be screened using a review the patient's risk factors and medical history. One-hour screening after a 50-g glucose load can be based on risk factors or applied universally. Because most patients have at least one risk factor, it is more common to administer the 50-g GCT to all pregnant patients at 24–28 weeks of gestation. Obese patients and those with previous GDM or known impaired glucose metabolism should undergo initial screening upon learning of the pregnancy.

The American College of Obstetricians and Gynecologists recommends a two-step screening approach to identify patients who have GDM. The American College Obstetricians and Gynecologists did not support the application of the newer one-step 75-g glucose screening, citing that this newer application leads to a significant increase in health care costs without proof of improvements in clinically significant maternal or neonatal outcomes. Therefore, the 50-g GCT is the most widely used screening test in pregnancy in the United States and is administered in the nonfasting state. Proposed cutoffs for this screening test are 130 mg/dL, 135 mg/dL, or 140 mg/dL. Those who receive positive screening test results for the 1-hour GCT undergo a 3-hour GTT with a 100-g glucose load. Typically, 1-hour GCT values of 200 mg/dL or more can be considered diagnostic of GDM; in such cases, a confirmatory 3-hour GTT is not required.

Sensitivity is defined as the number of patients who have a disease and receive a positive test result (a) divided by all the patients who have the disease ($a + c$) (Table 167–169-1). It shows the capacity of a test to correctly classify an individual who has a disease. A test with a high sensitivity has few false-negative results and will include most patients who have the disease. *Specificity* is defined as the number of patients who do not have disease and receive a negative test result (d) divided by the number of patients who do not have the disease ($b + d$). It shows the capacity of a test to correctly classify an individual who does not have a disease. A test with high specificity will have few false-positive results. *Positive predictive value* is defined as the number of patients who have a disease and receive a positive test result (a) divided by all those who received a positive test result ($a + b$). It gives the probability of the patient having the disease if the test result is positive. The *negative predictive value* is defined as the number of patients who have a disease and receive a negative test result (d) divided by all those who received a negative test result ($c + d$). It gives the probability of being disease-free if the test result is negative.

Sensitivity and specificity are noted to be 85% and 86%, respectively, for the 1-hour cutoff of 140 mg/dL and 99% and 77%, respectively, for the 1-hour cutoff of 130 mg/dL. Using a lower cutoff for 1-hour screening will cause more patients to screen positive, so the likelihood of identifying all the patients who have GDM increases. Therefore, the sensitivity increases. However, lowering the cutoff increases the number of patients who may be incorrectly considered as potentially having

TABLE 167–169-1. Calculating the Test Characteristics of a Screening Test

Test	Disease: Present	Disease: Absent	
Positive	*a* (= true positive)	*b* (= false positive)	Positive predictive value = $\frac{a}{(a+b)}$
Negative	*c* (= false negative)	*d* (= true negative)	Negative predictive value = $\frac{d}{(c+d)}$
	Sensitivity = $\frac{a}{(a+c)}$	Specificity = $\frac{d}{(b+d)}$	

GDM. Therefore, the specificity decreases. When the glucose screening cutoff is lowered from 140 mg/dL to 130 mg/dL, there will be more false-positive test results, so the positive predictive value will decrease. The negative predictive value will increase very slightly from 0.990 to 0.999.

Donovan L, Hartling L, Muise M, Guthrie A, Vandermeer B, Dryden DM. Screening tests for gestational diabetes: a systematic review for the U.S. Preventive Services Task Force. Ann Intern Med 2013;159: 115–22.

Gestational diabetes mellitus. Practice Bulletin No. 137. American College of Obstetricians and Gynecologists. Obstet Gynecol 2013;122:406–16.

Hartling L, Dryden DM, Guthrie A, Muise M, Vandermeer B, Donovan L. Benefits and harms of treating gestational diabetes mellitus: a systematic review and meta-analysis for the U.S. Preventive Services Task Force and the National Institutes of Health Office of Medical Applications of Research. Ann Intern Med 2013;159:123–9.

Mackeen AD, Trauffer P. Gestational diabetes. In: Berghella V, editor. Maternal–fetal evidence based guidelines. 2nd ed. New York (NY): Informa Healthcare; 2011. p. 47–54.

170–174

Modifiers to amend evaluation and management code

For each described patient (170–174), indicate which modifier (A–G) is appropriate to amend the evaluation and management (E/M) code.

(A) E/M service code only
(B) Modifier 22, increased procedural services
(C) Modifier 24, E/M service by the same physician or other qualified health care provider during a postoperative period
(D) Modifier 25, significant, separately identifiable E/M service by the same physician or other qualified health care provider on the same day of the procedure or other service
(E) Modifier 57, decision for surgery
(F) Procedure code only
(G) E/M service with procedure code

170. C. A 47-year-old woman, gravida 3, para 3, had a hysterectomy 8 weeks ago. She comes to your office reporting a breast lump. She has no family history of breast cancer. You perform an examination and order diagnostic mammography.

171. D. A 62-year-old woman, gravida 3, para 3, comes to your office with vaginal bleeding. You do a medical history and physical examination and recommend endometrial sampling, which you perform that day.

172. F. A 27-year-old woman, gravida 3, para 3, had cervical cytologic screening 3 weeks ago that showed a result of low-grade squamous intraepithelial lesion. She comes to your office today for a colposcopy and to discuss cervical cancer screening and the natural history of the human papillomavirus.

173. E. A 27-year-old woman, gravida 2, para 1, at 10 weeks of gestation previously underwent ultrasonography that showed an intrauterine gestational sac. She comes to your office now with heavy bleeding. You diagnose incomplete miscarriage and take her to the operating room to perform a dilation and curettage (D&C) the same day.

174. A. A 65-year-old woman, gravida 3, para 3, calls your office because of vaginal bleeding. You order ultrasonography that shows a thickened endometrial lining of 12 mm. During her appointment, you discuss her ultrasonographic findings, your recommendation for endometrial sampling, and your rationale.

Current Procedural Terminology (CPT) is the standard national coding system to describe procedures and services performed by physicians. The CPT code set identifies the cognitive, procedural, or diagnostic services provided to a patient. These codes are used for data collection, quality reviews, and communication with third-party payers and government agencies to accurately identify the services performed. The CPT's definition of its global surgical package can be found in the Surgical Guidelines section of CPT (Table 170–174-1). Global surgical packages include all necessary services furnished by the surgeon before, during, and after the procedure. According to Medicare and CPT, services outside the range of the global period are not bundled into the surgical package and are reported separately.

Evaluation and management service codes are used to report services provided in the diagnosis and treatment of illness, disease, and symptoms. In some circumstances, an E/M service and a procedure can be performed and reported during the same encounter. *Current Procedural Terminology* uses modifiers to indicate that a service or procedure has been altered by some specific circumstance but not altered such that the service or procedure itself has changed. Modifiers are two-character codes appended to the CPT code. *Current Procedural Terminology* and Medicare rules state that an E/M visit on the day of a procedure should be reported only if the patient's condition requires a significant, separately identifiable E/M service. All procedure codes include the evaluation services necessary to perform the procedure

TABLE 170–174-1. Comparison of Medicare and *Current Procedural Terminology* Global Surgical Packages

Types of Services	CPT Surgical Package	Medicare Surgical Packages		
		Major Surgery (90 days)	**Minor Surgery (0 days or 10 days)**	
	Preoperative Services Included in the Global Package			
Global Pre-op days	Day of or day before surgery	Day of or day before surgery	Day of surgery	
Related E/M Services*	Bill ONLY if decision for surgery made during visit (Modifier 57)	Bill ONLY if decision for surgery made during visit (Modifier 57)	Do not bill separately	
Related or unrelated significant, separately identifiable E/M services*	Bill separately (Modifier 25)	Bill separately (Modifier 25)	Bill separately (Modifier 25)	
	Intraoperative Services Included in the Global Package			
Anesthesia performed by surgeon	Bill ONLY for regional or general anesthesia	Do not bill separately for ANY anesthesia	Do not bill separately for ANY anesthesia	
Operation itself	All integral procedures included	All integral procedures included	All integral procedures included	
Complications treated by surgeon	Bill separately	Do not bill separately	Do not bill separately	
	Postoperative Services Included in the Global Package			
Global Post-op days	Not specified	90 days	0 day (Day of procedure)	10 days
Routine E/M services	Do not bill separately	Do not bill separately	Do not bill separately	Do not bill separately
Treatment of complications	Bill separately	Bill ONLY if provided in operating room (Modifier 78)	Do not bill separately	Bill ONLY if provided in operating room (Modifier 78)
Treatment of other conditions	Bill separately (modifier 24, 58, or 79)	Bill separately (modifier 24, 58, or 79)	Bill separately (modifier 24, 58, or 79)	

Abbreviation: CPT, *Current Procedural Terminology*; E/M, evaluation and management.

*Note: Significant and separately identifiable services can be reported both to CPT and Medicare (modifier 25).

Modifiers, as listed in the table, serve two functions: 1) to slightly alter the meaning of a CPT code or 2) to report additional information. The following modifiers may be required when reporting certain services:

24 Unrelated evaluation and management service by same physician during a postoperative period

25 Significant, separately identifiable evaluation and management service by same physician on same day of the procedure/other service

57 Decision for surgery

58 Staged of related procedure or service by the same physician during the postoperative period

78 Unplanned return to operating/procedure room by the same physician following initial procedure for a related procedure during the postoperative period

79 Unrelated procedure or service by same physician during the postoperative period

American Congress of Obstetricians and Gynecologists. 2016 coding manual: components of correct procedural coding. Washington, DC: American Congress of Obstetricians and Gynecologists; 2016.

and obtain consent. Therefore, the E/M service should be above and beyond the usual preoperative and postoperative care provided with that procedure. If distinct and separate services are performed, modifier 25 or modifier 57 is appropriate.

Only the procedure code should be reported if the patient is seen expressly for a procedure, if the decision to perform the procedure was made previously, and if the physician only provided services that are typically part of the procedure. Only the procedure code should be reported if the E/M service performed did not require significant history, physical examination, or decision making. The discussion of the indications is a part of counseling and consent and, therefore, is part of the global surgical package. However, to report the E/M service and the procedure code, the obstetrician–gynecologist or other health care provider must address signs, symptoms, and conditions before determining the need for the procedure; reporting the E/M and procedure codes also is warranted if the obstetrician–gynecologist or other health care provider's work is considered above and beyond the normal preprocedure and postprocedure work associated with that procedure, as supported by documentation in the medical record.

There are two primary definitions of the global package: the CPT definition and the Medicare definition. Most third-party payers follow either the CPT or Medicare global package definition. However, some third-party payers have developed their own definitions and apply their own payment policies, and these may differ from either CPT or Medicare guidelines. It is important to check with each individual payer regarding these guidelines.

Global periods are determined by the Centers for Medicare and Medicaid Services, and each procedure is assigned a 0-day, 10-day, or 90-day global period that encompasses the period during which services are included in the surgical package. Medicare major surgical procedures are assigned 90-day global periods beginning the day before the surgery and extending 90 days after the surgery; this period includes all intraoperative care as well as any in-hospital care and postoperative follow-up related to the procedure that does not require a return trip to the operating or procedure room. Examples of procedures that have a 90-day global period are surgical laparoscopy, cone biopsy or loop electrosurgical excision procedure, hysteroscopic sterilization, and D&C for failed pregnancies. Modifier 57 is appended for procedures that have a 90-day global period and should be used for major procedures.

Medicare minor surgical procedures that are assigned 10-day global periods (eg, D&C for nonobstetric indications or laparoscopic adnexal surgery) include only the day of the procedure plus the 10 days afterward. Most office-based procedures (eg, endometrial biopsy, colposcopy, diagnostic hysteroscopy) have 0-day global periods and include only the day of the procedure. If a patient is seen in your office and, after counseling, the decision is made to perform a procedure, modifier 25 is appended to the E/M visit code for procedures that have a 0-day or 10-day global period; this modifier should be used for minor procedures.

Postoperative care after a surgical procedure (eg, staple removal, wound checks, dressing changes at a routine postoperative visit) is included in the global surgical package. According to CPT guidelines, treatments resulting from surgical complications are not included as part of the global surgical package and should be coded using the appropriate CPT code(s) in addition to the supporting International Classification of Diseases, 10th Revision, Clinical Modification diagnosis code(s). Medicare includes treatments for surgical complications as part of the global package, and these services are not separately reported except in the following circumstances: visits unrelated to the diagnosis for which the surgical procedure was performed, treatment for the underlying condition or an added course of treatment that is not part of normal recovery from surgery, and treatment for postoperative complications requiring a return trip to the operating or procedure room (eg, evacuation of hematoma or treatment of a wound dehiscence). According to Medicare, if the patient returns to the operating room, the obstetrician–gynecologist or other qualified health care provider would report the appropriate CPT code appended with modifier 78 to indicate an unplanned return to the operating room for a related procedure during the postoperative period.

For patient encounters that are unrelated to the initial surgery and that are separately identifiable, as in the case of Patient 170, who was examined with a breast concern that was unrelated to her hysterectomy, modifier 24 is appended to the encounter. The encounter with Patient 171 provides an example of when modifier 25 should be appended to the E/M code because the health care provider does a history, performs an examination, and discusses options in addition to the minor procedure (0-day or 10 day-global surgical period). The E/M code is payer specific in this instance.

Patient 172 had a planned colposcopy. Encounters on the same day of the procedure include patient consent and discussion of the patient's reasons for the visit and are included in the global surgical package. The procedure code is billed without any modifiers. If the patient had come to your office only for counseling and no procedure at that time, no procedure code or modifier would be the appropriate E/M code. However, if the obstetrician–gynecologist or other health care provider had counseled the patient and also performed a colposcopy during the same appointment, the visit would be billed as an E/M service with procedure code.

Preoperative visits for a planned surgical procedure may be coded using an E/M code unless it is done within the global period (the day of or the day before a major surgical procedure). Patient 173, who had an incomplete miscarriage, represents a case where an unplanned procedure was done on the same day. In such cases, modifier 57, indicating an encounter with the decision for surgery, is appended to the E/M code reported with the major surgical procedure code (ie, 90-day global surgical period).

For Patient 174, the decision for the procedure was made during the time of the visit but no procedure or examination was performed. Therefore, the counseling and discussion are separately reported under E/M code only, and no modifier is required.

According to CPT, when the work necessary to provide the service(s) is substantially greater than what usually is required for the procedure, it may be identified by adding modifier 22 to the procedure code. The use of this code is not appropriate for E/M encounters. Modifier 22 may be appended only if the documentation supports the additional work as substantial and the reason for the additional work, such as the following:

- Increased intensity or time
- Increased technical difficulty of performing the procedure
- Severity of patient's condition
- Increased physical and mental effort required

If increased time was involved, the physician should specifically document the total time and how it compares with the typical time for the procedure. In most cases, the third-party payer will need to review the documentation to determine if the expanded services claim is justified.

American Congress of Obstetricians and Gynecologists. 2016 coding manual: components of correct procedural coding. Washington, DC: ACOG; 2016.

American Medical Association. CPT: current procedural terminology: 2016. Professional ed. Chicago (IL): AMA; 2016.

175–177

Patient safety

For each scenario (175–177), choose the best strategy (A–D) to ensure safe and effective care in the ambulatory setting.

(A) Electronic medical record
(B) Emergency drills
(C) Checklists
(D) Shared decision making

175. C. A busy outpatient gynecology office plans to start performing hysteroscopy and needs to ensure that the staff will be able to prepare and recover each patient safely and effectively.

176. B. An elderly patient comes in for a routine appointment and tells the front desk staff that she is feeling short of breath after walking from her car. The patient is asked to sit down while the front desk staff notifies a nurse that she has checked in. When the staff member returns, the patient is slumped over in the chair and unresponsive.

177. D. A 28-year-old woman, gravida 2, para 1, visits your office for a routine antepartum visit at 32 weeks of gestation. For her first delivery, she had planned on having a vaginal birth but delivered by cesarean delivery when she presented in active labor at term with the fetus in the breech presentation. She wants to discuss mode of delivery for her current pregnancy.

Obstetrician–gynecologists are natural leaders in the patient safety advocacy movement. Initial patient safety improvements have centered on the inpatient arenas of labor and delivery as well as the operating room. Standardizing patient safety in the outpatient setting has been more of a challenge because of the heterogeneity of office practice, the lack of a single regulating organization, and the difficulty in identifying applicable universal quality measures.

The American College of Obstetricians and Gynecologists (the College) recognizes that protocols and checklists have been shown to reduce patient harm through improved standardization and communication and should be recognized as guides to the management of a clinical situation or process of care that will apply to most patients. Although checklists and protocols should apply to most patients and situations, deviation from a protocol is allowable as long as there is documented reasoning and rationale. Checklists have long been used to ensure safety for highly reliable industries, such as aviation and the nuclear industry. Use of checklists, such as the Joint Commission's Universal Protocol, has been adopted in operating rooms to ensure adherence to such processes as documented informed consent, procedure-site verification, administration of preoperative antibiotics, and the use of venous thromboembolism prophylaxis in the perioperative period.

Performance of ambulatory surgery has many benefits for patients and can be more cost-effective, but because there are fewer regulations than in the inpatient setting, the potential for error is high. The use of checklists would be similarly useful for the standardization of safe care for patients undergoing office procedures such as hysteroscopy. It is the most useful option for Scenario 175.

The safe outpatient obstetrics and gynecology practice must be prepared to handle any number of possible, albeit rare, emergencies that may occur in pregnant patients or in women with comorbidities who are seeking routine gynecologic care. Examples of potential emergencies that may occur in the outpatient obstetrics and gynecology office include a precipitous delivery, hemorrhage, allergic reaction, or an acute medical event such as a seizure, stroke, or cardiac arrest. Emergency preparedness requires an assessment of the actual or potential risks related to the setting or patient population. Emergency response may require clinical obstetrician–gynecologists and other health care providers to step outside of their traditional roles to become a vital part of an efficient emergency response team. Necessary items such as a resuscitation cart should be readily and centrally located. The potential for an emergency event in the outpatient clinic is real, and because it is uncommon and unpredictable, the team does not have the opportunity to regularly test the response system. Conducting periodic drills enforces emergency protocols, team building, and the detection of issues related to the physical environment.

An encounter with an unstable or unresponsive patient, as in Scenario 176, should not be the first time that the office staff has to determine where the crash cart is or who to call for help. Emergency drills can prepare the entire care team for responding to rare but predictable emergencies.

The patient–physician relationship can be improved by the use of patient-centered interviewing, caring and effective communication skills, and shared decision making. Shared decision making is a process in which physicians and patients share information, express treatment preferences, and agree on a treatment plan. The National Institutes of Health Consensus Development Panel on vaginal birth after cesarean delivery recommends that the decision between a trial of labor or a planned repeat cesarean delivery occur after a conversation between the patient and the physician that incorporates risks, benefits, and patient preferences. This is an example of shared decision making and is the most appropriate strategy for Scenario 177.

There are many areas of outpatient care that have the potential to be made safer by the use of electronic medical records. These include a reduction of medication errors through embedded software to check for cross-reactions among multiple medications; the use of electronic prescribing to reduce errors in interpretation of handwriting; improved communication among various obstetrician–gynecologists and other health care providers with access to the same electronic record; and the ability to create tracking and reminder systems to facilitate follow-up of ordered laboratory tests, imaging, or referrals.

The College published its executive summary of the Presidential Task Force on Patient Safety in the Office Setting in 2010. In addition, the College has moved to improve patient safety in the outpatient setting through the creation of the Safety Certification in Outpatient Practice Excellence, a voluntary certification based on implementation of patient safety concepts and techniques in an obstetrics and gynecology office.

Clinical guidelines and standardization of practice to improve outcomes. Committee Opinion No. 629. American College of Obstetricians and Gynecologists. Obstet Gynecol 2015;125:1027–9.

Effective patient-physician communication. Committee Opinion No. 587. American College of Obstetricians and Gynecologists. Obstet Gynecol 2014;123:389–93.

Erickson TB, Kirkpatrick DH, DeFrancesco MS, Lawrence HC 3rd. Executive summary of the American College of Obstetricians and Gynecologists Presidential Task Force on Patient Safety in the Office Setting: reinvigorating safety in office-based gynecologic surgery. Obstet Gynecol 2010;115:147–51.

Patient safety in obstetrics and gynecology. ACOG Committee Opinion No. 447. American College of Obstetricians and Gynecologists. Obstet Gynecol 2009;114:1424–7.

178–181

Evaluation of incontinence

Determine the most cost-effective test (A–E) to establish a diagnosis for each patient (178–181).

(A) Urine culture
(B) Postvoid residual urine volume
(C) Cough stress test
(D) Urinalysis
(E) Multichannel urodynamics

178. C. A 37-year-old woman, gravida 3, para 3, who is 10 months postpartum complains that she cannot lose her pregnancy weight because she leaks urine whenever she tries to exercise.

179. D. A 52-year-old woman says she has not experienced dysuria but reports frequent urination and knows the location of the closest bathrooms off the freeway on her daily commute.

180. E. A 63-year-old woman with prior pelvic radiation reports ongoing leakage and urgency despite 3 months of antimuscarinic use.

181. A. A 72-year-old diabetic woman is brought in by the caretakers at her retirement community because of acute onset of leakage and frequency.

Urinary incontinence is quite common and affects approximately 10–70% of community-living women and up to 50% of female nursing-home residents. Incidence increases starting around middle age. Numerous etiologies of incontinence exist, some of which are not genitourinary (Box 178–181-1). Most cases of incontinence can be classified as stress (approximately 50%), urge (approximately 15%), and overflow or mixed (approximately 35% combined). Incontinence is often, although not always, associated with pelvic organ prolapse. Other risk factors for developing urinary incontinence include obesity, parity, vaginal delivery, and family history.

Despite the prevalence of incontinence, many women are not aware that loss of bladder control is abnormal and not just a routine part of getting older. Additionally, many women are unaware that incontinence is amenable to treatment, so only one half of symptomatic women seek care. Not all obstetrician–gynecologists and other health care providers routinely assess for incontinence, making it more difficult for women to obtain the care they need. In some studies, just over one half of primary care providers feel comfortable even inquiring about urinary incontinence, and only 20% feel comfortable diagnosing it. Being alert for common symptoms and specifically eliciting them with the use of focused questions can help uncover this common condition and the relative effect on a patient's life (Box 178–181-2).

The initial diagnosis of incontinence is made by history, physical examination, and laboratory testing. Standard initial evaluation in the office consists of urinalysis, postvoid residual urine volume, and cough stress test. Patient voiding diaries can be useful tools to add to the history assessment. These daily urinary diaries—used to record voiding frequency, nocturia, episodes of incontinence, and oral intake—have been found to correlate well with urodynamic diagnosis. Medical and surgical history taking is especially important in older patients or those with incontinence that is mixed or resistant to standard treatment. Older patients also are more likely to have chronic conditions or take medications that exacerbate incontinence. Although initial evaluation commonly includes a urinalysis, urine culture, postvoid residual urine volume, cough stress test, and complete urogenital examination, patient symptoms often point to a single test that may lead to the correct diagnosis.

Patient 178 describes symptoms most consistent with stress incontinence, so a cough stress test would be the single most useful test in her initial evaluation. After filling the bladder with water, the patient is asked to cough or strain. Leakage of urine is consistent with a positive cough stress test result and is suggestive of stress urinary incontinence.

Patient 179 describes classic symptoms of overactive bladder or urge incontinence. A urinalysis would be the single most important step to rule out hematuria or infection before starting lifestyle modification. Although in practice many obstetrician–gynecologists and other health care providers also would measure postvoid residual urine volume and begin empiric treatment with an antimuscarinic agent, simple evaluation with a urinalysis

BOX 178–181-1

Differential Diagnosis of Urinary Incontinence in Women

Genitourinary Etiology
- Filling and storage disorders
  - Urodynamic stress incontinence
  - Detrusor overactivity (idiopathic)
  - Detrusor overactivity (neurogenic)
  - Mixed types
- Fistula
  - Vesical
  - Ureteral
  - Urethral
- Infectious
  - Urinary tract infection
  - Vaginitis
- Congenital
  - Ectopic ureter
  - Epispadias

Nongenitourinary Etiology
- Functional
  - Neurologic
  - Cognitive
  - Psychologic
  - Physical impairment
- Environmental
- Pharmacologic
- Metabolic

Urinary incontinence in women. Practice Bulletin No. 155. American College of Obstetricians and Gynecologists. Obstet Gynecol 2015;126:e66–81.

BOX 178–181-2

Key Questions in Evaluating Patients for Urinary Incontinence

Do you leak urine when you cough, laugh, lift something, or sneeze? How often?*

Do you ever leak urine when you have a strong urge on the way to the bathroom? How often?†

How frequently do you empty your bladder during the day?†

How many times do you get up to urinate after going to sleep? Is it the urge to urinate that wakes you?†

Do you ever leak urine during sex?†

Do you wear pads that protect you from leaking urine? How often do you have to change them?‡

Did you ever find urine on your pads or clothes and were unaware of when the leakage occurred?‡

Does it hurt when you urinate?§

Do you ever feel that you are unable to completely empty your bladder?§

*To help identify the symptom of stress incontinence.

†To help diagnose overactive bladder.

‡To assess the severity of urine loss.

§To identify outlet obstruction, interstitial cystitis, or urinary tract infection.

Culligan PJ, Heit M. Urinary incontinence in women: evaluation and management. Am Fam Physician 2000;62: 2433,44, 2447, 2452.

would be an appropriate first test before starting conservative treatment with lifestyle modification.

Patient 180 would most likely benefit from referral to a specialist for multichannel urodynamics, given her treatment resistance, mixed incontinence, and history of radiation. Multichannel urodynamics testing allows for more complete evaluation of the bladder and urethra and the associated pressures and volumes with bladder filling, contractions, and urge.

Evaluation of Patient 181 should begin with a urine culture because acute incontinence in the elderly and institutionalized population is a common symptom of a urinary tract infection. Urinary tract infections in this population can easily lead to urosepsis and hospitalizations complicated by delirium, so prompt evaluation and treatment is recommended.

Jirschele K, Ross R, Goldberg R, Botros S. Physician attitudes toward urinary incontinence identification. Female Pelvic Med Reconstr Surg 2015;21:273–6.

Siddiqui NY, Levin PJ, Phadtare A, Pietrobon R, Ammarell N. Perceptions about female urinary incontinence: a systematic review. Int Urogynecol J 2014;25:863–71.

Urinary incontinence in women. Practice Bulletin No. 155. American College of Obstetricians and Gynecologists. Obstet Gynecol 2015;126:e66–81.

Well-woman visit. Committee Opinion No. 534. American College of Obstetricians and Gynecologists. Obstet Gynecol 2012;120:421–4.

Willis-Gray MG, Sandoval JS, Maynor J, Bosworth HB, Siddiqui NY. Barriers to urinary incontinence care seeking in White, Black, and Latina women. Female Pelvic Med Reconstr Surg 2015;21:83–6.

Wu JM, Matthews CA, Conover MM, Pate V, Jonsson Funk M. Lifetime risk of stress urinary incontinence or pelvic organ prolapse surgery. Obstet Gynecol 2014;123:1201–6.

Appendix A

Normal Values for Laboratory Tests*

Analyte	Conventional Units
Alanine aminotransferase, serum	8–35 units/L
Alkaline phosphatase, serum	15–120 units/L
Menopause	
Amniotic fluid index	3–30 mL
Amylase	20–300 units/L
Greater than 60 years old	21–160 units/L
Aspartate aminotransferase, serum	15–30 units/L
Bicarbonate	
Arterial blood	21–27 mEq/L
Venous plasma	23–29 mEq/L
Bilirubin	
Total	0.3–1 mg/dL
Conjugated (direct)	0.1–0.4 mg/dL
Newborn, total	1–10 mg/dL
Blood gases (arterial) and pulmonary function	
Base deficit	Less than 3 mEq/L
Base excess, arterial blood, calculated	–2 mEq/L to +3 mEq/L
Forced expiratory volume (FEV_1)	3.5–5 L Greater than 80% of predicted value
Forced vital capacity	3.5–5 L
Oxygen saturation (So_2)	95% or higher
Pao_2	80 mm Hg or more
Pco_2	35–45 mm Hg
Po_2	80–95 mm Hg
Peak expiratory flow rate	Approximately 450 L/min
pH	7.35–7.45
Pvo_2	30–40 mm Hg
Blood urea nitrogen	
Adult	7–18 mg/dL
Greater than 60 years old	8–20 mg/dL
CA 125	Less than 34 units/mL
Calcium	
Ionized	4.6–5.3 mg/dL
Serum	8.6–10 mg/dL
Chloride	98–106 mEq/L
Cholesterol	
Total	
Desirable	140–199 mg/dL
Borderline high	200–239 mg/dL
High	240 mg/dL or more
High-density lipoprotein	40–85 mg/dL
Low-density lipoprotein	
Desirable	Less than 130 mg/dL
Borderline high	140–159 mg/dL
High	Greater than 160 mg/dL
Total cholesterol-to-high-density lipoprotein ratio	
Desirable	Less than 3
Borderline high	3–5
High	Greater than 5
Triglycerides	
20 years and older	Less than 150 mg/dL
Younger than 20 years old	35–135 mg/dL

*Values listed are specific for adults or women, if relevant, unless otherwise differentiated.

(continued)

Normal Values for Laboratory Tests* (*continued*)

Analyte	Conventional Units
Cortisol, plasma	
8 AM	5–23 micrograms/dL
4 PM	3–15 micrograms/dL
10 PM	Less than 50% of 8 AM value
Creatinine, serum	0.6–1.2 mg/dL
Dehydroepiandrosterone sulfate	60–340 micrograms/dL
Erythrocyte	
Count	3,800,000–5,100,000/mm^3
Distribution width	10 plus or minus 1.5%
Sedimentation rate	
Wintrobe method	0–15 mm/hour
Westergren method	0–20 mm/hour
Estradiol-17β	
Follicular phase	30–100 pg/mL
Ovulatory phase	200–400 pg/mL
Luteal phase	50–140 pg/mL
Child	0.8–56 pg/mL
Ferritin, serum	18–160 micrograms/L
Fibrinogen	150–400 mg/dL
Follicle-stimulating hormone	
Premenopause	2.8–17.2 mIU/mL
Midcycle peak	15–35 mIU/mL
Postmenopause	24–170 mIU/mL
Child	0.1–7 mIU/mL
Glucose	
Fasting	70–105 mg/dL
2-hour postprandial	Less than 120 mg/dL
Random blood	65–110 mg/dL
Hematocrit	36–48%
Hemoglobin	12–16 g/dL
Fetal	Less than 1% of total
Hemoglobin A_{1c} (nondiabetic)	5.5–8.5%
Human chorionic gonadotropin	0–5 mIU/mL
Pregnant	Greater than 5 mIU/mL
17α-Hydroxyprogesterone	
Adult	50–300 ng/dL
Child	32–63 ng/dL
25-Hydroxyvitamin D	10–55 ng/mL
International Normalized Ratio	Greater than 1
Prothrombin time	10–13 seconds
Iron, serum	65–165 micrograms/dL
Binding capacity total	240–450 micrograms/dL
Lactate dehydrogenase, serum	313–618 units/L
Leukocytes	
Total	5,000–10,000/cubic micrometers
Differential counts	
Basophils	0–1%
Eosinophils	1–3%
Lymphocytes	25–33%
Monocytes	3–7%
Myelocytes	0%
Band neutrophils	3–5%
Segmented neutrophils	54–62%

*Values listed are specific for adults or women, if relevant, unless otherwise differentiated.

(continued)

Normal Values for Laboratory Tests* (*continued*)

Analyte	Conventional Units
Lipase	
60 years or younger	10–140 units/L
Older than 60 years	18–180 units/L
Luteinizing hormone	
Follicular phase	3.6–29.4 mIU/mL
Midcycle peak	58–204 mIU/mL
Postmenopause	35–129 mIU/mL
Child	0.5–10.3 mIU/mL
Magnesium	
Adult	1.6–2.6 mg/dL
Child	1.7–2.1 mg/dL
Newborn	1.5–2.2 mg/dL
Mean corpuscular	
mCH Hemoglobin	27–33 pg
mCHC Hemoglobin concentration	33–37 g/dL
mCV Volume	80–100 cubic micrometers
Partial thromboplastin time, activated	21–35 seconds
Phosphate, inorganic phosphorus	2.5–4.5 mg/dL
Platelet count	140,000–400,000/mm^3
Potassium	3.5–5.3 mEq/L
Progesterone	
Follicular phase	Less than 3 ng/mL
Luteal phase	2.5–28 ng/mL
On oral contraceptives	0.1–0.3 ng/mL
Secretory phase	5–30 ng/mL
Older than 60 years	0–0.2 ng/mL
1st trimester	9–47 ng/mL
2nd trimester	16.8–146 ng/mL
3rd trimester	55–255 ng/mL
Prolactin	0–17 ng/mL
Pregnant	34–386 ng/mL by 3rd trimester
Prothrombin time	10–13 seconds
Reticulocyte count	Absolute: 25,000–85,000 cubic micrometers 0.5–2.5% of erythrocytes
Semen analysis, spermatozoa	
Antisperm antibody	% of sperm binding by immunobead technique; greater than 20% = decreased fertility
Count	Greater than or equal to 20 million/mL
Motility	Greater than or equal to 50%
Morphology	Greater than or equal to 15% normal forms
Sodium	135–145 mEq/L
Testosterone, female	
Total	6–86 ng/dL
Pregnant	3–4 × normal
Postmenopause	One half of normal
Free	
20–29 years old	0.9–3.2 pg/mL
30–39 years old	0.8–3 pg/mL
40–49 years old	0.6–2.5 pg/mL
50–59 years old	0.3–2.7 pg/mL
Older than 60 years	0.2–2.2 pg/mL
Thyroid-stimulating hormone	0.2–3 microunits/mL
Thyroxine	
Serum free	0.9–2.3 ng/dL
Total	1.5–4.5 micrograms/dL

*Values listed are specific for adults or women, if relevant, unless otherwise differentiated.

(continued)

Normal Values for Laboratory Tests* (*continued*)

Analyte	Conventional Units
Triiodothyronine uptake	25–35%
Urea nitrogen, blood	
Adult	7–18 mg/dL
Older than 60 years	8–20 mg/dL
Uric acid, serum	2.6–6 mg/dL
Urinalysis	
Epithelial cells	0–3/HPF
Erythrocytes	0–3/HPF
Leukocytes	0–4/HPF
Protein (albumin)	
Qualitative	None detected
Quantitative	10–100 mg/24 hours
Pregnancy	Less than 300 mg/24 hours
Urine specific gravity	
Normal hydration and volume	1.005–1.03
Concentrated	1.025–1.03
Diluted	1.001–1.01

*Values listed are specific for adults or women, if relevant, unless otherwise differentiated.

Appendix B

BOX B-1

Edinburgh Postnatal Depression Scale

Instructions for users:

1. The mother is asked to underline the response that comes closest to how she has been feeling in the previous 7 days.
2. All 10 items must be completed.
3. Care should be taken to avoid the possibility of the mother discussing her answers with others.
4. The mother should complete the scale herself, unless she has limited English or has difficulty reading.
5. The instrument may be used at 6–8 weeks to screen postnatal women. The child health clinic, postnatal check-up, or a home visit may provide suitable opportunities for its completion.

Name:________________ Address:________________ Baby's age:________

As you recently had a baby, we would like to know how you are feeling. Please UNDERLINE the answer that comes closest to how you have felt IN THE PAST 7 DAYS, not just how you feel today.

Here is an example, already completed.

I have felt happy.

Yes, all the time
<u>Yes, most of the time</u>
No, not very often
No, not at all

This would mean: "I have felt happy most of the time" during the past week. Please complete the other questions in the same way.

In the past 7 days:

1. I have been able to laugh and see the funny side of things.
   As much as I always could
   Not quite as much now
   Definitely not so much now
   Not at all

2. I have looked forward with enjoyment to things.
   As much as I ever did
   Rather less than I used to
   Definitely less than I used to
   Hardly at all

*3. I have blamed myself unnecessarily when things went wrong.
   Yes, most of the time
   Yes, some of the time
   Not very often
   No, never

4. I have been anxious or worried for no good reason.
   No, not at all
   Hardly ever
   Yes, sometimes
   Yes, very often

*5. I have felt scared or panicky for no very good reason.
   Yes, quite a lot
   Yes, sometimes
   No, not much
   No, not at all

*6. Things have been getting on top of me.
   Yes, most of the time I haven't been able to cope at all
   Yes, sometimes I haven't been coping as well as usual
   No, most of the time I have coped quite well
   No, I have been coping as well as ever

*7. I have been so unhappy that I have had difficulty sleeping.
   Yes, most of the time
   Yes, sometimes
   Not very often
   No, not at all

*8. I have felt sad or miserable.
   Yes, most of the time
   Yes, quite often
   Not very often
   No, not at all

*9. I have been so unhappy that I have been crying.
   Yes, most of the time
   Yes, quite often
   Only occasionally
   No, not ever

*10. The thought of harming myself has occurred to me.
   Yes, quite often
   Sometimes
   Hardly ever
   Never

Response categories are scored 0, 1, 2, and 3 according to increased severity of the symptom.

*Items marked with an asterisk are reverse scored (ie, 3, 2, 1, and 0). The total score is calculated by adding together the scores for each of the 10 items.

 Translations of the scale, and guidance as to its use, may be found in Cox JL, Holden J. (2003) Perinatal Mental Health: A Guide to the Edinburgh Postnatal Depression Scale. London: Gaskell.

Appendix C

BOX C-1

Revised Diagnostic Criteria for Polycystic Ovary Syndrome

1990 Criteria (both 1 and 2)

1. Chronic anovulation and
2. Clinical and/or biochemical signs of hyperandrogenism and exclusion of other etiologies.

Revised 2003 criteria (2 out of 3)

1. Oligo-ovulation or anovulation,
2. Clinical and/or biochemical signs of hyperandrogenism,
3. Polycystic ovaries and exclusion of other etiologies (congenital adrenal hyperplasia, androgen-secreting tumors, Cushing syndrome)

Note: Thorough documentation of applied diagnostic criteria should be done (and described in research papers) for future evaluation.

Reprinted from Rotterdam ESHRE/ASRM-Sponsored PCOS Consensus Workshop Group, authors. Revised 2003 consensus on diagnostic criteria and long-term health risks related to polycystic ovary syndrome. Fertil Steril 2004;81:19–25. Copyright 2004, with permission from Elsevier.

TABLE C-1. Recommended Diagnostic Schemes for Polycystic Ovary Syndrome by Varying Expert Groups

Signs and Symptoms*	National Institutes of Health Criteria† 1990 (both are required for diagnosis)	Rotterdam Consensus Criteria‡ 2003 (two out of three are required for diagnosis)	Androgen Excess Society§ 2006 (hyperandrogenism plus one out of remaining two are required for diagnosis)
Hyperandrogenism‖	R	NR	R
Oligoamenorhhea or amenorrhea	R	NR	NR
Polycystic ovaries by ultrasound diagnosis	NR		NR

Abbreviations: NR, possible diagnostic criteria but not required to be present; R, required for diagnosis.

*All criteria recommend excluding other possible etiologies of these signs and symptoms and more than one of the factors present to make a diagnosis.

†Dunaif A, Givens JR, Haseltine FP, Merriam GR, editors. Polycystic ovary syndrome. Boston (MA): Blackwell Scientific Publications; 1992.

‡Revised 2003 consensus on diagnostic criteria and long-term health risks related to polycystic ovary syndrome. Rotterdam ESHRE/ASRM-Sponsored PCOS Consensus Workshop Group. Fertil Steril 2004;81:19–25.

§Azziz R, Carmina E, Dewailly D, Diamanti-Kandarakis E, Escobar-Morreale HF, Futterweit W, et al. Positions statement: criteria for defining polycystic ovary syndrome as a predominantly hyperandrogenic syndrome: an Androgen Excess Society guideline. Androgen Excess Society. J Clin Endocrinol Metab 2006;91:4237–45.

‖Hyperandrogenism may be either the presence of hirsutism or biochemical hyperandrogenemia.

Polycystic ovary syndrome. ACOG Practice Bulletin No. 108. American College of Obstetricians and Gynecologists. Obstet Gynecol 2009;114:936–49.

Appendix D

Table D-1. Common Hypercoagulable States

Abnormality	Prevalence (%) in the General Population	Prevalence (%) in Patients With Thrombosis	Testing Methods	Can Patients Be Tested During Pregnancy?	Is the Test Reliable During Acute Thrombosis?	Is the Test Reliable in Patients Using Anticoagulant therapy?
Factor V Leiden						
Heterozygous	5	20	Activated protein C resistance assay	No	Yes	Yes
Homozygous	0.02	—	DNA analysis	Yes	Yes	Yes
Prothrombin gene mutation *G20210A*	2–3	6	DNA analysis	Yes	Yes	Yes
Antiphospholipid antibody	1–2	5	Functional assay (eg, dilute Russell viper venom time) Anticardiolipin antibodies β_2-Glycoprotein-1 antibodies	Yes	Yes	Yes
Protein C deficiency	0.2–0.5	3	Protein C activity	Yes	No	No
Protein S deficiency	0.03–0.13	3.2	Protein S total and free antigen	Yes	No	No
Antithrombin-III deficiency	0.2–0.4	Less than 1	Antithrombin-III activity	Yes	No	No
Acquired hyperhomo-cysteinemia	—	8–25	Fasting plasma homocystine	Yes	Unclear	Yes
Methylenetetra-hydrofolate reductase 677T carriers (homozygous)	10	25	DNA analysis	Yes	Yes	Yes

Data from Rosendaal FR. Venous thrombosis: the role of genes, environment, and behavior. Hematology Am Soc Hematol Educ Program 2005; 1–12 *and* Kyle PA, Eichinger S. Deep vein thrombosis. Lancet 2005;365:1163–74.

Appendix E

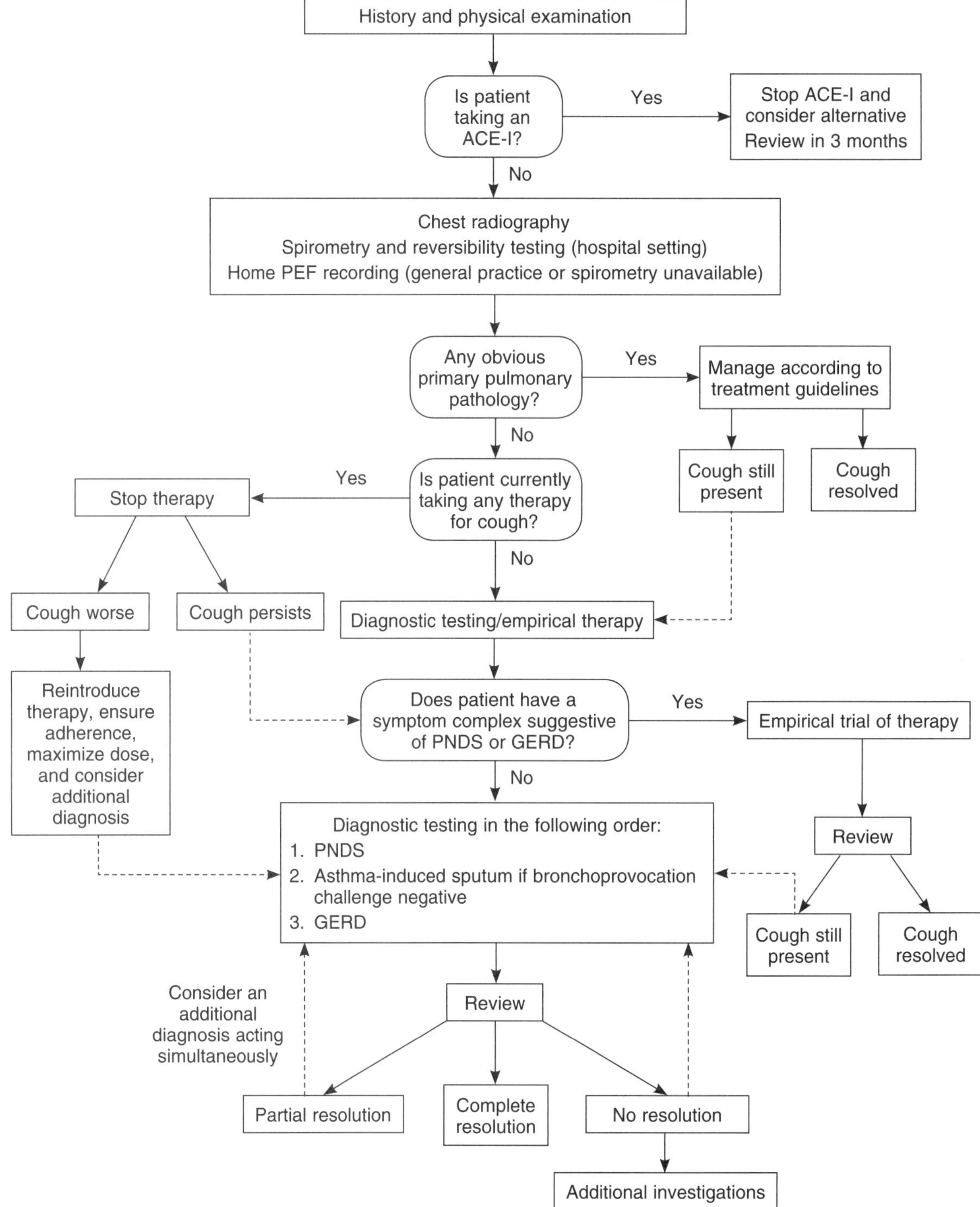

FIGURE E-1. Algorithm for evaluation of chronic cough in an adult. Abbreviations: ACE-I, angiotensin-converting enzyme inhibitor; GERD, gastroesophageal reflux disease; PEF, peak expiratory flow; PNDS, postnasal drip syndrome. (Morice AH, Fontana GA, Sovijarvi ARA, Pistolesi M, Chung KF, Widdicombe J, et al. The diagnosis and management of chronic cough. Eur Respir J 2004;24:481–92. This material has not been reviewed by European Respiratory Society prior to release; therefore, the European Respiratory Society may not be responsible for any errors, omissions or inaccuracies, or for any consequences arising there from, in the content. Reproduced with permission of the European Respiratory Society [copyright]: European Respiratory Journal Sep 2004, 24 (3) 481–92.

Appendix F

TABLE F-1. Risk Factors for Type I Uterine Corpus Cancer

Factors Influencing Risk	Estimated Relative Risk*
Older age	2–3
Residency in North America or Northern Europe	3–18
Higher level of education or income	1.5–2
White race	2
Nulliparity	3
History of infertility	2–3
Menstrual irregularities	1.5
Late age at natural menopause	2–3
Early age at menarche	1.5–2
Long-term use of unopposed estrogen	10–20
Tamoxifen use	2–3†
Obesity	2–5
Estrogen-producing tumor	>5
History of type 2 diabetes, hypertension, gallbladder disease, or thyroid disease	1.3–3
Lynch syndrome	6–20‡

*Relative risks depend on the study and referent group employed.

†Data from Tamoxifen and uterine cancer. Committee Opinion No. 601. American College of Obstetricians and Gynecologists. Obstet Gynecol 2014;123:1394–7.

‡Data from Bonadona V, Bonaiti B, Olschwang S, Grandjouan S, Huiart L, Longy M, et al. Cancer risks associated with germline mutations in MLH1, MSH2, and MSH6 genes in Lynch syndrome. French Cancer Genetics Network. JAMA 2011;305:2304–10.

Modified from Gershenson DM, McGuire WP, Gore M, Quinn MA, Thomas G, editors. Gynecologic cancer: controversies in management. Philadelphia (PA): Elsevier Churchill Livingstone; 2004.

Appendix G

Table G-1. Risk Classification for Venous Thromboembolism in Patients Undergoing Surgery Without Prophylaxis

Level of Risk	Definition	Successful Prevention Strategies
Low	Surgery lasting less than 30 minutes in patients younger than 40 years with no additional risk factors	No specific prophylaxis; early and "aggressive" mobilization
Moderate	Surgery lasting less than 30 minutes in patients with additional risk factors; surgery lasting less than 30 minutes in patients aged 40–60 years with no additional risk factors; major surgery in patients younger than 40 years with no additional risk factors	Low-dose unfractionated heparin (5,000 units every 12 hours), low-molecular-weight heparin (2,500 units dalteparin or 40 mg enoxaparin daily), graduated compression stockings, or intermittent pneumatic compression device
High	Surgery lasting less than 30 minutes in patients older than 60 years or with additional risk factors; major surgery in patients older than 40 years or with additional risk factors	Low-dose unfractionated heparin (5,000 units every 8 hours), low-molecular-weight heparin (5,000 units dalteparin or 40 mg enoxaparin daily), or intermittent pneumatic compression device
Highest	Major surgery in patients older than 60 years plus prior venous thromboembolism, cancer, or molecular hypercoagulable state	Low-dose unfractionated heparin (5,000 units every 8 hours), low-molecular-weight heparin (5,000 units dalteparin or 40 mg enoxaparin daily), or intermittent pneumatic compression device/graduated compression stockings + low-dose unfractionated heparin or low-molecular-weight heparin Consider continuing prophylaxis for 2–4 weeks after discharge.

Modified from Geerts WH, Pineo GF, Heit JA, Bergqvist D, Lasses MR, Colwell CW, et al. Prevention of venous thromboembolism: the Seventh ACCP Conference on Antithrombotic and Thrombolytic Therapy. CHEST 2004; 126(suppl):338S–400S. Copyright 2004, with permission from Elsevier.

Appendix H

BOX H-1

Classification of Underweight, Overweight, and Obese Patients

Category	Body Mass Index*
Underweight	Less than 18.5
Normal weight	18.5–24.9
Overweight	25–29.9
Obese	Equal to or more than 30
Class I obesity	30–34.9
Class II obesity	35–39.9
Class III obesity	More than 40

*Body mass index is calculated as weight in kilograms divided by height in meters squared (kg/m^2).

Index

NOTE: Numbers refer to questions, not pages.

NOTE: Numbers refer to questions, not pages.

NOTE: Numbers refer to questions, not pages.

NOTE: Numbers refer to questions, not pages.

NOTE: Numbers refer to questions, not pages.

NOTE: Numbers refer to questions, not pages.

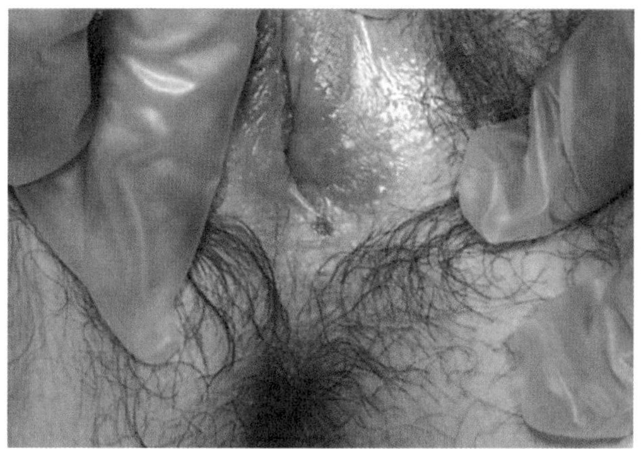

FIGURE 9-1. Reprinted from Lamb CA, Lamb EI, Mansfield JC, Sankar KN. Sexually transmitted infections manifesting as proctitis. Frontline Gastroenterol 2013;4:32–40. DOI: 10.1136/flgastro-2012-100274.

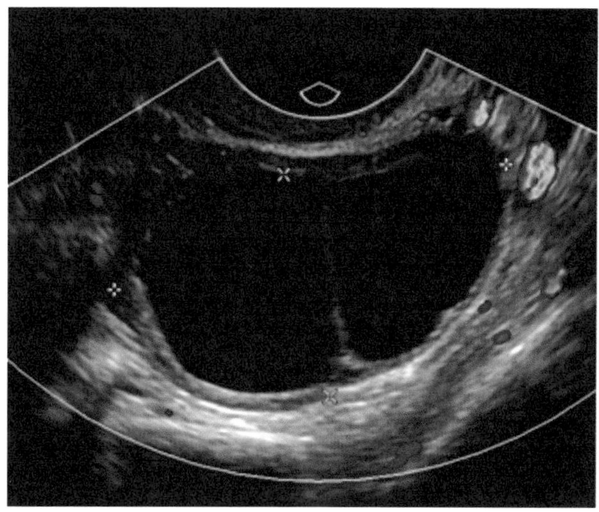

FIGURE 25-1. Used with the permission of Jeffrey Dungan, MD.

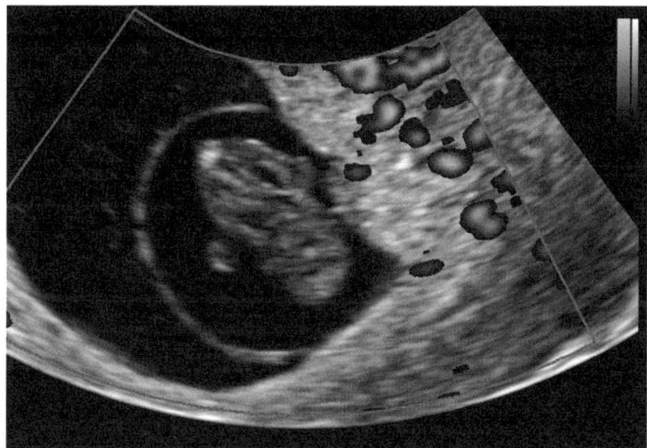

FIGURE 33-1. Used with the permission of Jeffrey Dungan, MD.

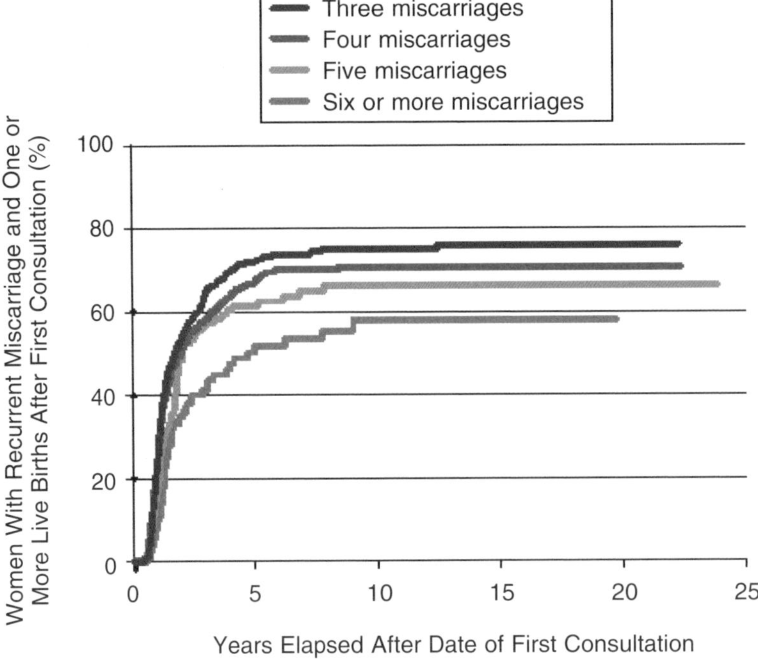

FIGURE 33-2. Kaplan–Meier plot showing percentage of women in the recurrent miscarriage cohort who have had at least one live birth after first consultation. (Reprinted from Lund M, Kamper-Jorgensen M, Nielsen HS, Lidegaard O, Andersen AM, Christiansen OB. Prognosis for live birth in women with recurrent miscarriage: what is the best measure of success? Obstet Gynecol 2012;119:37–43.)

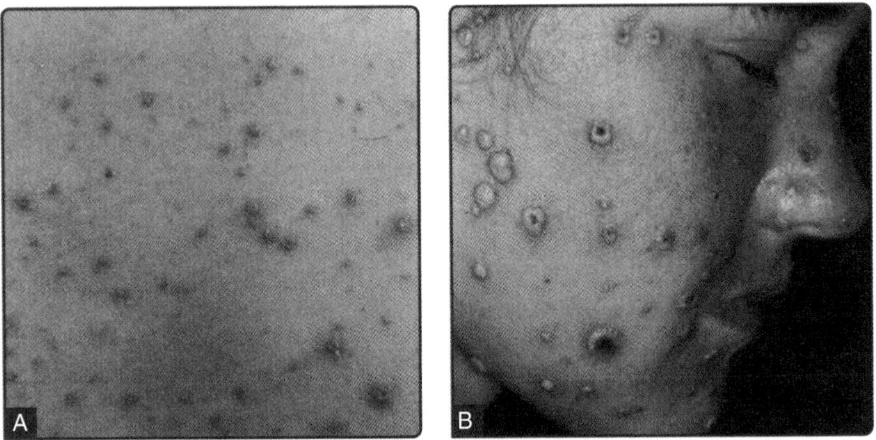

FIGURE 41-1. Varicella. **A.** A full spectrum of lesions—that is, erythematous papules, vesicles ("dewdrops on rose petals"), crusts, and erosions at sites of excoriation—is seen in a child with a typical case of varicella. **B.** A wider range of lesions, including many large pustules, is seen in a 21-year-old female who was febrile as well as "toxic" and had varicella pneumonitis. (Reprinted from Schmader KE, Oxman MN. Varicella herpes zoster. In: Goldsmith LA, Katz SI, Gilchrest BA, Paller AS, Leffell DJ, Wolff K, editors. Fitzpatrick's dermatology in general medicine. 8th ed. New York (NY): McGraw-Hill Medical; 2012. p. 2383–2401. Copyright 2016 with permission of McGraw-Hill Education.)

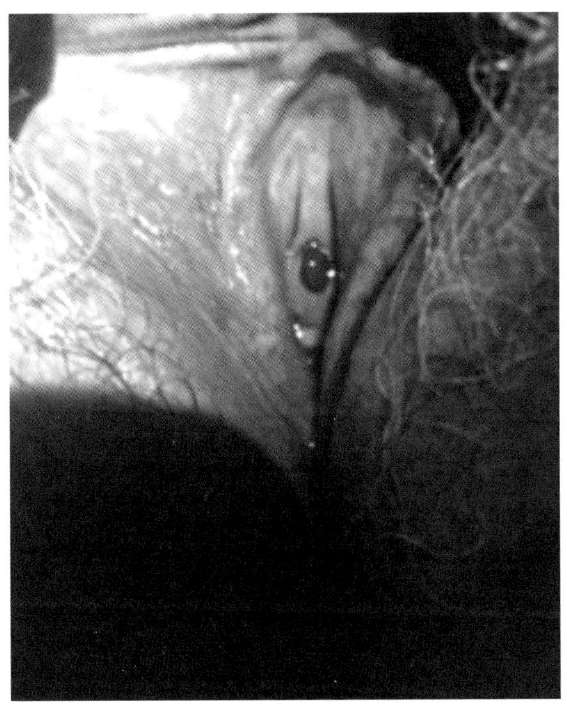

FIGURE 62-1. Used with the permission of Keisha Jones, MD.

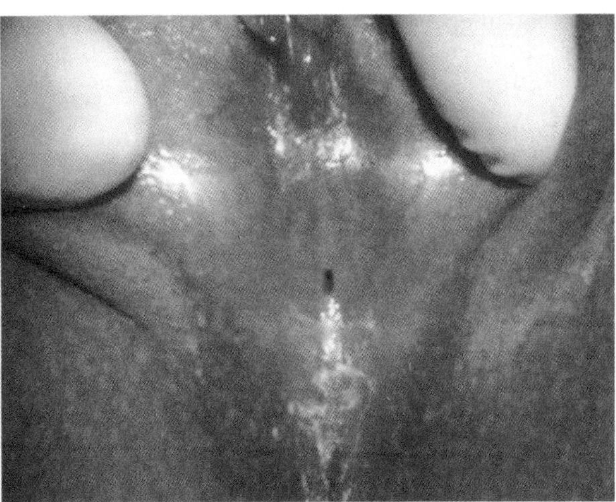

FIGURE 74-1. Reprinted from McInerny TK, Adam HM, Campbell DE, Kamat DM, Kelleher NJ, editors. American Academy of Pediatrics textbook of pediatric care. Elk Grove Village, IL: American Academy of Pediatrics; 2009.

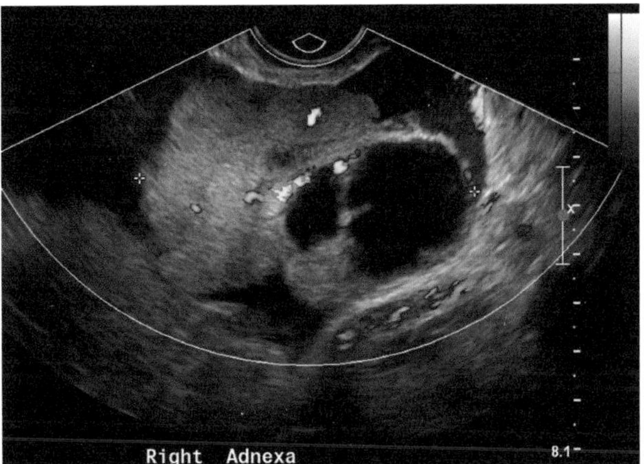

FIGURE 105-1. Used with the permission of Jeffrey Dungan, MD.

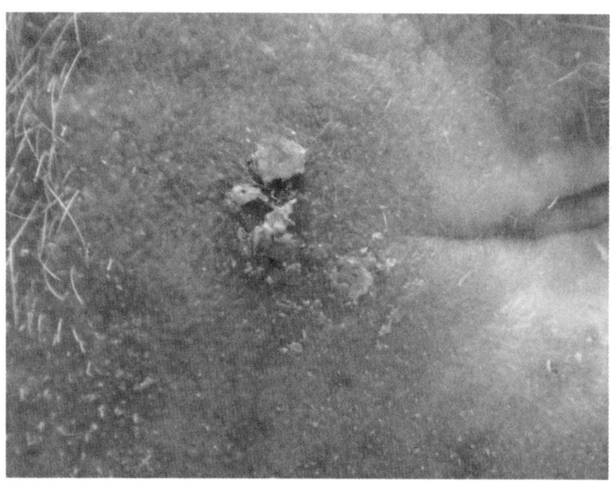

FIGURE 122-1. Actinic keratosis. (Reprinted from Ibrahim SF, Brown MD. Actinic keratoses: a comprehensive update. J Clin Aesthet Dermatol. 2009 Jul; 2(7): 43–8. Copyright 2009 Matrix Medical Communications. All rights reserved.)

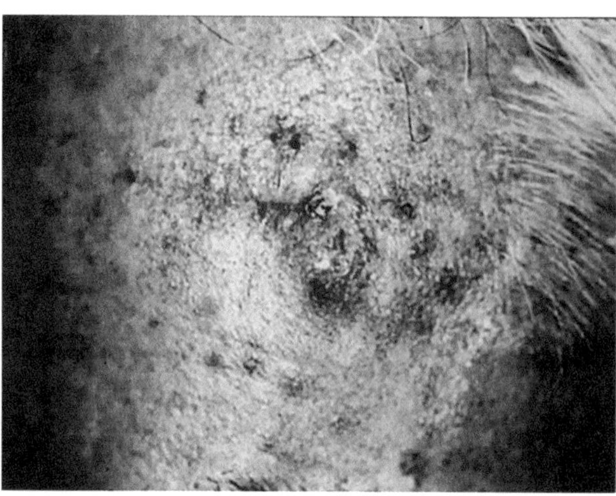

FIGURE 122-2. Squamous cell carcinoma. (Reprinted from Grossman D, Leffell DJ. Squamous cell carcinoma. In: Goldsmith LA, Katz SI, Gilchrest BA, Paller AS, Leffell DJ, Wolff K, editors. Fitzpatrick's dermatology in general medicine. 8th ed. New York (NY): McGraw-Hill Medical; 2012. p. 1283–1292. Copyright 2016 with permission of McGraw-Hill Education.)

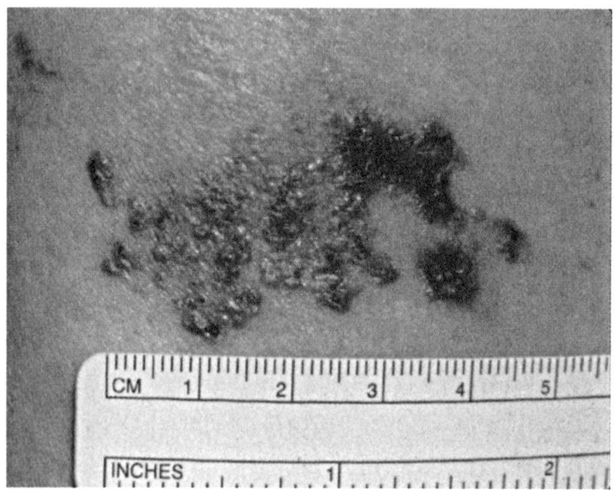

FIGURE 122-3. Basal cell carcinoma (Reprinted from Carucci JA, Leffell DJ, Pettersen JS. Basal cell carcinoma. In: Goldsmith LA, Katz SI, Gilchrest BA, Paller AS, Leffell DJ, Wolff K, editors. Fitzpatrick's dermatology in general medicine. 8th ed. New York (NY): McGraw-Hill Medical; 2012. p. 1293–1303. Copyright 2016 with permission of McGraw-Hill Education.)

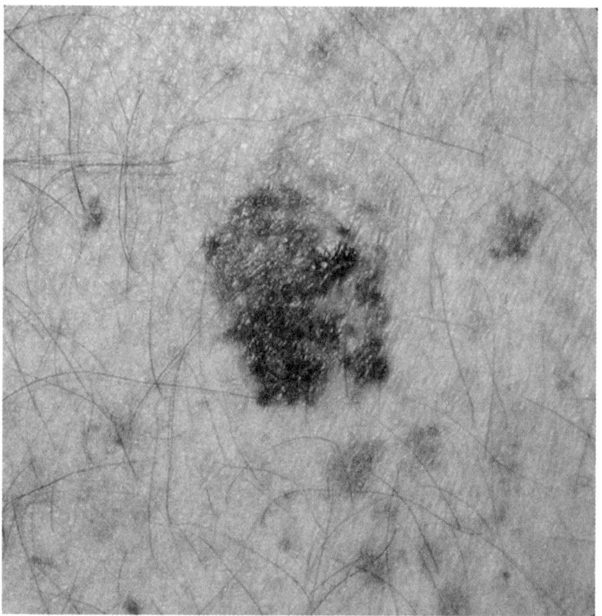

FIGURE 122-4. Melanoma. (Reprinted from Bailey EC, Sober AJ, Tsao H, Mihon Jr MC, Johnson TM. Cutaneous melanoma. In: Goldsmith LA, Katz SI, Gilchrest BA, Paller AS, Leffell DJ, Wolff K, editors. Fitzpatrick's dermatology in general medicine. 8th ed. New York (NY): McGraw-Hill Medical; 2012. p. 1416–1444. Copyright 2016 with permission of McGraw-Hill Education.)

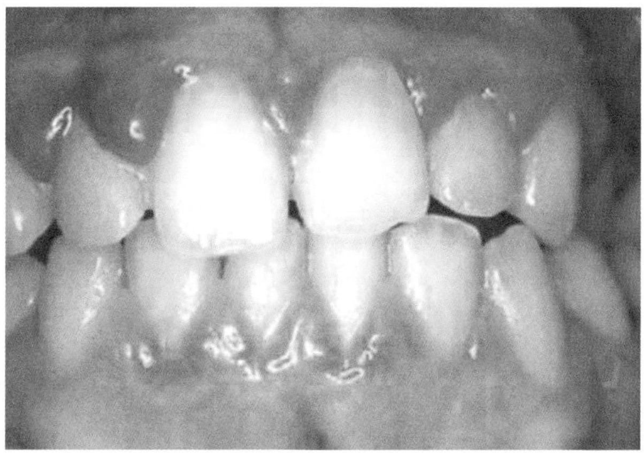

FIGURE 124-1. Photograph of moderate-to-severe periodontal disease. (Used with the permission of Steven Offenbacher, DDS, PhD.)

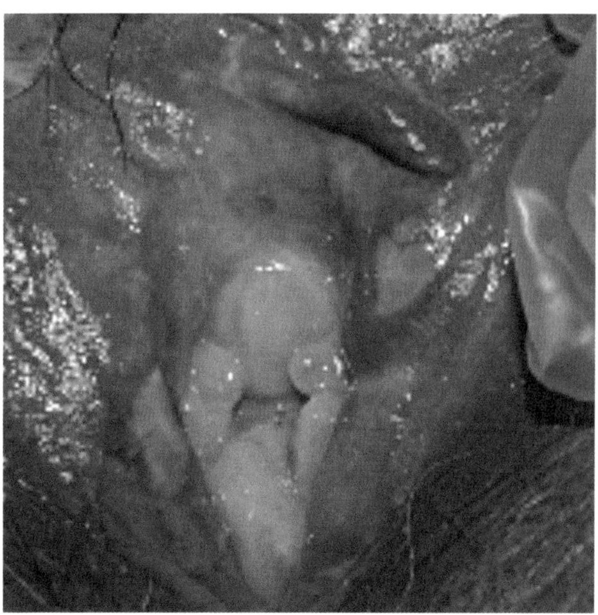

FIGURE 162–166-1. Used with the permission of Roxanne Vrees, MD.

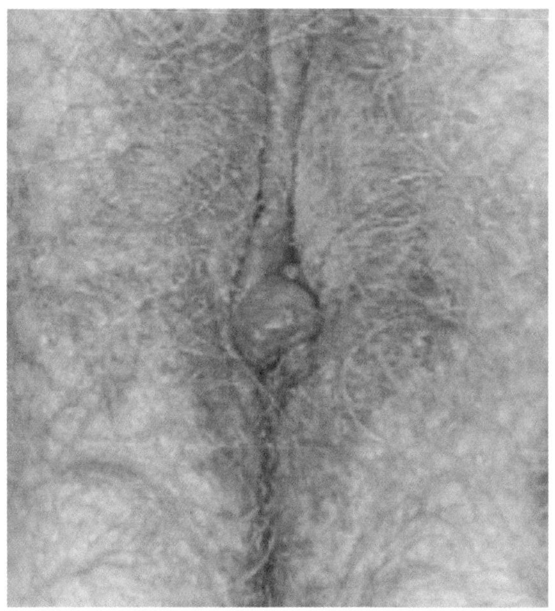

FIGURE 162–166-2. Used with the permission of Roxanne Vrees, MD.

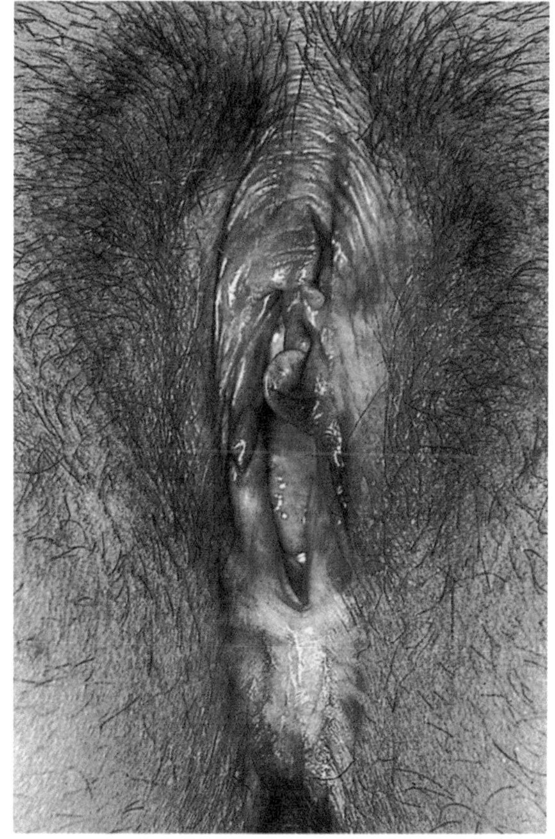

FIGURE 162–166-3. The perineal body in this photograph has the most extensive involvement. (Reprinted from Parish LC, Brenner S, Ramos-e-Silva M, editors. Women's dermatology: from infancy to maturity. New York (NY): Parthenon Publishing Group; 2001.)

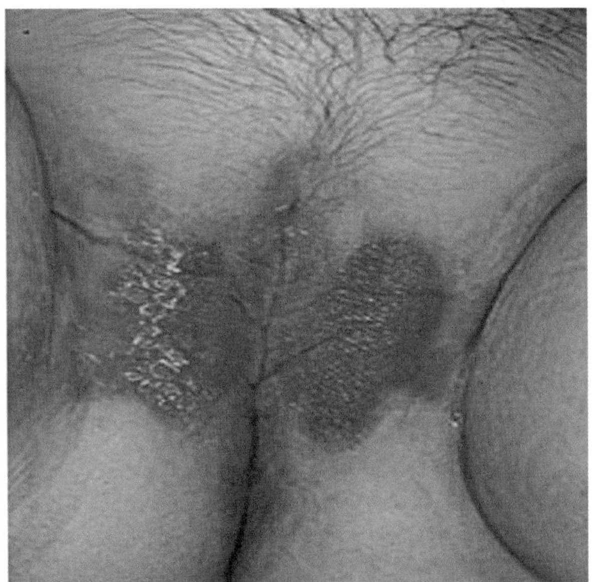

FIGURE 162–166-4. Used with the permission of Roxanne Vrees, MD.

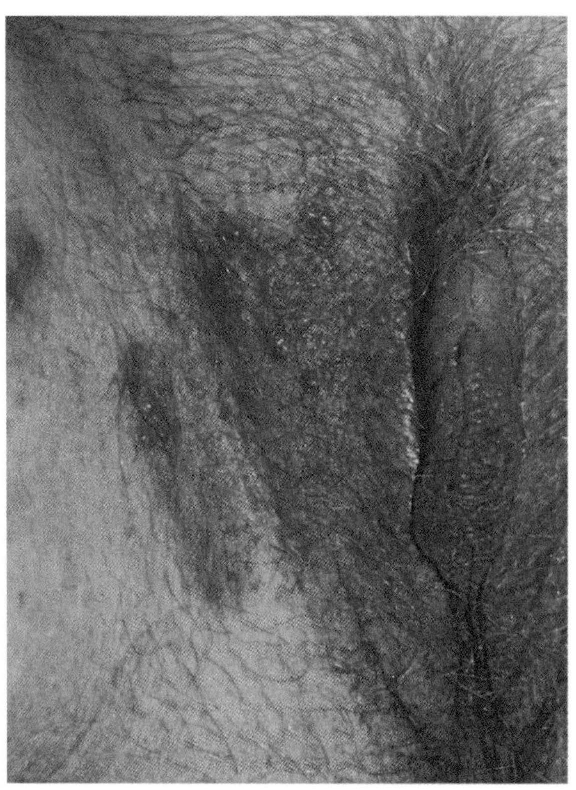

FIGURE 162–166-5. Reprinted from Edwards L. Red plaques and patches. In: Edwards L, Lynch, PJ, editors. Genital dermatology atlas. 2nd ed. Philadelphia (PA): Lippincott Williams & Wilkins; 2011. p. 57–83.